UPDATE ON ESSENTIAL HYPERTENSION

Edited by **Lizbeth Salazar-Sánchez**

Update on Essential Hypertension
http://dx.doi.org/10.5772/61565
Edited by Lizbeth Salazar-Sánchez

Contributors

Guang-Hui Dong, Li-Wen Hu, Xiao-Wen Zeng, Lizbeth Salazar-Sanchez, Juan Jose Madrigal Sanchez, Edel Paredes, Ligia Vera Gamboa, Nina Valadez Gonzalez, Norma Pavia Ruz, Pedro Gonzalez-Martinez, Anne-Maj Samuelsson, Ramón Rodrigo, Roberto Brito, Jaime González, Hans Hendrik Schäfer, GianLuca Colussi, Cristiana Catena, Marileda Novello, Leonardo A. Sechi, Narcisa Tribulova, Tamara Egan Benova, Barbara Szeiffova Bacova, Csilla Viczenczova, Aborlo Nkporbu, Princewill Stanley, Carlos Jose Rodriguez, TanYa M. Gwathmey

Published by InTech

Janeza Trdine 9, 51000 Rijeka, Croatia

Publishing Process Manager Edi Lipovic

Technical Editor SPi Global

Cover InTech Design team

First published September, 2016

Printed in Croatia

Additional hard copies can be obtained from orders@intechopen.com

Update on Essential Hypertension , Edited by Lizbeth Salazar-Sánchez

p. cm.

Print ISBN 978-953-51-2614-0
Online ISBN 978-953-51-2615-7

For EU product safety concerns:
IN TECH d.o.o., Prolaz Marije Krucifikse Kozulić 3, 51000 Rijeka, Croatia,
info@intechopen.com or visit our website at intechopen.com.

Meet the editor

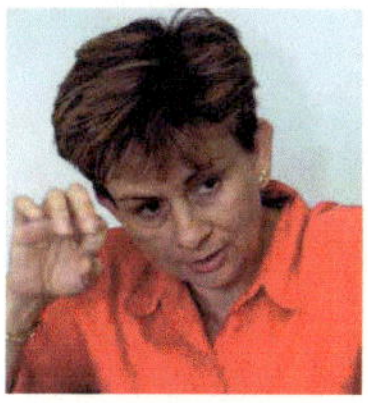

Lizbeth Salazar-Sanchez, MD obtained her PhD with Magnum Cum Lauden, at the Ernst-Moritz-Arndt-Universität, Greifswald, Germany, in 2002. She got her Masters Degree in Microbiology (1996) and Hematology Specialization (1991) with honors at the University of Costa Rica. In 2003, she has been awarded the National Prize Research Award "the Clodomiro Picado Twight" for her excellent work in the field of molecular markers and cardiovascular disease; she got the Humboldt Cathedratic in 2013 and she obtained the Mesoamerican Prize Research of the Mesoamerican Group in 2014. Since 2014 she is a director of the Medical School of Medicine and Director of the Medical Postgraduate Program of the University of Costa Rica. Dr. Salazar-Sanchez is a member of many scientific societies, such as the Central America Research Network of Alumni DAAD, International Society of Homeostasis and Thrombosis, Scientific Committee of the Medical College of Costa Rica, among others. With her long career and professional and scientific works in molecular medicine, she has as well excelled in the clinical aspect in her field.

Contents

Preface IX

Section 1 Update in Hypertension 1

Chapter 1 **Introductory chapter: Essential Hypertension in the Twenty-First Century...What is Next? 3**
Lizbeth Salazar-Sánchez and Krystell Oviedo-Flores

Chapter 2 **Essential Hypertension in Children: New Mechanistic Insights 9**
Anne-Maj Sofia Samuelsson

Chapter 3 **Oxidative Stress and Essential Hypertension 27**
Ramón Rodrigo, Roberto Brito and Jaime González

Chapter 4 **Omega-3 Polyunsaturated Fatty Acids in Blood Pressure Control and Essential Hypertension 49**
GianLuca Colussi, Cristiana Catena, Marileda Novello and Leonardo A. Sechi

Chapter 5 **Psychiatric Comorbidity in Essential Hypertension 71**
Aborlo Kennedy Nkporbu and Princewill Chukwuemeka Stanley

Section 2 Hypertension Highlights 101

Chapter 6 **Ambient Particulate Matter Air Pollution Exposure and Hypertension 103**
Wen-Wen Bao and Guang-Hui Dong

Chapter 7 **ACE I/D (Rs1799752), MTHFR C677T (Rs1801133), and CCR5 D32 (Rs333) Genes and their Association with Hypertension and Diabetic Nephropathy in Urban Areas of Costa Rica, Nicaragua, and Mexico 113**
Lizbeth Salazar-Sanchez, Juan Jose Madrigal-Sanchez, Pedro Gonzalez-Martinez, Edel Paredes, Ligia Vera-Gamboa, Norma Pavia Ruz and Nina Valadez-Gonzalez

Chapter 8 **Relevance of Personalized Health Care in Patients with Arterial Hypertension: Where are we now? 131**
Carmen Binder, Hans Hendrik Schäfer, Edelgard Kaiser, Martin Hund and Thomas Dieterle

Chapter 9 **Myocardial Connexin-43 is Implicated in the Prevention of Malignant Arrhythmia in Rats Suffering from Essential Hypertension 185**
Tamara Egan Benova, Barbara Szeiffova Bacova, Csilla Viczenczova, Miroslav Barancik and Narcis Tribulova

Chapter 10 **Hypertension and Hypertension-Related Disparities in Underrepresented Minorities 209**
Carlos J. Rodriguez

Preface

Essential hypertension is a quantitative characteristic that is important for correlating with the rate of the morbidity and mortality in the developed and developing countries. The etiology of essential hypertension is complex; it is a major contributor to cardiovascular disease, a leading cause of death in many countries. For this reason, there exists a commitment of many health organizations worldwide to continue initiatives of research in hypertension. Now it is clear that multiple factors interact in this development. To prevent hard end points, early definitive diagnosis and optimum therapy play a significant role. This work, authored by renowned researchers in the field of Hypertension Research, details the state of the art in new knowledge related with essential hypertension. Novel advanced topics are present in a sole document, as well as hypertension in children; the contribution in the psychiatric comorbidities associated with hypertension; the role of the oxidative stress at different levels, and mechanisms of omega-3 in protection against hypertension-related organ damage are described. Other topics included in the book are genetics-associated studies; the role of pollution in essential hypertension; personalized healthcare in a hypertensive patient; and hypertension and hypertension-related disparities between ethnic groups, so that essential hypertension continuous to be one of the hottest topics in contemporary medicine.

This book is dedicated to my parents Carlos e Isabel and to my daughter Brenda.

Lizbeth Salazar-Sanchez
Medicine School, University of Costa Rica,
San Jose, Costa Rica

Section 1

Update in Hypertension

Introductory chapter: Essential Hypertension in the Twenty-First Century...What is Next?

Lizbeth Salazar-Sánchez and Krystell Oviedo-Flores

Additional information is available at the end of the chapter

http://dx.doi.org/10.5772/64260

1. Introduction: historical concerns about blood pressure determination

The history of hypertension measurements begins in the late 1800s, with the introduction of the sphygmomanometer, an instrument to measure blood pressure with a noninvasive device.

At that time, some practitioners were still skeptical about the clinical importance of determining blood pressure. Others considered it as a valuable tool for diagnosis and began with early descriptions of the variability of blood pressure among individuals [1].

Additionally, the life insurance industry in the United States played also an important role in the recognition of an association between blood pressure level and cardiovascular morbidity and mortality. In the first half of the twentieth century, the use of the sphygmomanometer was indispensable in life insurance examinations because insurance companies required it for the applicants. The Actuarial Society of American published a report in 1939 about the relationship between blood pressure and mortality from cardiovascular and renal diseases. However, the clinical significance of high blood pressure during this time was not well understood, and essential hypertension was considered as a compensatory feature of blood pressure to ensure adequate perfusion of the target organs. This is the explanation why many clinicians were reluctant to treat high blood pressure because essential hypertension was considered a control mechanism to assure tissue perfusion, only to be controlled or regulated, even when there was increasing evidence of the association of cardiovascular disease and mortality with high blood pressure [2].

The two first clinical trials from the Veterans Administration Cooperative Studies evidenced the benefits of lowering blood pressure with antihypertensive treatment, published in 1967 and 1971, respectively. The design of both studies served as a prototype for future clinical trials. Furthermore, on a report in 1979, the Actuarial Society of American concluded that mortality ratios rose with an increase in blood pressure in both men and women; they stated that overweight (35–45% above the average weight) increased mortality considerably in men with high blood pressure. Coronary disease, cerebral hemorrhage, left ventricular hypertrophy, and renal disease were among the causes of death identified, and mortality of these causes rose as blood pressure increased [2]. Since then, many studies showed that reduction in high blood pressure reduces cardiovascular morbidity and mortality for hypertension and served as evidence for early recommendations for antihypertensive therapy [3].

2. Epidemiologic transition: infectious diseases are replaced by cardiovascular diseases

During 1940s and 1950s, after World War II, the health priority became the control of infectious diseases, because they were the major contributors to morbidity and mortality at that time. As a consequence, the efforts in public health to control and prevent infectious diseases resulted in the decline in mortality rates and average life expectancy increase. During the twentieth century, an epidemiologic transition was evident in developed countries, in which infectious disease pandemics were replaced as a major cause of death by chronic degenerative diseases, such as cardiovascular diseases [4].

Since mortality rate for cardiovascular disease had been increasing progressively, the National Health Institute, in USA (now known as the National Heart, Lung, and Blood Institute) decided to conduct an ambitious project in 1948: the Framingham Heart Study. The researchers of the project recruited more than 5000 men and women who had not suffered symptoms of cardiovascular disease or had a cardiovascular event—heart attack or stroke, and analyzed them over a long period of time [5, 6]. As a prospective longitudinal epidemiologic study, its objective was to characterize the population subject to cardiovascular disease. The original cohort was followed up over decades, enrolling a second and a third generation to the original cohort. Since 1951, several articles were published based on research results of the Framingham Study, obtained by the careful monitoring of the study population, which led to the identification of the major coronary heart disease risk factors—high blood pressure, high cholesterol levels, smoking, obesity, diabetes, physical inactivity, closely related to other factors such as blood triglyceride and HDL cholesterol levels, age, gender, and psychosocial issues.

3. Essential hypertension: definition and etiology

Essential hypertension, also known as primary or idiopathic hypertension, is the presence of high blood pressure not explainable by secondary causes, representing 95% of all cases of high blood pressure. Secondary causes of hypertension are aldosteronism, renal disease, pheochromocytoma, hyperthyroidism, etc. [7].

Essential hypertension is a quantitative characteristic, defined by its strong positive correlation between blood pressure and risk of cerebral or cardiac, events and kidney disease. The etiology of essential hypertension is complex, and it is possible that multiple factors interact and produce hypertension. Furthermore, it has become notorious that a genetic susceptibility and the interaction of environmental factors, such as stress, diet, and physical activity play a relevant role in the pathogenesis of hypertension, as suggested in 1949 by Page in his mosaic theory to explain the possible mechanisms involved in the etiology of hypertension (**Figure 1**) [8]. The development of essential hypertension is composed of a primary process, in which vasoconstriction raises blood pressure initially, followed by a secondary amplifying process, in which the difference in blood pressure rises throughout life. This primary event can be in the perinatal and early postnatal life, a phenomenon known as 'intrauterine programming', important in long-term effects on the subsequent development of high blood pressure, with possible onset of hypertension during childhood and adolescence.

In developed countries, there is a probability of 90% of becoming hypertensive during the lifetime. Risk factors often cluster with other cardiovascular risk factors in individuals with an unhealthy lifestyle, including the sedentary lifestyle, smoking, stressful life of industrialized societies and Western diet patterns. Among dietary factors, it has been demonstrated that excessive salt intake, high alcohol consumption, low intake of potassium and calcium are related to hypertension. On the other hand, an increased consumption of polyunsaturated fatty acids of the omega-3 family has shown to have a hypotensive effect and reduces the cardiovascular risk.

Furthermore, blood pressure is affected by several environmental factors such as ambient temperature, air pollution, and noise. In addition, the repeated or prolonged exposure to these factors leads consequently to an increased sympathetic and adrenal activity [9]. Likewise, stress related situations, such as job strain, emotional distress, and social environment can cause hypertension through repeated blood pressure elevation and increased secretion of vasoconstrictive hormones.

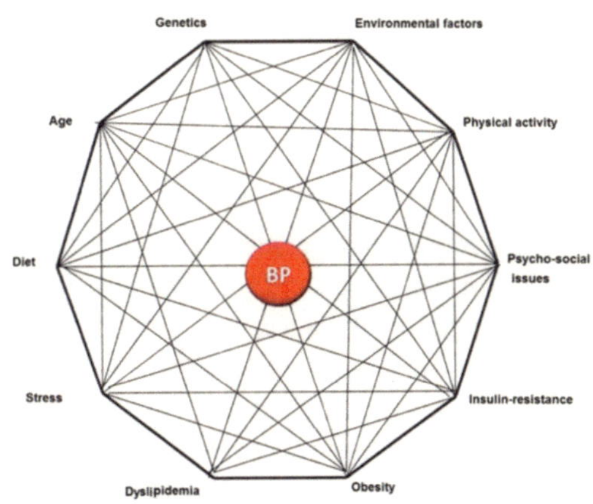

Figure 1. Interactions of factors in essential hypertension development, modified from the original Paige's mosaic theory of blood pressure regulation [8]. There is a circuitry of several factors interacting in an individual that may lead to the development of essential hypertension, such as genetic background, diet, physical activity, psychosocial factors, environmental factors, obesity, insulin resistance, dyslipidemia and stress.

Recognition of a genetic basis in hypertension is deduced from epidemiological and family studies, such as the Framingham Study [10]. Genetic alterations and polymorphisms in inherited 'essential' hypertension have also been identified. As a result, the individual response to the environmental factors mentioned above is variable, because the effect of an allelic variation of any gene depends on the environment in which the gene is expressed. In summary, it becomes clear that various factors contribute to blood pressure elevation in essential hypertension in susceptible individuals.

4. Twenty-first century challenges: genetic strategies and personalized medicine

Hypertension is a major contributor to cardiovascular disease, a leading cause of death in many countries. For this reason, there exists a commitment of many health organizations worldwide, to continue initiatives of research in hypertension. In the last twenty years, the use of experimental animal models for hypertension-related research has provided information in various aspects of the disease, which includes etiology, pathophysiology, complications, and treatment. In addition, comparative mapping techniques allow comparison of the syntenic genomic regions between rodents and the human genome. Recently, the identification of the role of cardiovascular genetic determinants of hypertension through linkage analyses and genome-wide scan studies permits a better understanding of the complex genetic architecture of the disease [11]. Numerous genes have been identified, including the genes from the renin-angiotensin-aldosterone system, the epithelial sodium channel, the adrenergic receptor, endogenous adducin, etc.

Furthermore, pharmacogenetics association studies in hypertensive patients are a useful tool helping to individualize therapy, by predicting patient response to a treatment, chosen to provide greatest clinical efficacy with the lowest risk of adverse effects.

5. Conclusion

During the twenty-first century, it has been a challenge to find the genetic etiology of human essential hypertension. Many studies on genetics and pharmacogenomics of hypertension have served as the basis, facilitating results of the role of candidate genes. However, as high blood pressure results from a complex interplay of diverse environmental and genetic factors, the replication of many studies has been problematic. The application of genetic data to the current therapeutic guidelines must be encouraged because provided evidence from several studies has not readily been translated into personalized medicine. The heterogeneity and complexity of the genetic network that in interaction with the environment controls the physiological mechanisms involved in blood pressure regulation has hampered the clinical application of animal genetic results to humans [12]. Additional discoveries in hypertension pharmacogenomics are expected to be obtained from genome-wide association studies. In order to translate the findings of candidate gene studies and genome-wide association studies to the clinical practice, more efficient genetic testing, denser mapping techniques, full utilization of animal models and increased collaboration among research groups need to be improved.

Author details

Lizbeth Salazar-Sánchez[1*] and Krystell Oviedo-Flores[1,2]

*Address all correspondence to: lizbeth.salazar@gmail.com

1 Medicine School, University of Costa Rica, San Pedro Montes de Oca, San José, Costa Rica

2 University of Salamanca, Salamanca, Spain

References

[1] Fisher JW. "The diagnostic value of the sphygmomanometer in examinations for life insurance". JAMA. 1914; 63: 1752–1754.

[2] Kotchen T. "Historical trends and milestones in hypertension research: a model of the process of translational research". Hypertension. 2011; 58: 522–538.

[3] Messerli FH, Williams B, Ritz E. "Essential hypertension". Lancet. 2007; 370: 591–603.

[4] McKeown R. "The epidemiologic transition: changing patterns of mortality and population dynamics". Am J Lifestyle Med. 2009; 3(1 Suppl): 19S–26S.

[5] Dawber TR, Kannel WB, Revotskie N, Stokes JI, Kagan A, Gordon T. "Some factors associated with the development of coronary heart disease. Six years' follow-up experience in the Framingham study". Am J Public Health 1959; 49(10): 1349–1356.

[6] Dawber TR, Kannel WB. An epidemiologic study of heart disease: the Framingham study. Nutr Rev. 1958; 16(1): 1–4.

[7] Carretero OA, Oparil S. "Essential hypertension part I: definition and etiology". Circulation. 2000; 101: 329–335.

[8] Page IH. The mosaic theory. In: Page IH, editor. Hypertension Mechanisms. New York: Grune and Stratton; 1987. pp. 910–923.

[9] Brook RD, Weder A, Rajagopalan S. "Environmental hypertensionology" the effects of environmental factors on blood pressure in clinical practice and research. J Clin Hypertens (Greenwich). 2011; 13: 836–842.

[10] Pausova Z, Trembla J, Hamet P. "Gene-environment interactions in hypertension". Curr Hypertens Rep. 1999, 1: 42–50 (Current Science Inc.).

[11] Harrison M, Maresso K, Broeckel U. "Genetic determinants of hypertension: an update". Curr Hypertens Rep. 2008; 10:488–495.

[12] Manunta P, Ferrandi M, Cusi D, Ferrari P, Staessen J, Bianchi G. "Personalized therapy of hypertension: the past and the future". Curr Hypertens Rep. 2016; 18: 24.

Chapter 2

Essential Hypertension in Children: New Mechanistic Insights

Anne-Maj Sofia Samuelsson

Additional information is available at the end of the chapter

http://dx.doi.org/10.5772/62652

Abstract

Paediatric hypertension is on the rise accompanied by concomitant increase of childhood obesity. The origin of paediatric hypertension however remains unknown. New epidemiological evidence suggests that environmental insult in utero or postnatally may lead to hypertension later in life. Independent associations have been reported between maternal obesity and cardiometabolic disorders in the offspring. In the first part, I will focus on functionally mechanistic pathways of essential hypertension with an attempt to elucidate the rather complex interplay of autonomic dysfunction, leptin, melanocortin-4 receptor (MC4R), inflammation, genetic and epigenetic predispositions. In the second part, the standalone risk factors will be integrated in a flow chart in attempt to understand the deeper meaning of this regulatory machinery in paediatric hypertension. I will refer to the pathophysiology of early sympathetic-mediated hypertension arising from maternal obesity. Maternal diet-induced obesity in rodents permanently resets the responsiveness to leptin-induced SNS in rat offspring via the hypothalamic paraventricular nucleus (PVN)-MC4R pathway. The stimulus that mediates Leptin-SNS-MC4R activity and promotes hypertension is still unknown and remains as a key for future investigations. Future research needs to identify effective preventive measures in the pregnant mother and child to reduce the risk of paediatric hypertension and prevent future cardiovascular disease.

Keywords: essential hypertension, maternal obesity, leptin, melanocortin system, sympathetic activity, hypothalamus

1. Introduction

Hypertension in children and adolescence is becoming an increasing health problem. The prevalence of pre-hypertension is approximately 14% in boys and 6% in girls (age 8–17 years)

[1, 2], and the prevalence of hypertension is estimated to be 3–4% (age 3–18 years) [3, 4]. One in three of the hypertensive children develops end-organ damage, including ventricular hypertrophy [5], chronic kidney disease [6] and vascular changes [7] and cognitive impairment [8, 9], all predictors for premature morbidity and mortality. Accumulating evidence supports the theory that elevated blood pressure levels in adolescence are a precursor of elevated blood pressure in adulthood, and an important risk factor for future cardiovascular diseases [10]. Another factor is the coexistent epidemic of childhood obesity, which in the US rose from 5 to 11% from the 1960s to the 1990 [11, 12], becoming a concomitant cardiovascular risk factor. Childhood BMI has strong positive concordance with blood pressure [13]. Children who are overweight demonstrate 4.5 and 2.3 times higher risk of developing increased systolic blood pressure and diastolic blood pressure, respectively [14], consistent findings were obtained by Sorof et al. [15] with a three-fold prevalence of childhood hypertension in obese versus lean at school age. Blood pressure in children may also vary by age, sex, race and height [4] but not as solid as BMI, all these inclusion criteria of risk being underdiagnosed [3]. Children within the "normotensive" range of blood pressure demonstrate elevated left ventricular mass [16] and greater risk of developing hypertension in adulthood [17]. Thus, blood pressure in children diverges from adults in that an underestimation of risk may cause severe cardiovascular diseases in adulthood [18]. Recent report indicates that more than 90% of children evaluated for hypertension have no underlying cause identified [19], which suggests that prevalence of essential hypertension is increasing. This revives the discussion of the aetiology and pathogenesis research of essential hypertension to identify important targets of prevention.

2. Pathophysiology of childhood hypertension

The origin of paediatric hypertension evolves a cluster of metabolic and haemodynamic disorders identifies as a polyfactorial disease. Unfavourable metabolic profiles, such as hyperinsulineaemia and dyslipidaemia, at an young age with abnormalities of vascular structure and function leads to adverse cardiovascular outcome [12, 20, 21]. The adverse metabolic profile may originate from an unbalanced autonomic nervous system (ANS). ANS is known as the major adaptor for stress responses which regulate the two neural efferent pathways the parasympathetic and sympathetic system [22]. Long-term increase to stress may lead to increased sympathetic activity and decreased parasympathetic activity, contributing to obesity, insulin resistance, dyslipidaemia and hypertension [23–25]. Dysregulation of ANS may therefore predict metabolic abnormalities [26, 27] and hypertension [22]. In children, these associations have barely been investigated. Childhood obesity has been associated with lower parasympathetic activity [28–31], but more conflicting results regarding the influence of the sympathovagal balance and sympathetic hyperactivity [31–33]. Possible confounding factors and differences in methodology and sample size might explain these differences. Latchman et al. [32] showed that normotensive obese 9-year-old children exhibited reduced baroreflex sensitivity, parasympathetic control as well as increased sympathetic control compared with normotensive lean children. Thus, suggest that autonomic dysfunction may precede the hypertension in obese children. Obesity is associated with increased sympathetic nervous system (SNS) activity, with impaired heart rate variability [34]. The resting heart rate is positively correlated with sub-capsular skinfold thickness in children [35]. Similar findings have been obtained in early origin of cardiometabolic disease. Foetuses born to obese mothers demonstrate increased foetal sympathetic activation [36], which may predict long-term cardiovascular outcome.

3. Maternal obesity and offspring cardiovascular complications

A large body of epidemiological literature supports the link between an adverse intrauterine environment and disease in later life, showing inverse association between low birth weights (poor nutrition) with subsequent hypertension [37–40]. Similar findings have been demonstrated in animal models of maternal malnutrition and uterine growth restriction (IUGR) [41]. Despite the worldwide obesity epidemic, relative few studies have investigated the influence of maternal obesity on offspring health, with only recent emerging human data suggesting detrimental effects with preterm mortality in the offspring [42]. Epidemiological study demonstrates associations between maternal BMI and increased systolic blood pressure (SBP) in 7-year-old children [43]. The Amsterdam Born Children and their Development (ABCD) study recently reported that maternal pre-pregnancy BMI, in 3074 women, was positively associated with childhood diastolic blood pressure (DBP) and SBP at the age of 5–6 [44]. In the Jerusalem perinatal study (JPS), both gestational weight gain (GWG) and pre-pregnancy BMI were related to cardiovascular risk factors including SBP and DBP in adult offspring, at the age of 32 [45]. A stronger association for maternal pre-pregnancy BMI than paternal BMI with adverse cardiometabolic health in offspring suggests a direct intrauterine mechanisms, instead of life-style-related characteristics or genetic factors [46]. However, the causation is difficult to establish in human cohort studies. Interestingly, a recent study demonstrated an increased risk for cardiovascular mortality in children born to obese mothers, and this association remained after removing the child BMI [42]. Thus, suggests a direct effect of maternal obesity on child cardiovascular function, independent of childhood obesity [42]. The WHO Global Burden of Disease database currently identifies a rapid rise in maternal obesity in the past two decades. In the US, 64% of women of reproductive age are overweight and 35% are obese [47], with a similar pattern in Europe [48] and the rest of the world [49–51]. Obese pregnant women not only develop a higher risk of preeclampsia, preterm labour, stillbirth, caesarean deliveries, there are also a higher incidence of developing diabetes and hypertension in the offspring [52]. The increasing rate of maternal obesity may therefore provide a major challenge to future generations' health. Children born to obese mothers not only are prone to develop obesity but also essential hypertension which is the primary risk factor for developing other cardiovascular diseases leading to premature death. Whilst further randomised controlled clinical trials of improved design are indicated, there is an important task to revisit the basic science of autonomic function using experimental models that mimics the human condition of essential hypertension.

3.1. Autonomic dysfunction and paediatric hypertension

The autonomic nervous system (ANS) has two principal divisions, the parasympathetic pathway and the sympathetic pathway which acts either in synergy or in opposition synergy. The autonomic system continuously controls heart rate and blood pressure, respiratory rate and gut motility, body temperature and other essential functions. The autonomic function interacts with the primitive brain, including the limbic system (memory function), brain stem and hypothalamus [53]. Neurons within hypothalamic nuclei, particularly the paraventricular nucleus (PVN) and dorsomedial hypothalamus (DMN), make direct or indirect connection with sympathetic and parasympathetic preganglionic neurons and interfere with autonomic balance, sympathetic hyperactivity and neurogenic hypertension [53]. Early stages of hypertension, particularly in children, are defined by autonomic dysfunction [54]. Excessive sympathetic activity and/or withdrawal of parasympathetic balance are assessed by HR variability (HRV), using the ratio of low to high frequency (LF/HF) power. Pioneering studies conducted by Urbina et al. showed altered HRV in 39 male adolescences and reported trends of higher LF/HF ratio with higher BP, but did not reach statistical significance [65]. In a larger cohort, Sorof et al. [20] reported increased HR and BP variability in obese children with isolated systolic hypertension assessed by office HR/BP measurement and ambulatory blood pressure monitoring (ABPM). Interestingly, obese hypertensive children had higher HR than non-obese hypertensive children, suggesting that obesity is independently related with SNS activation [20]. These initial findings of SNS hyperactivity in hypertensive children, measured by indirect methods, were later confirmed by direct measurement of sympathetic activity using microneurography [55]. Zhou et al. [56] demonstrated altered vagal and sympathetic activity in hypertensive children, with a greater influence of systolic blood pressure (SBP) than diastolic blood pressure (DBP) on HRV [57]. Genovesi et al. [58] demonstrated baroreflex impairment, in both hypertensive and pre-hypertensive children. Autonomic dysfunction is therefore considered a critical feature in pre-hypertensive children which may predict future cardiovascular health. In children with arterial hypertension, the increase of sympathetic activity during sleep correlate with increase left ventricular mass and left ventricular mass index [59]. Moreover, HRV can predict the severity of children with pulmonary arterial hypertension [60]. This is particular worrisome as historical reference data on child HRV by Massin et al. [61] with current child HRV in Germany [62] showed change in children's ANS in the last 15 years. These changes constitute reduced vagal activity and a shift towards sympathetic dominance [62]. The authors suggest that these changes might be related to the rise in childhood obesity, with a negative association between BMI and ANS activity [62]. The historical samples of Kauzuma et al. [63], however, featured a comparable overweight rate (17%), but still reported much lower mean sympathetic activity. Additional factors including physical inactivity or nutrient composition may influence ANS [64, 65]. Maternal BMI, which recently been associated with the offspring ANS activity, may be another important determinant [66]. Several different mechanisms leading to and maintaining central sympathetic hyperactivity in essential hypertension have been identified. An impaired vagal heart rate control exerted by arterial baroreflex impaired volume-sensitive cardiopulmonary reflex, arterial chemoreceptors as well as humoral factors such as leptin and angiotensin II with direct central sympathoexcitatory effects have all been shown to play at least partial roles in essential hypertension.

3.2. Leptin and childhood obesity and hypertension

Experimental models of maternal obesity in sheep, non-human primate and rodents provide evidence for the adverse influence on offspring cardiovascular function [67]. In rodents, the perinatal exposure to metabolic milieu of maternal obesity may permanently change the central pathways involved in blood pressure regulation [66]. Leptin, an adipocyte-derived hormone, promotes weight loss by reducing appetite and increasing energy expenditure through hypothalamic sympathetic stimulation to brown adipose tissue [68] and kidney [69] which results in increased arterial pressure [70]. This has been confirmed in chronic infusion of leptin in rats developing increased blood pressure [71]. Transgenic mice overexpressing leptin develops overt obesity with elevations of blood pressure [72]. Selective leptin resistance of the appetite and weight reducing effect of leptin [73], and preservation of the sympathetic action of leptin, been implicated in obesity-related hypertension [74]. In humans, high plasma leptin concentration has been associated with arterial pressure [75] and muscle sympathetic nerve activity [76]. Leptin is also thought to have a neurotrophic role in the development of the hypothalamus [77], and altered neonatal leptin profiles secondary to maternal obesity are associated with permanently altered brain hypothalamic structure and function. In rodent studies, maternal obesity confers persistent sympathoexcitatory hyper-responsiveness and hypertension acquired in the early stages of development [78]. Unrevealing the mechanisms controlling hypothalamic development may help to identify the nature of the hypothalamic dysfunction and develop future therapies. High leptin in cord blood from foetuses of obese mothers [79] might cause permanent changes of the hypothalamic circuits leading to heightened leptin-induced sympathetic activity and blood pressure in juvenile offspring, prior to obesity and metabolic dysfunction [70].

3.3. The role of the central melanocortin system

The melanocortin system is an essential pathway in central regulation of metabolic and cardiovascular function. Central pro-opiomelanocortin (POMC) containing neurons in the arcuate nucleus (ARC) of the hypothalamus and the brain stem (e.g. nucleus of the tractus solitaries, NTS) project to other brain regions involved in energy homeostasis but also cardiovascular regulation [80]. The POMC neurons stimulate melanocortin receptor subtype 3 (MC3R) and 4 (MC4R) and reduce appetite and increase energy expenditure, SNS activity and BP [80]. Mutation of the melanocortin-4 receptor (MC4R) or pro-opiomelanocortin (POMC) gene estimates for 5–6% of early onset obesity in human [81]. Pharmacological blockade of MC4R causes pronounced obesity in rodents [82], whereas activation of MC4R promotes weight loss by reducing appetite and increase energy expenditure [83, 84]. Conversely, chronic MC4R activation causes sustained increased in BP despite reducing food intake and promoting weight loss [85]. MC4R-deficient rodents demonstrate reduced SNS activity and BP, independent of obesity [86]. Similar observations have been shown in humans, and MC4R deficiency leads to obesity but exhibits lower BP and reduced 24-h noradrenaline excretion compared with obese subjects with normal MC4R function [87, 88]. We and others have also demonstrated a critical role for the POMC-neurons MC4R axis in mediating appetite-suppressing and blood pressure effects of leptin [89, 90]. Rahmouni et al.

[89] showed that acute effect of leptin-induced hypophagia and renal SNS activity which were attenuated and abolished in heterozygous and homozygous MC4R knockout mice, respectively. Intact POMC neurons-MC4R axis is also required in chronic leptin-induced SNS activity and BP regulation [91]. MC4R antagonism markedly reduced BP in juvenile offspring born to obese dams (OffOb) [90] and spontaneous hypertensive rats (SHR) [92] two experimental models of hypertension that is associated with increased SNS activity in the absence of obesity [70, 93]. MC4R antagonism also attenuates or abolishes the acute pressor responses to leptin that raises BP by SNS stimulation [92]. Collectively, these observations suggest that the MC4R plays a key role in contributing to elevated BP in several forms of hypertension that accompany SNS overactivity. Greatest abundance of MC4R is the paraventricular nucleus of the hypothalamus (PVN), lateral hypothalamus (LH), the amygdala, the NTS and the preganglionic sympathetic neurons, which are all important sites for regulation of autonomic function [80]. Although the specific contribution of MC4R in distinct CNS nuclei in mediating the actions of the brain melanocortin system on energy balance, appetite and glucose homeostasis has been the subject of intense investigation, the particular regions of the brain, where MC4R is the most important in regulation of SNS activity and BP, are still unclear. We have recently shown that the activation of MC4R in the PVN (using sim-cre genetic-modified mice) demonstrated increased BP in offspring of obese dams that were protected in the MC4R-mutated mice; suggest an important role for MC4R in PVN in contributing to early onset hypertension [90]. One study has also observed that specific neuronal populations including cholinergic preganglionic parasympathetic and sympathetic neurons are involved in MC4R-mediated hypertension [94]. The specific stimuli that mediate the effect of MC4R to evoke sustained increases in SNS activity to cardiovascular-relevant tissue and promote chronic increase in BP are still unknown and remain an important area for future investigations.

3.4. Common genetic traits in paediatric hypertension

There has been a great progress in elucidating molecular targets for hypertension from monogenic disorders [95]. Among the most significant findings has been from single-gene disorders with primary effect on blood pressure that acts via common pathway alterations including renin-angiotensin and melanocortin system [95]. Recent genome-wide association studies (GWASs), conducted mostly in Europeans, have identified >30 genomic loci associated with systolic/diastolic BP [96], including candidate genes angiotensinogen [97], angiotensin-converting enzyme (ACE) [98], and alpha 2 adrenergic receptor genes (ADRA2A) [98]. The GWAS analysis is, however, inconsistent between populations, with a great gene-environment interaction, that significantly contributes to the increased risk of hypertension [99]. Obesity is one of the most dominant risk factor of childhood hypertension with a common genetic traits in FTO [100] and downstream of MC4R [101]. Hypertension has been associated with the risk allele A for FTO rs9939609 and the risk allele C for MC4R rs17782313, independent of BMI [102, 103]. Recent study by Sun et al. demonstrated an association of the FTO rs9939609 and MC4R rs17782313 genes with nocturnal blood pressure in the Chinese Han population [104]. The effect sizes are, however, small for each individual genetic variant, typically 1 mmHg for SBP and 0.5 mmHg for DBP [105]. Even collectively, the 30 variants tested in one experiment explain only 1–2% of SBP and DBP variance [105]. Heritability of hypertension is estimated to be between 30 and 40% which is approximately 25 times larger than the phenotypic variation and disease risk currently explained by GWAS SNPs. The observation that only little of the total heritability can be currently be explained by the GWAS has led to the term "missing heritability" [106]. It is expected that many more yet undiscovered loci, possible including variants in the rare allele spectrum that might have larger effects sizes, will contribute to explain the missing heritability [106]. It has been suggested that epigenetic changes may account for the missing heritability determinants of complex diseases, such as hypertension.

3.5. Epigenetic traits in experimental model of hypertension

Recent years have shown a dramatic interest in the epigenetic trait of human disease. Phenotypic variation is regulated independent of changes in DNA sequence, such as DNA methylation, histone modification, chromatin remodelling and the action of small noncoding RNAs (microRNA) [107]. These epigenetic modifications change the accessibility of gene promoter sequence (by methyl donor) and binding domain [107]. Several animal studies have characterise epigenetic modification influenced by the intrauterine environment (maternal stress, nutrition and behaviour) [107]. In cardiovascular disease, recent studies of low-protein diet during pregnancy showed early onset hypertension in the offspring [108]. The renin-angiotensin system showed to be a main target as angiotensin receptor (AT1R) antagonist reversed the hypertension in the offspring [108]. Consistent with these finding, offspring showed a hypomethylated AT1R gene promoter along with the increased expression of AT1R [109], suggesting a role for specific AT1R hypomethylation in regulating elevated blood pressure in this model. Similar epigenetic modification has been shown in the hypothalamic POMC neurons in a rat model of neonatal overfeeding [110]. Hypothalamic POMC showed hypermethylated in the overfed neonates and consequently influence the set point of the melanocortin system which is critical for metabolic and cardiovascular regulation [110]. Fewer studies of epigenetic changes have been conducted in primates, and there is little direct evidence relating this to humans. One study showed a correlation of epigenetic RXRA (retinoid X receptor alpha—induces transcription of PPARs) promoter methylation with increased adiposity in children of mothers with lower carbohydrate intake in two independent cohorts [111]. Although this fails to confirm a causal relationship, it may provide an objective marker in identifying children at risk of obesity and hypertension-induced cardiac hypertrophy [112].

3.6. The role of central inflammation

Several reports have demonstrated enhanced inflammatory profile with paediatric hypertension [113, 114]. The C-reactive protein (CRP) which normally is involved in innate immune responses is heightened both in hypertensive and pre-hypertensive obese children, suggesting that systemic low-grade inflammation may precede hypertension [115]. This has been further confirmed in animal models of hypertension. Spontaneous hypertensive rats (SHR) a genetic model of essential hypertension demonstrate increased renal infiltration of lymphocytes and macrophages and activation of nuclear factor –kappa B (NF-kB) in 3-week-old pre-hypertensive rats [116]. Serum CRP has also been associated with cardiovascular risk factors in children including BP variability [117], intima media thickness [118], arterial stiffness [119], left ventricular hypertrophy [120]. Obese children and adolescence also demonstrate elevated serum concentration of pro-inflammatory cytokines interleukin-6 (IL-6) IL-1β and ICAM-1 (intercellular cell adhesion molecule-1) with increased ambulatory BP [121]. The pro-inflammatory cytokines may also be increased due to obesity alone, independent of essential hypertension [122]. However, the highest concentration of these molecules was found in children with co-existing hypertension [114]. Mounting evidence suggests that the pro-inflammatory condition in mother may induce inflammation-induced hypertension in their offspring [123]. An overactive immune response during pregnancy, as shown in obese pregnancy [124], can lead to chronic neuro-inflammation in the foetus [125]. Activated microglia, resident immune cells in the brain, increases pro-inflammatory cytokines release from the PVN, which stimulate preganglionic nerve fibres and sympathetic nerve activity (SNA) [126]. Vice versa, SNA has a direct impact on microglia via adrenergic receptors [127] or indirect via regulating distribution and production of lymphocytes, or modulating the release of pro-inflammatory peptides. SNA is also involved in inflammatory cell recruitment and redistribution, and SNA mobilise inflammatory cells from spleen and bone marrow [128]. In addition, parasympathetic nervous system has anti-inflammatory effects [129]. Vagal afferents sense peripheral inflammation and feedback via the cholinergic anti-inflammatory pathway [129]. There are also important direct effects of cytokines and angiotensin II on the brain that certainly could contribute to SNA [129, 130]. Catheter-base renal denervation is a promising therapeutic approach to treat hypertension [131], and recent animal studies suggest

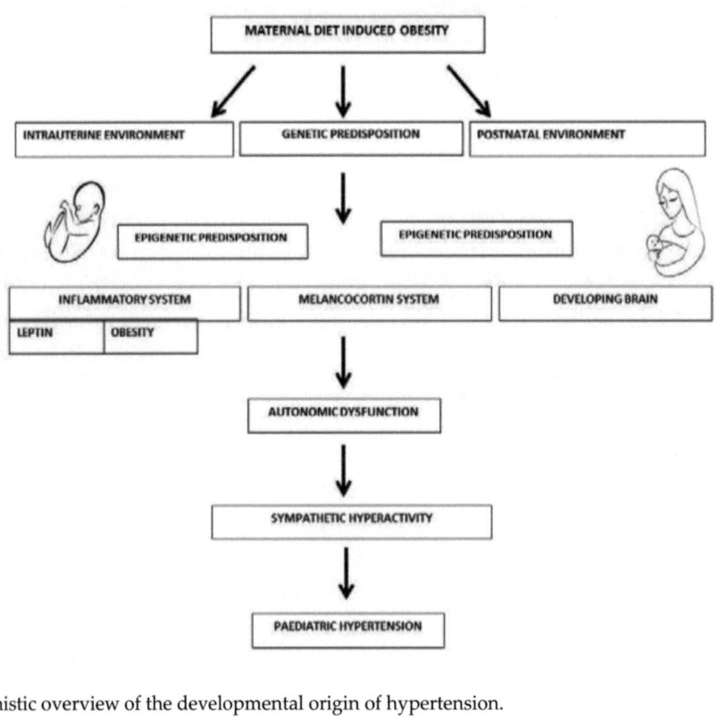

Figure 1. Mechanistic overview of the developmental origin of hypertension.

http://dx.doi.org/10.5772/62652

an improvement of renal inflammation with reduced renal macrophages and levels of cortical TNF-alpha and suggest a potential target for renal injury and dysfunction [132]. Minocyclin treatment, an anti-inflammatory antibiotic that crosses the blood brain barrier, has shown to prevent autonomic dysfunction and hypertension in experimental models of hypertension [126]. The reduction in blood pressure was associated with "de-activation" of the microglia in the PVN [126]. Overall, all these studies suggest a potentially important link between inflammation, melanocortin system, developing brain and autonomic dysfunction in the environmental and genetic predisposition of hypertension arising from maternal diet-induced obesity (**Figure 1**).

4. Future research and intervention strategies

Paediatric hypertension has been gaining significant attention in the last decade, mainly due to the increased prevalence worldwide. The estimated prevalence of paediatric hypertension is from 1 to 10%, with a steady rise over time. Alarming rate of childhood obesity and metabolic syndrome with the precondition of maternal obesity may worsen the future cardiovascular morbidity and mortality. This could be hypothetically prevented by early diagnosis and management in children before they even develop the pathophysiological progression state of hypertension. In fact, certain drugs may fail to reduce sympathetic hyperactivity as other stimuli of SNA have become predominant in elevating SNA, which are independent of the standard antihypertensive strategies. The progress and impact of preventive blood pressure screening for children could also inhibit adult hypertension and cardiovascular disease. Therefore, increased alertness to paediatric hypertension including several risk parameters (genetic, maternal, inflammatory, adiposity) and standardise sequential ABPM monitoring to avoid "white-coat" and "masked" hypertension in the diagnosis could improve future statistics in adverse cardiovascular outcome. Research effort should continue with the goal to clarify the aetiology, complexity and inheritable factors of paediatric hypertension. Research efforts should also focus on optimal treatment of these children and on effective preventive measures starting in the pregnant mother to the child at a young age.

Author details

Anne-Maj Sofia Samuelsson

Address all correspondence to: anne-maj.samuelsson@kcl.ac.uk

Division of Women's Health, King's College London, Women's Health Academic Centre KHP, London, UK

References

[1] Ostchega Y., et al., *Trends of elevated blood pressure among children and adolescents: data from the National Health and Nutrition Examination Survey1988–2006*. Am J Hypertens, 2009. 22(1): pp. 59–67.

[2] Din-Dzietham R., et al., *High blood pressure trends in children and adolescents in national surveys, 1963 to 2002*. Circulation, 2007. 116(13): pp. 1488–96.

[3] Hansen M.L., Gunn P.W., and Kaelber D.C., *Underdiagnosis of hypertension in children and adolescents*. JAMA, 2007. 298(8): pp. 874–9.

[4] McCrindle B.W., *Assessment and management of hypertension in children and adolescents*. Nat Rev Cardiol, 2010. 7(3): pp. 155–63.

[5] Kavey R.E., *Left ventricular hypertrophy in hypertensive children and adolescents: predictors and prevalence*. Curr Hypertens Rep, 2013. 15(5): pp. 453–7.

[6] Hadtstein C. and Schaefer F., *Hypertension in children with chronic kidney disease: pathophysiology and management*. Pediatr Nephrol, 2008. 23(3): pp. 363–71.

[7] Urbina E.M., *Abnormalities of vascular structure and function in pediatric hypertension*. Pediatr Nephrol, 2015.

[8] Cha S.D., et al., *The effects of hypertension on cognitive function in children and adolescents*. Int J Pediatr, 2012. 2012: p. 891094.

[9] Lande M.B., Kupferman J.C., and Adams H.R., *Neurocognitive alterations in hypertensive children and adolescents*. J Clin Hypertens (Greenwich), 2012. 14(6): pp. 353–9.

[10] Chen X. and Wang Y., *Tracking of blood pressure from childhood to adulthood: a systematic review and meta-regression analysis*. Circulation, 2008. 117(25): pp. 3171–80.

[11] Ogden C.L., et al., *Prevalence of overweight among preschool children in the United States, 1971 through 1994*. Pediatrics, 1997. 99(4): p. E1.

[12] Bridger T., *Childhood obesity and cardiovascular disease*. Paediatr Child Health, 2009. 14(3): pp. 177–82.

[13] Verma M., Chhatwal J., and George S.M., *Obesity and hypertension in children*. Indian Pediatr, 1994. 31(9): pp. 1065–9.

[14] Freedman D.S., et al., *The relation of overweight to cardiovascular risk factors among children and adolescents: the Bogalusa Heart Study*. Pediatrics, 1999. 103(6 Pt 1): pp. 1175–82.

[15] Sorof J.M., et al., *Isolated systolic hypertension, obesity, and hyperkinetic hemodynamic states in children*. J Pediatr, 2002. 140(6): pp. 660–6.

[16] Goonasekera C.D. and Dillon M.J., *Measurement and interpretation of blood pressure*. Arch Dis Child, 2000. 82(3): pp. 261–5.

[17] Bao W., et al., *Essential hypertension predicted by tracking of elevated blood pressure from childhood to adulthood: the Bogalusa Heart Study*. Am J Hypertens, 1995. 8(7): pp. 657–65.

[18] *Update on the 1987 Task Force Report on High Blood Pressure in Children and Adolescents: a working group report from the National High Blood Pressure Education Program. National High Blood Pressure Education program working group on Hypertension control in Children and Adolescents*. Pediatrics, 1996. 98(4 Pt 1): pp. 649–58.

[19] Kapur G., et al., *Secondary hypertension in overweight and stage 1 hypertensive children: a Midwest Pediatric Nephrology Consortium report*. J Clin Hypertens (Greenwich), 2010. 12(1): pp. 34–9.

[20] Sorof J. and Daniels S., *Obesity hypertension in children: a problem of epidemic proportions*. Hypertension, 2002. 40(4): pp. 441–7.

[21] Wang Y. and Lim H., *The global childhood obesity epidemic and the association between socio-economic status and childhood obesity*. Int Rev Psychiatry, 2012. 24(3): pp. 176–88.

[22] Guyenet P.G., *The sympathetic control of blood pressure*. Nat Rev Neurosci, 2006. 7(5): pp. 335–46.

[23] Licht C.M., et al., *Increased sympathetic and decreased parasympathetic activity rather than changes in hypothalamic-pituitary-adrenal axis activity is associated with metabolic abnormalities*. J Clin Endocrinol Metab, 2010. 95(5): pp. 2458–66.

[24] Straznicky N.E., et al., *Mediators of sympathetic activation in metabolic syndrome obesity*. Curr Hypertens Rep, 2008. 10(6): pp. 440–7.

[25] Joyner M.J., Charkoudian N., and Wallin B.G., *Sympathetic nervous system and blood pressure in humans: individualized patterns of regulation and their implications*. Hypertension, 2010. 56(1): pp. 10–6.

[26] Lichty B.D., et al., *Dysregulation of HOX11 by chromosome translocations in T-cell acute lymphoblastic leukemia: a paradigm for homeobox gene involvement in human cancer*. Leuk Lymphoma, 1995. 16(3–4): pp. 209–15.

[27] Berntson G.G., et al., *Cardiac autonomic balance versus cardiac regulatory capacity*. Psychophysiology, 2008. 45(4): pp. 643–52.

[28] Nagai N., et al., *Autonomic nervous system activity and the state and development of obesity in Japanese school children*. Obes Res, 2003. 11(1): pp. 25–32.

[29] Kaufman C.L., et al., *Relationships of cardiac autonomic function with metabolic abnormalities in childhood obesity*. Obesity (Silver Spring), 2007. 15(5): pp. 1164–71.

[30] Yakinci C., et al., *Autonomic nervous system functions in obese children*. Brain Dev, 2000. 22(3): pp. 151–3.

[31] Vrijkotte T.G., et al., *Cardiac autonomic nervous system activation and metabolic profile in young children: the ABCD Study*. PLoS One, 2015. 10(9): p. e0138302.

[32] Latchman P.L., et al., *Impaired autonomic function in normotensive obese children*. Clin Auton Res, 2011. 21(5): pp. 319–23.

[33] Graziano P.A., et al., *Cardiovascular regulation profile predicts developmental trajectory of BMI and pediatric obesity*. Obesity (Silver Spring), 2011. 19(9): pp. 1818–25.

[34] Riva P., et al., *Obesity and autonomic function in adolescence*. Clin Exp Hypertens, 2001. 23(1–2): pp. 57–67.

[35] Voors A.W., Webber L.S., and Berenson G.S., *Resting heart rate and pressure-rate product of children in a total biracial community: the Bogalusa Heart Study*. Am J Epidemiol, 1982. 116(2): pp. 276–86.

[36] Ojala T., et al., *Fetal cardiac sympathetic activation is linked with maternal body mass index*. Early Hum Dev, 2009. 85(9): pp. 557–60.

[37] Barker D.J., et al., *Growth in utero, blood pressure in childhood and adult life, and mortality from cardiovascular disease*. BMJ, 1989. 298(6673): pp. 564–7.

[38] Primatesta P., Falaschetti E., and Poulter N.R., *Birth weight and blood pressure in childhood: results from the Health Survey for England*. Hypertension, 2005. 45(1): pp. 75–9.

[39] Belfort M.B., et al., *Size at birth, infant growth, and blood pressure at three years of age*. J Pediatr, 2007. 151(6): pp. 670–4.

[40] Barker D.J. and Osmond C., *Infant mortality, childhood nutrition, and ischaemic heart disease in England and Wales*. Lancet, 1986. 1(8489): pp. 1077–81.

[41] Ojeda N.B., Grigore D., and Alexander B.T., *Developmental programming of hypertension: insight from animal models of nutritional manipulation*. Hypertension, 2008. 52(1): pp. 44–50.

[42] Reynolds R.M., et al., *Maternal obesity during pregnancy and premature mortality from cardiovascular event in adult offspring: follow-up of 1 323 275 person years*. BMJ, 2013. 347: p. f4539.

[43] Wen X., et al., *Prenatal factors for childhood blood pressure mediated by intrauterine and/or childhood growth?* Pediatrics, 2011. 127(3): pp. e713–21.

[44] Gademan M.G., et al., *Maternal prepregnancy body mass index and their children's blood pressure and resting cardiac autonomic balance at age 5 to 6 years*. Hypertension, 2013. 62(3): pp. 641–7.

[45] Hochner H., et al., *Associations of maternal prepregnancy body mass index and gestational weight gain with adult offspring cardiometabolic risk factors: the Jerusalem Perinatal Family Follow-up Study*. Circulation, 2012. 125(11): pp. 1381–9.

[46] Gaillard R., et al., *Childhood cardiometabolic outcomes of maternal obesity during pregnancy: the Generation R Study*. Hypertension, 2014. 63(4): pp. 683–91.

[47] Flegal K.M., et al., *Prevalence of obesity and trends in the distribution of body mass index among US adults, 1999–2010.* JAMA, 2012. 307(5): pp. 491–7.

[48] Heslehurst N., et al., *A nationally representative study of maternal obesity in England, UK: trends in incidence and demographic inequalities in 619 323 births, 1989–2007.* Int J Obes (Lond), 2010. 34(3): pp. 420–8.

[49] Miller M., et al., *Preventing maternal and early childhood obesity: the fetal flaw in Australian perinatal care.* Aust J Prim Health, 2014. 20(2): pp. 123–7.

[50] Martorell R., et al., *Obesity in Latin American women and children.* J Nutr, 1998. 128(9): pp. 1464–73.

[51] Balarajan Y. and Villamor E., *Nationally representative surveys show recent increases in the prevalence of overweight and obesity among women of reproductive age in Bangladesh, Nepal, and India.* J Nutr, 2009. 139(11): pp. 2139–44.

[52] Leddy M.A., Power M.L., and Schulkin J., *The impact of maternal obesity on maternal and fetal health.* Rev Obstet Gynecol, 2008. 1(4): pp. 170–8.

[53] McCorry L.K., *Physiology of the autonomic nervous system.* Am J Pharm Educ, 2007. 71(4): p. 78.

[54] Feber J., et al., *Autonomic nervous system dysregulation in pediatric hypertension.* Curr Hypertens Rep, 2014. 16(5): pp. 426.

[55] Smith P.A., et al., *Sympathetic neural mechanisms in white-coat hypertension.* J Am Coll Cardiol, 2002. 40(1): pp. 126–32.

[56] Zhou Y., et al., *Cardiovascular risk factors significantly correlate with autonomic nervous system activity in children.* Can J Cardiol, 2012. 28(4): pp. 477–82.

[57] Gui-Ling X., et al., *Association of high blood pressure with heart rate variability in children.* Iran J Pediatr, 2013. 23(1): pp. 37–44.

[58] Genovesi S., et al., *Analysis of heart period and arterial pressure variability in childhood hypertension: key role of baroreflex impairment.* Hypertension, 2008. 51(5): pp. 1289–94.

[59] Kowalewski M., et al., *Heart rate variability and left ventricular mass in slim children and young adults with hypertension.* Kardiol Pol, 2005. 63(6): pp. 605–10; discussion 611–2.

[60] Latus H., et al., *Heart rate variability is related to disease severity in children and young adults with pulmonary hypertension.* Front Pediatr, 2015. 3: p. 63.

[61] Massin M. and von Bernuth G., *Normal ranges of heart rate variability during infancy and childhood.* Pediatr Cardiol, 1997. 18(4): pp. 297–302.

[62] De Bock F., et al., *Do our children lose vagus activity? Potential time trends of children's autonomic nervous system activity.* Int J Cardiol, 2013. 170(2): pp. e30–2.

[63] Kazuma N., et al., *Heart rate variability in normotensive healthy children with aging*. Clin Exp Hypertens, 2002. 24(1–2): pp. 83–9.

[64] Young J.B., Weiss J., and Boufath N., *Effects of dietary monosaccharides on sympathetic nervous system activity in adipose tissues of male rats*. Diabetes, 2004. 53(5): pp. 1271–8.

[65] Urbina E.M., et al., *Ethnic (black-white) contrasts in heart rate variability during cardiovascular reactivity testing in male adolescents with high and low blood pressure: the Bogalusa Heart Study*. Am J Hypertens, 1998 Feb. 11(2): pp. 196–202.

[66] Taylor P.D., Samuelsson A.M., and Poston L., *Maternal obesity and the developmental programming of hypertension: a role for leptin*. Acta Physiol (Oxf), 2014. 210(3): pp. 508–23.

[67] Nathanielsz P.W., Poston L., and Taylor P.D., *In utero exposure to maternal obesity and diabetes: animal models that identify and characterize implications for future health*. Clin Perinatol, 2007. 34(4): pp. 515–26.

[68] Collins S., et al., *Role of leptin in fat regulation*. Nature, 1996. 380(6576): p. 677.

[69] Haynes W.G., et al., *Receptor-mediated regional sympathetic nerve activation by leptin*. J Clin Investig, 1997. 100(2): pp. 270–8.

[70] Samuelsson A.M., et al., *Evidence for sympathetic origins of hypertension in juvenile offspring of obese rats*. Hypertension, 2010. 55(1): pp. 76–82.

[71] Shek E.W., Brands M.W., and Hall J.E., *Chronic leptin infusion increases arterial pressure*. Hypertension, 1998. 31(1 Pt 2): pp. 409–14.

[72] Aizawa-Abe M., et al., *Pathophysiological role of leptin in obesity-related hypertension*. J Clin Invest, 2000. 105(9): pp. 1243–52.

[73] Halaas J.L., et al., *Physiological response to long-term peripheral and central leptin infusion in lean and obese mice*. Proc Natl Acad Sci USA, 1997. 94(16): pp. 8878–83.

[74] Rahmouni K., et al., *Selective resistance to central neural administration of leptin in agouti obese mice*. Hypertension, 2002. 39(2 Pt 2): pp. 486–90.

[75] Agata J., et al., *High plasma immunoreactive leptin level in essential hypertension*. Am J Hypertens, 1997. 10(10 Pt 1): pp. 1171–4.

[76] Monroe M.B., et al., *Relation of leptin and insulin to adiposity-associated elevations in sympathetic activity with age in humans*. Int J Obes Relat Metab Disord, 2000. 24(9): pp. 1183–7.

[77] Bouret S.G. and Simerly R.B., *Minireview: leptin and development of hypothalamic feeding circuits*. Endocrinology, 2004. 145(6): pp. 2621–6.

[78] Kirk S.L., et al., *Maternal obesity induced by diet in rats permanently influences central processes regulating food intake in offspring*. PLoS One, 2009. 4(6): p. e5870.

[79] Okereke N.C., et al., *The effect of gender and gestational diabetes mellitus on cord leptin concentration*. Am J Obstet Gynecol, 2002. 187(3): pp. 798–803.

[80] da Silva A.A., et al., *The brain melanocortin system, sympathetic control, and obesity hypertension*. Physiology (Bethesda), 2014. 29(3): pp. 196–202.

[81] Vaisse C., et al., *Melanocortin-4 receptor mutations are a frequent and heterogeneous cause of morbid obesity*. J Clin Investig, 2000. 106(2): pp. 253–62.

[82] Hagan M.M., et al., *Role of the CNS melanocortin system in the response to overfeeding*. J Neurosci, 1999. 19(6): pp. 2362–7.

[83] Fan W., et al., *Role of melanocortinergic neurons in feeding and the agouti obesity syndrome*. Nature, 1997. 385(6612): pp. 165–8.

[84] Li G., et al., *Unabated anorexic and enhanced thermogenic responses to melanotan II in diet-induced obese rats despite reduced melanocortin 3 and 4 receptor expression*. J Endocrinol, 2004. 182(1): pp. 123–32.

[85] Kuo J.J., Silva A.A., and Hall J.E., *Hypothalamic melanocortin receptors and chronic regulation of arterial pressure and renal function*. Hypertension, 2003. 41(3 Pt 2): pp. 768–74.

[86] Tallam L.S., et al., *Melanocortin-4 receptor-deficient mice are not hypertensive or salt-sensitive despite obesity, hyperinsulinemia, and hyperleptinemia*. Hypertension, 2005. 46(2): pp. 326–32.

[87] Greenfield J.R., et al., *Modulation of blood pressure by central melanocortinergic pathways*. N Engl J Med, 2009. 360(1): pp. 44–52.

[88] Martinelli C.E., et al., *Obesity due to melanocortin 4 receptor (MC4R) deficiency is associated with increased linear growth and final height, fasting hyperinsulinemia, and incompletely suppressed growth hormone secretion*. J Clin Endocrinol Metab, 2011. 96(1): pp. E181–8.

[89] Rahmouni K., et al., *Role of melanocortin-4 receptors in mediating renal sympathoactivation to leptin and insulin*. J Neurosci, 2003. 23(14): pp. 5998–6004.

[90] Samuelsson A.M., *New perspectives on the origin of hypertension; the role of the hypothalamic melanocortin system*. Exp Physiol, 2014. 99(9): pp. 1110–5.

[91] Tallam L.S., da Silva A.A., and Hall J.E., *Melanocortin-4 receptor mediates chronic cardiovascular and metabolic actions of leptin*. Hypertension, 2006. 48(1): pp. 58–64.

[92] da Silva A.A., et al., *Endogenous melanocortin system activity contributes to the elevated arterial pressure in spontaneously hypertensive rats*. Hypertension, 2008. 51(4): pp. 884–90.

[93] Dickhout J.G. and Lee R.M., *Blood pressure and heart rate development in young spontaneously hypertensive rats*. Am J Physiol, 1998. 274(3 Pt 2): pp. H794–800.

[94] Sohn J.W., et al., *Melanocortin 4 receptors reciprocally regulate sympathetic and parasympathetic preganglionic neurons*. Cell, 2013. 152(3): pp. 612–9.

[95] Lifton R.P., Gharavi A.G., and Geller D.S., *Molecular mechanisms of human hypertension*. Cell, 2001. 104(4): pp. 545–56.

[96] Munroe P.B., Barnes M.R., and Caulfield M.J., *Advances in blood pressure genomics*. Circ Res, 2013. 112(10): pp. 1365–79.

[97] Jeunemaitre X., et al., *Molecular basis of human hypertension: role of angiotensinogen*. Cell, 1992. 71(1): pp. 169–80.

[98] Staessen J.A., et al., *The deletion/insertion polymorphism of the angiotensin converting enzyme gene and cardiovascular-renal risk*. J Hypertens, 1997. 15(12 Pt 2): pp. 1579–92.

[99] Lieb W., et al., *Genetic predisposition to higher blood pressure increases coronary artery disease risk*. Hypertension, 2013. 61(5): pp. 995–1001.

[100] Frayling T.M., et al., *A common variant in the FTO gene is associated with body mass index and predisposes to childhood and adult obesity*. Science, 2007. 316(5826): pp. 889–94.

[101] Loos R.J., et al., *Common variants near MC4R are associated with fat mass, weight and risk of obesity*. Nat Genet, 2008. 40(6): pp. 768–75.

[102] Pausova Z., et al., *A common variant of the FTO gene is associated with not only increased adiposity but also elevated blood pressure in French Canadians*. Circ Cardiovasc Genet, 2009. 2(3): pp. 260–9.

[103] Qi L., et al., *The common obesity variant near MC4R gene is associated with higher intakes of total energy and dietary fat, weight change and diabetes risk in women*. Hum Mol Genet, 2008. 17(22): pp. 3502–8.

[104] Sun Y., et al., *Combined effects of FTO rs9939609 and MC4R rs17782313 on elevated nocturnal blood pressure in the Chinese Han population*. Cardiovasc J Afr. 2016 Jan-Feb. 27(1): pp. 21–4. doi: 10.5830/CVJA-2015-064. Epub 2015 Aug 31.

[105] International Consortium for Blood Pressure Genome-Wide Association Studies, et al., *Genetic variants in novel pathways influence blood pressure and cardiovascular disease risk*. Nature, 2011. 478(7367): pp. 103–9.

[106] Manolio T.A., et al., *Finding the missing heritability of complex diseases*. Nature, 2009. 461(7265): pp. 747–53.

[107] Sookoian S., et al., *Fetal metabolic programming and epigenetic modifications: a systems biology approach*. Pediatr Res, 2013. 73(4 Pt 2): pp. 531–42.

[108] Sherman R.C. and Langley-Evans S.C., *Early administration of angiotensin-converting enzyme inhibitor captopril, prevents the development of hypertension programmed by intrauterine exposure to a maternal low-protein diet in the rat*. Clin Sci (Lond), 1998. 94(4): pp. 373–81.

[109] Bogdarina I., et al., *Epigenetic modification of the renin-angiotensin system in the fetal programming of hypertension*. Circ Res, 2007. 100(4): pp. 520–6.

[110] Plagemann A., et al., *Hypothalamic proopiomelanocortin promoter methylation becomes altered by early overfeeding: an epigenetic model of obesity and the metabolic syndrome.* J Physiol, 2009. 587(Pt 20): pp. 4963–76.

[111] Godfrey K.M., et al., *Epigenetic gene promoter methylation at birth is associated with child's later adiposity.* Diabetes, 2011. 60(5): pp. 1528–34.

[112] Zhu J., et al., *Retinoid X receptor agonists inhibit hypertension-induced myocardial hypertrophy by modulating LKB1/AMPK/p70S6K signaling pathway.* Am J Hypertens, 2014. 27(8): pp. 1112–24.

[113] Lopez-Jaramillo P., et al., *Inter-relationships between body mass index, C-reactive protein and blood pressure in a Hispanic pediatric population.* Am J Hypertens, 2008. 21(5): pp. 527–32.

[114] Glowinska-Olszewska B., Tolwinska J., and Urban M., *Relationship between endothelial dysfunction, carotid artery intima media thickness and circulating markers of vascular inflammation in obese hypertensive children and adolescents.* J Pediatr Endocrinol Metab, 2007. 20(10): pp. 1125–36.

[115] Chrysohoou C., et al., *Association between prehypertension status and inflammatory markers related to atherosclerotic disease: the ATTICA Study.* Am J Hypertens, 2004. 17(7): pp. 568–73.

[116] Rodriguez-Iturbe B., et al., *Evolution of renal interstitial inflammation and NF-kappaB activation in spontaneously hypertensive rats.* Am J Nephrol, 2004. 24(6): pp. 587–94.

[117] Kim K.I., et al., *Association between blood pressure variability and inflammatory marker in hypertensive patients.* Circ J, 2008. 72(2): pp. 293–8.

[118] Reinehr T., et al., *Intima media thickness in childhood obesity: relations to inflammatory marker, glucose metabolism, and blood pressure.* Metabolism, 2006. 55(1): pp. 113–8.

[119] Kampus P., et al., *The relationship between inflammation and arterial stiffness in patients with essential hypertension.* Int J Cardiol, 2006. 112(1): pp. 46–51.

[120] Assadi F., *Relation of left ventricular hypertrophy to microalbuminuria and C-reactive protein in children and adolescents with essential hypertension.* Pediatr Cardiol, 2008. 29(3): pp. 580–4.

[121] Syrenicz A., et al., *Relation of low-grade inflammation and endothelial activation to blood pressure in obese children and adolescents.* Neuro Endocrinol Lett, 2006. 27(4): pp. 459–64.

[122] Sacheck J., *Pediatric obesity: an inflammatory condition?* JPEN J Parenter Enteral Nutr, 2008. 32(6): pp. 633–7.

[123] Diaz J.J., et al., *C-reactive protein is elevated in the offspring of parents with essential hypertension.* Arch Dis Child, 2007. 92(4): pp. 304–8.

[124] Bugatto F., et al., *Second-trimester amniotic fluid proinflammatory cytokine levels in normal and overweight women*. Obstet Gynecol, 2010. 115(1): pp. 127–33.

[125] Harry G.J., *Neuroinflammation: a need to understand microglia as resident cells of the developing brain*. Neurotoxicology, 2012. 33(3): pp. 558–9.

[126] Shi P., et al., *Brain microglial cytokines in neurogenic hypertension*. Hypertension, 2010. 56(2): pp. 297–303.

[127] Nance D.M. and Sanders V.M., *Autonomic innervation and regulation of the immune system (1987–2007)*. Brain Behav Immun, 2007. 21(6): pp. 736–45.

[128] Zubcevic J., et al., *Functional neural-bone marrow pathways: implications in hypertension and cardiovascular disease*. Hypertension, 2014. 63(6): pp. e129–39.

[129] Pavlov V.A. and Tracey K.J., *The vagus nerve and the inflammatory reflex—linking immunity and metabolism*. Nat Rev Endocrinol, 2012. 8(12): pp. 743–54.

[130] Harwani S.C., et al., *Neurohormonal modulation of the innate immune system is proinflammatory in the prehypertensive spontaneously hypertensive rat, a genetic model of essential hypertension*. Circ Res, 2012. 111(9): pp. 1190–7.

[131] Davis M.I., et al., *Effectiveness of renal denervation therapy for resistant hypertension: a systematic review and meta-analysis*. J Am Coll Cardiol, 2013. 62(3): pp. 231–41.

[132] Veelken R., et al., *Autonomic renal denervation ameliorates experimental glomerulonephritis*. J Am Soc Nephrol, 2008. 19(7): pp. 1371–8.

Chapter 3

Oxidative Stress and Essential Hypertension

Ramón Rodrigo, Roberto Brito and Jaime González

Additional information is available at the end of the chapter

http://dx.doi.org/10.5772/64079

Abstract

Experimental evidence supports a pathogenic role of free radicals or reactive oxygen species (ROS) in the mechanism of hypertension. Indeed, vascular ROS produced in a controlled manner are considered important physiological mediators, functioning as signaling molecules to maintain vascular integrity by regulating endothelial function and vascular contraction-relaxation. However, oxidative stress can be involved in the occurrence of endothelial dysfunction and related vascular injury. Thus, ROS activity could trigger pathophysiological cascades leading to inflammation, monocyte migration, lipid peroxidation, and increased deposition of extracellular matrix in the vascular wall, among other events. In addition, impairment of the antioxidant capacity associates with blood pressure elevation, indicating potential role of antioxidants as therapeutic antihypertensive agents. Nevertheless, although increased ROS biomarkers have been reported in patients with essential hypertension, the involvement of oxidative stress as a causative factor of human essential hypertension remains to be established. The aim of this chapter is to provide a novel insight into the mechanism of essential hypertension, including a paradigm based on the role played by oxidative stress.

Keywords: essential hypertension, oxidative stress, antioxidants, endothelial dysfunction, nitric oxide

1. Introduction

Hypertension is a major risk factor for cardiovascular disease [1]. Recently, a growing body of evidence has involved oxidative stress in the mechanism of development of hypertension. Indeed, reactive oxygen species (ROS) contribute to regulating the biological processes occurring in the vascular wall, both in normal physiological conditions, as well as in the occurrence of hypertension [2–4]. Available evidence of the contribution of oxidative stress in the pathogenesis of human hypertension includes enhancement of ROS production, together with decreased bioavailability of both nitric oxide (NO) and antioxidants. The first-formed ROS is superoxide anion radical, which is produced from NADPH oxidase (NOX), an enzyme subjected to regulation by hormones such as angiotensin II (AT-II), endothelin-1 (ET-1), and urotensin II (UT-II), among others. Furthermore, mechanical stimuli known to occur in blood pressure elevation further contribute to increased ROS production. It is of interest to mention that increased intracellular calcium concentration may result from ROS-induced vasoconstriction, thus enhancing the development of hypertension [2]. The regulation of vasomotor tone depends upon a delicate balance between vasoconstrictor and vasodilator forces, the latter being likely to be modulated by oxidative stress. This view has stimulated the interest for searching novel antihypertensive therapies aimed to decrease ROS generation and/or increase NO bioavailability. The present study was aimed to present an update of the available studies related to the role of oxidative stress in the mechanism of development of blood pressure elevation, as well as the role of antioxidants in the prevention or treatment of this derangement.

2. Pathophysiology of hypertension

2.1. Endothelial dysfunction

The response to cardiovascular risk factors is expressed in alterations of endothelial function, a chronic inflammatory process characterized by loss of antithrombotic factors and an increase in vasoconstrictor and prothrombotic products, thus elevating the risk of cardiovascular events. Consequently, an impairment of the ability of endothelium to induce vasodilation leads to hypertension. Recently, it has been argued that ROS play a key role in this pathological process.

2.2. Role of vascular oxidative stress in hypertension

The occurrence of oxidative stress is due to an imbalance between ROS generation and the antioxidant potential in the body, the latter being overwhelmed by the increased ROS concentration in the steady state. It should be noted that although ROS are mediators of normal biological effects related to vascular function at the cell level, the increased levels of these species can give rise to pathological changes, as those observed in cardiovascular disease. ROS behave as redox-sensitive blood pressure modulators [5–7]. Accordingly, increased ROS concentration has been demonstrated both in patients with essential hypertension and in various animal models of hypertension [8–12]. In addition, this derangement is accompanied by a decreased antioxidant potential [13]. Therefore, these data provide evidence of the involvement of vascular oxidative stress in the mechanism of development of essential hypertension [2, 3, 14]. Furthermore, a strong association between blood pressure and oxidative stress-related parameters has been found, such as plasma 8-isoprostane levels [15]. Interestingly, studies performed in mice models having genetic deficiency in ROS-generating enzymes showed that these animals had lower blood pressure than control with wild-type mice [16, 17]. Moreover, at the cellular level, it has been reported that ROS production is enhanced in cultured vascular smooth muscle cells (VSMC) isolated from both hypertensive rats and isolated arteries of hypertensive human patients; these findings are associated with amplified, redox-dependent signaling and reduced antioxidant bioactivity [18]. These reports could support the view that the modulation of oxidative stress could be expressed in blood pressure lowering in the case of known antihypertensive agents, such as β-adrenergic blockers, angiotensin-converting enzyme (ACE) inhibitors, angiotensin receptor antagonists, and calcium channel blockers [19, 20].

2.2.1. *Vascular ROS sources*

There are various ROS sources formed in blood vessels, from both enzymatic and non-enzymatic origin. Together with the mitochondrion, the major enzymatic sources comprise NADPH oxidase (NOX), xanthine oxidase (XO), and uncoupled NO synthase.

2.2.1.1. *NADPH oxidase*

In the vascular wall, as well as in the kidney, superoxide anion is mainly produced enzymatically through NOX activity; consequently, the upregulation of this enzyme exerts an important pathogenic role in the development of renal dysfunction and vascular damage [12, 21]. The enhanced activity of NOX in hypertension is achieved through mechanical and humoral signals, with AT-II being the most studied stimulus. However, it is important to remark that ET-1 and UT-II cooperatively participate in NOX activation. In addition, NOX-derived superoxide anion is able to inactivate NO, thus producing peroxynitrite anion. The latter induces downregulation of prostacyclin synthase, further allowing the development of hypertension. Finally, oxidative stress leads to eNOS uncoupling [16, 22]. Therefore, several effects contribute to the impairment of endothelial function related to oxidative stress. In summary, increased superoxide anion, decreased NO bioavailability, and decreased prostacyclin synthesis contribute to the impairment of endothelium-dependent vasodilation. Thus, NOX activation in the vascular wall results in several effects contributing to the mechanism of development of hypertension [23].

2.2.1.2. *Uncoupled endothelial NO synthase*

The vascular tone is modulated by vasoconstriction-vasodilation balance, and NO bioavailability constitutes an important component of the latter process. The NO production is partly dependent upon the activity of eNOS. However, other factors, such as L-arginine and tetrahydrobiopterin (BH4) availability, are also required as substrate and coupling factor, respectively. Deficiency or oxidation of either of these two factors will result in decreased NO production. The initial ROS source is NOX-dependent superoxide generation. Furthermore, peroxynitrite is formed through the reaction between NO and superoxide [24]. The activity and function of eNOS are changed due to the peroxidant ability generated by peroxynitrite, and this enzyme produces more superoxide instead of NO [22, 25]. This vicious cycle results in BH4 oxidation, thereby promoting eNOS uncoupling and enhancement in ROS production.

2.2.1.3. *Xanthine oxidase*

This enzyme system provides an important endothelial source of superoxide in the vascular wall [23, 26]. XO-catalyzed reactions lead to oxygen reduction to produce superoxide from purine metabolism. It has been reported that spontaneously hypertensive rats demonstrate increased levels of both endothelial XO activity and ROS production, together with increased arteriolar tone [21]. Furthermore, it was suggested that XO may contribute to end-organ damage in hypertension [27].

2.2.1.4. *Mitochondrial dysfunction*

The mitochondrion could behave as both a ROS source and target. Superoxide is produced in the intermembrane space, but it is rapidly carried to the cytoplasm [28]. Either ubiquinol or coenzyme Q could be a source of superoxide when these mitochondrial components are partially reduced; but these molecules behave as antioxidants when they are fully reduced [29]. Superoxide produced by mammalian mitochondria in vitro mostly comes from complex I. This high rate of complex I-dependent superoxide production can be very effectively decreased through mild uncoupling. In addition, it was found that patients with hypertension show reduced activity of antioxidant enzymes [30].

2.2.2. *Role of vascular wall components*

In response to mechanical and hormonal stimuli, the endothelium releases agents participating in the regulation of vasomotor tone. Particularly relevant is the ability of endothelium to exert a protective role through the generation of vasorelaxing factors. In addition, pathophysiological conditions result in increased released of endothelium-derived vasoconstricting factors, such as ET-1, AT-II, UT-II, superoxide anions, vasoconstrictor prostaglandins, and thromboxane A2, all of them capable of producing vasoconstrictor effects. It should be mentioned that VSMC contribute to modulating blood pressure not solely in short-term regulation of the blood vessel diameter, but also in the structural remodeling occurring during long-term adaptation, both processes being mediated by ROS. It is of interest considering that the adventitia can also participate in the development of hypertension, which is achieved through ROS contribution in either reduction of NO bioavailability or vascular remodeling.

2.2.3. *Role of vascular hormones and factors*

2.2.3.1. *Nitric oxide*

NO plays a key role as a paracrine regulator of vascular tone. It is involved in the physiological regulation responsible for the maintenance of the health of vascular endothelium through processes such as inhibition of leukocyte-endothelial cell adhesion, VSMC proliferation and migration, and platelet aggregation. The effect of decreased NO bioavailability is particularly relevant, leading to reduction of vasodilatory capacity in the vasculature, thereby providing a mechanism of hypertension. The formation of NO from the substrates oxygen and L-arginine is catalyzed by the enzyme eNOS, being the predominant isoform of NOS family in the vascular wall. This enzyme can be rapidly activated by receptor-mediated agonist stimulation, shear stress, and allosteric modulators [31]. It is of interest to mention that NO diffuses easily to the adjacent VSMC, thus binding to receptors such as soluble guanylyl cyclase. The numerous NO biological properties include not only vasorelaxing and antiproliferative actions but also antagonizing the effects of AT-II, endothelins and ROS, among other vasoconstrictors. Though L-arginine, a substrate for eNOS, could be considered as a promising factor in preserving NO formation, it failed to prevent blood pressure elevation and left ventricle remodeling in a model based on chronic treatment with the methyl ester of N-nitro-L-arginine (L-NAME), an inhibitor of eNOS [32]. Furthermore, NO-deficient hypertension was completely prevented by the ACE inhibitor captopril, yet without improving NOS activity. Another reported effect for NO consists of its ability to exert an ACE downregulation effect. NO half-life can be prolonged by thiols, as these compounds protect NO from oxidation and are able to form nitrosothiols [33, 34]. It should be remarked that reduced NO levels can be the result of its combination with superoxide to form peroxynitrite, a compound capable of enhancing oxidative stress by oxidizing BH4, destabilizing eNOS, and producing more superoxide [22, 24, 25]. The importance of the balance between NO and AT-II in the regulation of the sympathetic tone has been reported.

2.2.3.2. *Renin-angiotensin system*

There is cumulated evidence supporting that the renin-angiotensin system (RAS) contributes to the development of cardiovascular disease. The production of AT-II, a potent vasoactive peptide, occurs in vascular beds having important ACE activity. Increased AT-II production above normal levels is able to induce vascular remodeling and endothelial dysfunction, as well as increases in levels of blood pressure. At the cell level, AT-II acts as a potent NOX activator, thus leading to enhancement of ROS production [35, 36]. It was reported that the expression of NOX subunits, oxidase activity, and ROS production are all increased in rat and mice models of hypertension achieved by AT-II infusion [37]. In addition, the effect of AT-II is not only confined to increasing NADPH oxidase activity but also upregulating SOD, likely as a compensation mechanism against ROS increase. Consequently, ROS levels and oxidative stress biomarkers may appear normal despite the occurrence of an oxidative challenge. However, the consequences of oxidative stress will be apparent when ROS production becomes overwhelming and the compensatory mechanisms are inadequate, thus explaining the pathophysiological consequences [38]. Pharmacological inhibition of ACE by captopril and enalapril prevented blood pressure rise in young spontaneously hypertensive rats. The hypotensive effect of captopril is higher than that of enalapril, which could be due to the antioxidant role of its thiol group [39]. Interestingly, NO not only antagonizes the vascular effects of AT-II on blood pressure, cell growth, and renal sodium excretion but also downregulates the synthesis of ACE and AT1 receptors. In addition, upregulation of eNOS expression has been reported as a consequence of ACE inhibition [40]. Recently, a relationship through Ca2+/calmodulin-dependent protein kinase II has been proposed to link the actions of AT-II and ROS in cardiovascular pathological conditions [41].

2.2.3.3. *Acetylcholine*

The endothelium-dependent vasodilation by acetylcholine (Ach) in vascular vessels occurs mainly via NO production. NO rapidly diffuses to the underlying VSMC, thereby inducing relaxation in these cells. Under oxidative stress conditions, a diminution in NO bioavailability should be expected, thus leading to significantly reduced ACh-mediated vasodilation [40].

2.2.3.4. *Endothelin-1*

Vascular endothelium, among others vascular tissues, produces potent vasoconstrictor isopeptides known as endothelins. ET-1 is the major endothelin generated by endothelial cells, and is probably the most important in cardiovascular physiology and disease. It has been demonstrated that large concentration of exogen ET-1 acts as potent vasoconstrictor capable of altering arterial pressure. ET-1 mediates its effect through two receptors, ETA and ETB. ETA exerts its effects via activation of NOX, XO, lipoxygenase, uncoupled NOS, and mitochondrial respiratory chain enzymes. ETB induces relaxation on endothelial cells [42]. The vasoconstricting action of ET-1 is counteracted by vasodilators such as prostacyclin (PGI2) and/or NO, and it has been seen that many factors that stimulate ET-1 synthesis (e.g. thrombin, AT-II) also cause the release of the vasodilators above mentioned. Several studies reported in primary hypertension demonstrate an increased ET-1 vasoconstrictor tone, apparently dependent on decreased endothelial ETB-mediated NO production, contributing to NO bioavailability impairment.

2.2.3.5. *Urotensin-II*

UT-II is the most potent vasoconstrictor identified [43]. It acts through the activation of NOX. UT receptors have been identified in several other organs besides vascular bed, suggesting that vasoconstriction is not its only effect [44, 45]. UT-II has also been shown to act as a potent vasodilator in some models [46]. Nevertheless, the role of UT-II in disease is not fully elucidated yet.

2.2.3.6. *Norepinephrine*

VSMC is innervated primarily by the sympathetic nervous system through three types of adrenergic receptors: $\alpha1$, $\alpha2$ and $\beta2$. VSMC proliferation is stimulated by norepinephrine. Interestingly, blood pressure is increased by over-expression of inducible nitric oxide synthase (iNOS) through central activation of the sympathetic nervous system, mainly mediated by an increase in oxidative stress [5].

2.2.3.7. *Prostaglandins*

PGI2 is considered one of the most important vasodilators depending on the endothelium and relaxes the vascular musculature. A large amount of substances that generate an increase in PGI2 release have been described, such as thrombin, arachidonic acid, histamine, and serotonin. Prostaglandin H2 is formed by the prostaglandin H2 synthase, which uses arachidonic acid as a substrate. Then, prostaglandin H2 is converted to PGI2, a vasoactive molecule.

Oxidative stress-related conditions, such as hypertension, impair the PGI2-mediated vasodilation. It has been demonstrated that peroxynitrite inhibits the enzymatic activity of prostacyclin synthase. Thus, the isoform prostaglandin H2 synthase-2 may mediate vascular dysfunction under such conditions.

2.2.3.8. Homocysteine

It has been proposed that homocysteine plays an important role in the pathophysiology of primary hypertension [3]. An increase in homocysteinemia augments the proliferation of VSCM, thus altering the elasticity of vascular wall; it generates an oxidative stress state and diminishes NO bioavailability, thus impairing vasodilation. All the mechanisms exposed contribute to elevated blood pressure [47]. Homocysteine could also lead to endothelium oxidative damage [3]. The administration of vitamins B6, B12, and folic acid has been proposed as a potential adjuvant treatment in hypertension, probably by correcting the increased homocysteinemia [3, 48]. Despite the above mentioned, further randomized controlled trials are required to establish the efficacy of these therapeutic agents in the treatment of hypertension.

A hypothesis for the role of vascular oxidative stress in hypertension is depicted in **Figure 1**.

Besides the key role of ROS production in the vasculature and its relation to hypertension, it has been demonstrated that hypertensive stimuli, such as high salt and AT-II, also increase the production in the kidney and the central nervous system, contributing either to generate hypertension or to the untoward sequels of this disease [49, 50]

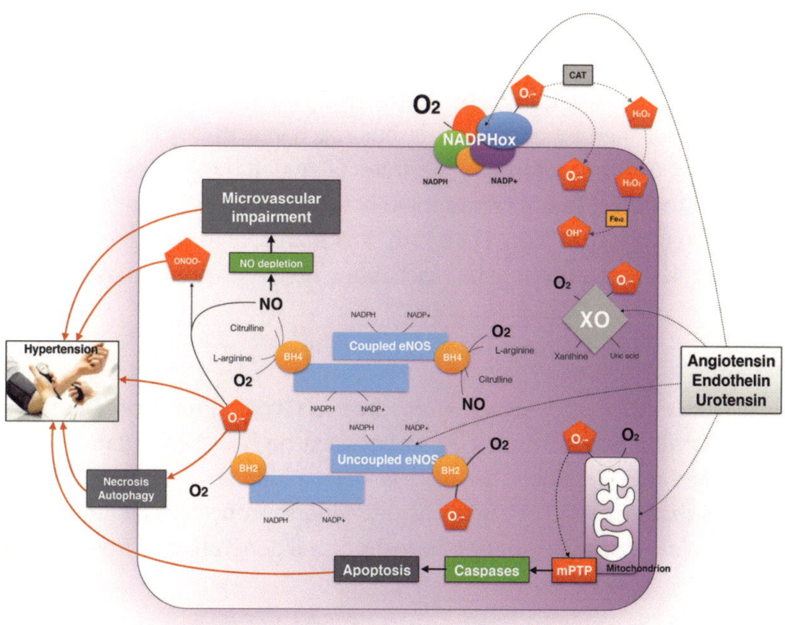

Figure 1. Schematic summary of the role of vascular oxidative stress in the pathogenesis of hypertension. NO: nitric oxide, eNOS: nitric oxide synthase, BH4: tetrahydrobiopterin, and mPTP: mitochondrial permeability transition pore.

3. Antioxidants in hypertension

This section refers to the antihypertensive role of endogenous and exogenous antioxidants that have demonstrated their ability to alter the blood vessels' function and to participate in the main redox reactions involved in the pathophysiology of hypertension.

3.1. Vitamin C

Vitamin C (or ascorbate) is a potent and widely used antioxidant, characteristically water-soluble. It has been described that this antioxidant could act as an enzyme modulator on the vascular wall, upregulating eNOS and downregulating NOX [51]. An inverse relationship between vitamin C plasma levels and arterial pressure in both healthy and hypertensive population has been demonstrated in several studies [15]. Antioxidant supplementation improves vascular function and reduces blood pressure in both experimental models [52, 53] and in patients [54, 55]. Ascorbate may improve vasodilation, probably by increasing NO bioavailability [56–58]. Vitamin C could protect BH4 from oxidation, which leads to an increase in the enzymatic activity of eNOS.

Despite the rationale of using vitamin C as an antihypertensive molecule, several clinical trials with methodological differences (including number of patients and follow-up) have yielded inconsistent outcomes [59–64]. The absence of antihypertensive effect observed in trials using the administration of ascorbate could be due to the lack of consideration of its pharmacological characteristics, mainly pharmacokinetics. It was determined in experimental conditions that the antihypertensive effect of ascorbate is reachable at a plasma concentration of 10 mM [57]. This concentration allows ascorbate to efficiently compete against the reaction between NO and superoxide, which is increased in oxidative stress–related conditions such as hypertension. The plasma level mentioned earlier is not reachable through oral administration of vitamin C. Daily oral doses of vitamin C between 60 and 100 mg are sufficient for the renal ascorbate threshold to occur. Plasma is completely saturated at doses of 400 mg daily, leading to a steady state level of 80 μM [65]. Therefore, it is plausible to propose that the antihypertensive effect of ascorbate would only be reachable with a high-dose infusion.

3.2. Vitamin E

Vitamin E is a lipid-soluble antioxidant which has received significant attention during the last decades. An epidemiological association between high dietary vitamin E intake and a lower incidence of cardiovascular disease has been established [58]. A growing body of evidence indicates that vitamin E, besides its antioxidant properties, could act as a biological modifier and is also capable of regulating mitochondrial generation of free radicals in a dose-dependent manner.

Interestingly, some studies fail to demonstrate the beneficial effects of vitamin E in cardiovascular disease patients [66–69]. Moreover, one trial proving vitamin E supplementation showed an increase in blood pressure and cardiac frequency in type 2 diabetes patients [70]. Probably, vitamin E by itself is unlikely to achieve enough levels to counteract all components of oxidative stress acting in primary hypertension [71].

3.3. Association of vitamins C and E

Alfa-tocopheroxyl radical is reduced in vivo by ascorbate; therefore vitamin C may be needed for achieving the beneficial effects of vitamin E [72]. In fact, both antioxidants may act synergistically to generate appropriate conditions for NO synthesis in endothelium [73]. Therefore, the association between vitamins C and E provides a reinforcement of their biological properties in a synergistic manner and could lead to a significant antihypertensive effect; however, further studies are required [74].

Despite the fact that some short-term studies have demonstrated that the supplementation of both antioxidants reduces blood pressure [60, 63, 64, 75], long-term clinical trials have failed to support this hypothesis. However, most of these studies have some serious methodological bias, mainly lack of rigorous exclusion criteria [76].

3.4. Allopurinol

XO has been proposed as an important enzymatic source of free radicals in the endothelium [24]. It produces uric acid by catalyzing the two final steps of purine metabolism. It has been demonstrated that XO activity is positively correlated with arteriolar tone and blood pressure [77, 78]. Moreover, allopurinol, an XO inhibitor, is capable of improving endothelial function in some experimental models. Treatment with allopurinol decreased blood pressure in a young people-based study [79], hypertensive murine models [80], and CKD patients [81]. Despite the evidence supplied by small studies, a small number of randomized controlled trials have not demonstrated benefit using XO inhibitors [82].

3.5. Selenium

Selenium is an essential trace element and a key part of several proteins. Its antioxidant properties are carried out mainly by selenocysteine residues, which are an integral constituent of glutathione peroxidase (GSH-Px), thioredoxin reductases (TR), and selenoprotein P [83]. It has been proposed that the maintenance of full GSH-Px and TR activity by proper selenium dietary intake could be useful for the prevention of cardiovascular disease. From a molecular point of view, selenium is capable of preventing the activity of nuclear factor kappa B (NF-κB) [84], conferring selenium anti-inflammatory and antioxidant properties. The inhibition of NF-kB is probably the result of the binding of selenium to the factor thiols [85].

Several trials have proved the antioxidant properties of selenium [84, 86–91]. Low-dose selenium showed to provide significant protection of coronary endothelium against oxidative damage in humans [83]. In spontaneously hypertensive rats, selenium supplementation was associated with an increased antioxidant response and protection against cardiac oxidative injury, as well as a reduction in disease severity and mortality [92]. Besides, in hypertensive pregnancies, reduced selenium levels are associated with a decrease in GSH-Px activity [93].

Therefore, it is plausible to propose that selenium deficiency could be an independent risk factor of cardiovascular disease, including hypertension [94].

3.6. N-acetylcysteine

N-acetylcysteine (NAC) is a sulfhydryl group donor that holds great attention for its antioxidant properties and potential benefits in cardiovascular disease. In salt-sensitive hypertension, NAC is capable of improving renal dysfunction and decreasing blood pressure [95]. The antihypertensive effect of NAC is mainly due to NO-dependent mechanisms and is probably mediated by the inhibition of oxidative stress [96]. NAC effectively prevents BH4 oxidation by the increased superoxide present in primary hypertension [97]. Besides this, NAC can protect against oxidative injury directly by scavenging ROS and inhibiting lipid peroxidation [98, 99].

3.7. Polyphenols

Polyphenols have been defined as the most abundant antioxidants in human diet. They exert several protective mechanisms, including ROS scavenging, iron chelating and modulation of antioxidant enzymes [100, 101]. NAC also possibly increases the endothelium-NO production [102, 103]. In this regard, NO levels increase after the consumption of polyphenols by humans [104]. Polyphenols improve endothelial function by increasing glutathione and inhibiting pro-oxidant enzymes such as NOX and XO [105]. Despite this, some studies using polyphenols and antioxidant vitamins have shown an increase in blood pressure [106]. Therefore, the evidence is still insufficient to establish polyphenols as a first-line treatment in hypertension.

A summary of the antioxidant approaches as clinical interventions on essential hypertension is presented in **Table 1**.

Details of study	Results	Reference
Intrabrachial vitamin C (2.4 mg/100 mL forearm tissue per minute). Randomized, placebo-controlled trial	In hypertensive patients but not in control subjects, vitamin C increased the impaired vasodilation to acetylcholine	[107]
Intra-arterial infusion of vitamin C at 24 mg/min for 10 minutes. Randomized trial	Forearm blood flow response to acetylcholine was significantly enhanced with intra-arterial infusion of vitamin C in hypertensive group before antihypertensive treatment	[108]
Oral administration of 500, 1000, or 2000 mg of vitamin C once daily. Randomized, double-blind, placebo-controlled trial	Significant diminution of mean systolic blood pressure and diastolic blood pressure, with no differences between the increasing doses of vitamin C	[109]
Chronic supplementation of 600mg/daily of vitamin C. Randomized, placebo-controlled trial	Reduced systolic blood pressure and pulse pressure in ambulatory elderly patients, but not in adult group	[110]
Included 29 trials of vitamin C supplementation. Meta-analysis	In short-term trials, vitamin C supplementation reduces systolic and diastolic blood pressure	[111]

Details of study	Results	Reference
Oral supplementation: 1g vitamin C + 400 UI vitamin E or placebo for 8 weeks. Randomized double-blind placebo-controlled trial	Specific association between oxidative stress-related parameters and blood pressure. Patients with essential hypertension had significantly lower systolic, diastolic, and mean arterial blood pressure	[112]
ACE inhibitors + NAC (600 mg t.i.d.) or ACE inhibitors only. Randomized, controlled trial, crossover study	Significant decrease in systolic and diastolic blood pressure with the combination of ACE inhibitors and NAC compared to ACE inhibitors-only	[113]
Intra-arterial administration: NAC (48 g/min) or vitamin C (18 mg/min). Cross-over randomized study	Intra-arterial administration of NAC had no effect on endothelium-dependent vasodilation. Intra-arterial vitamin C improved endothelium-dependent vasodilation	[114]
Vitamin C supplement daily. Either 50 or 500 mg, for 5 years. Randomized double-blind controlled trial	Neither systolic nor diastolic blood pressure was significantly related with the serum vitamin C concentration	[115]

Table 1. Clinical trials accounting for strategies using antioxidants in essential hypertension.

4. Conclusions and perspectives

There is a growing amount of evidence supporting the view that oxidative stress is involved and plays a key role in the pathophysiology of primary hypertension. In this regard, ROS act as mediators of the major physiological vasoconstrictors, increasing intracellular calcium concentration. In this review, we propose an integrative view of how oxidative stress is involved in the genesis of hypertension, mainly by reducing bioavailability of NO.

Antioxidant therapy can curtail the development of hypertension in animal models, but remains controversial in humans. Possible confounding factors in patients include co-existing pathologies and treatments and lack of selection of treatments according to ROS levels, among others. However, the dietary intake of antioxidants and polyphenols could have an effect on the primary prevention or reduction of hypertension. Though existing molecular basis and in-vitro evidence support the use of diverse antioxidants, clinical evidence continues to be controversial. It is necessary to perform basic/clinical trials that augment the current findings, which could eventually help to elucidate the role of antioxidants as novel therapy for essential hypertension. It is important to mention that the potential role of antioxidants in treatment of hypertension probably is reachable only at early stages of the disease, when endothelial dysfunction predominates over structural vascular damage.

In summary, oxidative stress plays a key role in the pathophysiology of hypertension, and antioxidants appear to be a promising treatment or co-adjuvant therapy, but further well-designed and conducted trials are required to establish them as a major alternative of pharmacology agents.

Author details

Ramón Rodrigo*, Roberto Brito and Jaime González

*Address all correspondence to: rrodrigo@med.uchile.cl

Molecular and Clinical Pharmacology Program, Institute of Biomedical Sciences, University of Chile, Santiago, Chile

References

[1] Yusuf S, Hawken S, Ounpuu S, Dans T, Avezum A, Lanas F et al. Effect of potentially modifiable risk factors associated with myocardial infarction in 52 countries (the INTERHEART Study): case control study. Lancet 2004;364:937–952. DOI: 10.1016/s0140-6736(04)17018-9

[2] Paravicini TM, Touyz RM. Redox signalling in hypertension. Cardiovasc Res 2006;71:247–258. DOI: 10.1016/j.cardiores.2006.05.001

[3] Rodrigo R, Passalacqua W, Araya J, Orellana M, Rivera G. Implications of oxidative stress and homocysteine in the pathophysiology of essential hypertension. J Cardiovasc Pharmacol 2003;42:453–461. DOI: 10.1097/00005344-200310000-00001

[4] Lassègue B, Griendling K. Reactive oxygen species in hypertension, an update. Am J Hypertens 2004;17:852–860.

[5] Kimura S, Zhang GX, Nishiyama A, Shokoji T, Yao L, Fan YY et al. Mitochondria-derived reactive oxygen species and vascular MAP kinases: comparison of angiotensin II and diazoxide. Hypertension 2005;45:438–444. DOI: 10.1161/01.hyp.0000157169.27818.ae

[6] Hool LC, Corry B. Redox control of calcium channels: from mechanisms to therapeutic opportunities. Antioxid Redox Signal 2007;9:409–435. DOI: 10.1089/ars.2006.1446

[7] Yoshioka J, Schreiter ER, Lee RT. Role of thioredoxin in cell growth through interactions with signaling molecules. Antioxid Redox Signal 2006;8:2143–2145. DOI: 10.1089/ars.2006.8.2143

[8] Lacy F, Kailasam MT, O'Connor DT, Schmid-Schonbein GW, Parmer RJ. Plasma hydrogen peroxide production in human essential hypertension: role of heredity, gender, and ethnicity. Hypertension 2000;36:878–884. DOI: 10.1161/01.hyp.36.5.878

[9] Stojiljkovic MP, Lopes HF, Zhang D, Morrow JD, Goodfriend TL, Egan BM. Increasing plasma fatty acids elevates F2-isoprostanes in humans: implications for the cardiovascular risk factor cluster. J Hypertens 2002;20:1215–1221. DOI: 10.1097/00004872-200206000-00036

[10] Redon J, Oliva MR, Tormos C, Giner V, Chaves J, Iradi A et al. Antioxidant activities and oxidative stress byproducts in human hypertension. Hypertension 2003;41:1096–1101. DOI: 10.1161/01.hyp.0000068370.21009.38

[11] Tanito M, Nakamura H, Kwon YW, Teratani A, Masutani H, Shioji K et al. Enhanced oxidative stress and impaired thioredoxin expression in spontaneously hypertensive rats. Antioxid Redox Signal 2004;6:89–97. DOI: 10.1089/152308604771978381

[12] Touyz RM. Reactive oxygen species, vascular oxidative stress, and redox signaling in hypertension: what is the clinical significance? Hypertension 2004;44:248–252. DOI: 10.1161/01.hyp.0000138070.47616.9d

[13] Briones AM, Touyz RM. Oxidative stress and hypertension: current concepts. Curr Hypertens Rep 2010;12:135–142. DOI: 10.1007/s11906-010-0100-z

[14] Bengtsson SH, Gulluyan LM, Dusting GJ, Drummond GR. Novel isoforms of NADPH oxidase in vascular physiology and pathophysiology. Clin Exp Pharmacol Physiol 2003;30:849–854. DOI: 10.1046/j.1440-1681.2003.03929.x

[15] Rodrigo R, Prat H, Passalacqua W, Araya J, Guichard C, Bächler JP. Relationship between oxidative stress and essential hypertension. Hypertens Res 2007;30:1159–1167. DOI: 10.1291/hypres.30.1159

[16] Landmesser U, Dikalov S, Price SR, McCann L, Fukai T, Holland SM et al. Oxidation of tetrahydrobiopterin leads to uncoupling of endothelial cell nitric oxide synthase in hypertension. J Clin Invest 2003;111:1201–1209. DOI: 10.1172/jci14172

[17] Gavazzi G, Banfi B, Deffert C, Fiette L, Schappi M, Herrmann F et al. Decreased blood pressure in NOX1-deficient mice. FEBS Lett 2006;580:497–504. DOI: 10.1016/j.febslet.2005.12.049

[18] Touyz RM, Schiffrin EL. Increased generation of superoxide by angiotensin II in smooth muscle cells from resistance arteries of hypertensive patients: role of phospholipase D-dependent NAD(P)H oxidase-sensitive pathways. J Hypertens 2001;19:1245–1254. DOI: 10.1097/00004872-200107000-00009

[19] Ghiadoni L, Magagna A, Versari D, Kardasz I, Huang Y, Taddei S et al. Different effect of antihypertensive drugs on conduit artery endothelial function. Hypertension 2003;41:1281–1286. DOI: 10.1161/01.hyp.0000070956.57418.22

[20] Yoshida J, Yamamoto K, Mano T, Sakata Y, Nishikawa N, Nishio M et al. AT1 receptor blocker added to ACE inhibitor provides benefits at advanced stage of hypertensive diastolic heart failure. Hypertension 2004;43:686–691. DOI: 10.1161/01.hyp.0000118017.02160.fa

[21] Feairheller DL, Brown MD, Park JY, Brinkley TE, Basu S, Hagberg JM et al. Exercise training, NADPH oxidase p22phox gene polymorphisms, and hypertension. Med Sci Sports Exerc 2009;41:1421–1428. DOI: 10.1249/mss.0b013e318199cee8

[22] Zou MH, Cohen RA, Ullrich V. Peroxynitrite and vascular endothelial dysfunction in diabetes mellitus. Endothelium 2004;11:89–97. DOI: 10.1080/10623320490482619

[23] Lassègue B, Clempus RE. Vascular NAD(P)H oxidases: specific features, expression, and regulation. Am J Physiol Regul Integr Comp Physiol 2003;285:277–297.

[24] Kuzkaya N, Weissmann N, Harrison DG, Dikalov S. Interactions of peroxynitrite, tetrahydrobiopterin, ascorbic acid, and thiols: implications for uncoupling endothelial nitric-oxide synthase. J Biol Chem 2003;278:22546–22554. DOI: 10.1074/jbc.m302227200

[25] Laursen JB, Somers M, Kurz S, McCann L, Warnholtz A, Freeman BA et al. Endothelial regulation of vasomotion in apoE-deficient mice: implications for interactions between peroxynitrite and tetrahydrobiopterin. Circulation 2001;103:1282–1288. DOI: 10.1161/01.cir.103.9.1282

[26] Viel EC, Benkirane K, Javeshghani D, Touyz RM, Schiffrin EL. Xanthine oxidase and mitochondria contribute to vascular superoxide anion generation in DOCA-salt hypertensive rats. Am J Physiol Heart Circ Physiol 2008;295:281–288. DOI: 10.1152/ajpheart.00304.2008

[27] Laakso JT, Teräväinen TL, Martelin E, Vaskonen T, Lapatto R. Renal xanthine oxidoreductase activity during development of hypertension in spontaneously hypertensive rats. J Hypertens 2004;22:1333–1340. DOI: 10.1097/01.hjh.0000125441.28861.9f

[28] Han D, Antunes F, Canali R, Rettori D, Cadenas E. Voltage-dependent anion channels control the release of the superoxide anion from mitochondria to cytosol. J Biol Chem 2003;278:5557–5563. DOI: 10.1074/jbc.m210269200

[29] Eto Y, Kang D, Hasegawa E, Takeshige K, Minakami S. Succinate-dependent lipid peroxidation and its prevention by reduced ubiquinone in beef heart submitochondrial particles. Arch Biochem Biophys 1992;295:101–106. DOI: 10.1016/0003-9861(92)90493-g

[30] Zhou L, Xiang W, Potts J, Floyd M, Sharan C, Yang H et al. Reduction in extracellular superoxide dismutase activity in African-American patients with hypertension. Free Radic Biol Med 2006;41:1384–1391. DOI: 10.1016/j.freeradbiomed.2006.07.019

[31] Michel JB, Feron O, Sase K, Prabhakar P, Michel T. Caveolin versus calmodulin. Counterbalancing allosteric modulators of endothelial nitric oxide synthase. J Biol Chem 1997;272:25907–25912. DOI: 10.1074/jbc.272.41.25907

[32] Simko F, Luptak I, Matuskova J, Krajcirovicova K, Sumbalova Z, Kucharska J et al. L-arginine fails to protect against myocardial remodelling in L-NAME-induced hypertension. Eur J Clin Invest 2005;35:362–368. DOI: 10.1111/j.1365-2362.2005.01507.x

[33] Zhang Y, Hogg N. S-Nitrosothiols: cellular formation and transport. Free Radic Biol Med 2005;38:831–838. DOI: 10.1016/j.freeradbiomed.2004.12.016

[34] Sládková M, Kojsová S, Jendeková L, Pechánová O. Chronic and acute effects of different antihypertensive drugs on femoral artery relaxation of L-NAME hypertensive rats. Physiol Res 2007;56:85–91.

[35] Touyz RM. Reactive oxygen species and angiotensin II signaling in vascular cells – implications in cardiovascular disease. Braz J Med Biol Res 2004;37:1263–1273. DOI: 10.1590/s0100-879x2004000800018

[36] Hitomi H, Kiyomoto H, Nishiyama A. Angiotensin II and oxidative stress. Curr Opin Cardiol 2007;22:311–315. DOI: 10.1097/hco.0b013e3281532b53

[37] Landmesser U, Cai H, Dikalov S, McCann L, Hwang J, Jo H et al. Role of p47(phox) in vascular oxidative stress and hypertension caused by angiotensin II. Hypertension 2002;40:511–515. DOI: 10.1161/01.hyp.0000032100.23772.98

[38] Taniyama Y, Griendling K. Reactive oxygen species in the vasculature: molecular and cellular mechanisms. Hypertension 2003;42:1075–1081. DOI: 10.1161/01.hyp.0000100443.09293.4f

[39] Pechánová O. Contribution of captopril thiol group to the prevention of spontaneous hypertension. Physiol Res 2007;56:41–48.

[40] Bitar MS, Wahid S, Mustafa S, Al-Saleh E, Dhaunsi GS, Al-Mulla F. Nitric oxide dynamics and endothelial dysfunction in type II model of genetic diabetes. Eur J Pharmacol 2005;511:53–64. DOI: 10.1016/j.ejphar.2005.01.014

[41] Wen H, Gwathmey JK, Xie LH. Oxidative stress-mediated effects of angiotensin II in the cardiovascular system. World J Hypertens 2012;2:34–44. DOI: 10.5494/wjh.v2.i4.34

[42] Gomez-Alamillo C, Juncos LA, Cases A, Haas JA, Romero JC. Interactions between vasoconstrictors and vasodilators in regulating hemodynamics of distinct vascular beds. Hypertension 2003;42:831–836. DOI: 10.1161/01.hyp.0000088854.04562.da

[43] Djordjevic T, BelAiba RS, Bonello S, Pfeilschifter J, Hess J, Görlach A. Human urotensin II is a novel activator of NADPH oxidase in human pulmonary artery smooth muscle cells. Arterioscler Thromb Vasc Biol 2005;25:519–525. DOI: 10.1161/01.atv.0000154279.98244.eb

[44] Matsushita M, Shichiri M, Imai T, Iwashina M, Tanaka H, Takasu N et al. Co-expression of urotensin II and its receptor (GPR14) in human cardiovascular and renal tissues. J Hypertens 2001;19:2185–2190. DOI: 10.1097/00004872-200112000-00011

[45] Jegou S, Cartier D, Dubessy C, Gonzalez BJ, Chatenet D, Tostivint H et al. Localization of the urotensin II receptor in the rat central nervous system. J Comp Neurol 2006;495:21–36. DOI: 10.1002/cne.20845

[46] Stirrat A, Gallagher M, Douglas SA, Ohlstein EH, Berry C, Kirk A et al. Potent vasodilator responses to human urotensin-II in human pulmonary and abdominal resistance arteries. Am J Physiol Heart Circ Physiol 2001;280:925–928.

[47] Rodrigo R, Passalacqua W, Araya J, Orellana M, Rivera G. Homocysteine and essential hypertension. J Clin Pharmacol 2003;43:1299–1306. DOI: 10.1177/0091270003258190

[48] Harrison DG, Gongora MC. Oxidative stress and hypertension. Med Clin North Am 2009;93:621–635. DOI: 10.1016/j.mcna.2009.02.015

[49] Sachse A, Wolf G. Angiotensin II-induced reactive oxygen species and the kidney. J Am Soc Nephrol 2007;18:2439–2446. DOI: 10.1681/asn.2007020149

[50] Zimmerman MC, Lazartigues E, Sharma RV, Davisson RL. Hypertension caused by angiotensin II infusion involves increased superoxide production in the central nervous system. Circ Res 2004;95:210–216. DOI: 10.1161/01.res.0000135483.12297.e4

[51] Ulker S, McKeown PP, Bayraktutan U. Vitamins reverse endothelial dysfunction through regulation of eNOS and NAD(P)H oxidase activities. Hypertension 2003;41:534–539. DOI: 10.1161/01.hyp.0000057421.28533.37

[52] Nishikawa Y, Tatsumi K, Matsuura T, Yamamoto A, Nadamoto T, Urabe K. Effects of vitamin C on high blood pressure induced by salt in spontaneously hypertensive rats. J Nutr Sci Vitaminol (Tokyo) 2003;49:301–309. DOI: 10.3177/jnsv.49.301

[53] Reckelhoff JF, Kanji V, Racusen LC, Schmidt AM, Yan SD, Marrow J et al. Vitamin E ameliorates enhanced renal lipid peroxidation and accumulation of F2-isoprostanes in aging kidneys. Am J Physiol 1998;274:767–774.

[54] Chen X, Touyz RM, Park JB, Schiffrin EL. Antioxidant effects of vitamins C and E are associated with altered activation of vascular NADPH oxidase and superoxide dismutase in stroke-prone SHR. Hypertension 2001;38:606–611. DOI: 10.1161/hy09t1.094005

[55] Atarashi K, Ishiyama A, Takagi M, Minami M, Kimura K, Goto A et al. Vitamin E ameliorates the renal injury of Dahl Salt-sensitive rats. Am J Hypertens 1997;10:116–119.

[56] Vita JA, Frei B, Holbrook M, Gokce N, Leaf C, Keaney JF Jr. L-2-Oxothiazolidine-4-carboxylic acid reverses endothelial dysfunction in patients with coronary artery disease. J Clin Invest 1998;101:1408–1414. DOI: 10.1172/jci1155

[57] Jackson TS, Xu A, Vita JA, Keaney JF Jr. Ascorbate prevents the interaction of superoxide and nitric oxide only at very high physiological concentrations. Circ Res 1998;83:916–922. DOI: 10.1161/01.res.83.9.916

[58] Duffy SJ, Gokce N, Holbrook M, Hunter LM, Biegelsen ES, Huang A et al. Effect of ascorbic acid treatment on conduit vessel endothelial dysfunction in patients with hypertension. Am J Physiol Heart Circ Physiol 2001;280:528–534.

[59] Duffy SJ, Gokce N, Holbrook M, Huang A, Frei B, Keaney JF Jr et al. Treatment of hypertension with ascorbic acid. Lancet 1999;354:2048–2049. DOI: 10.1016/s0140-6736(99)04410-4

[60] Fotherby MD, Williams JC, Forster LA, Craner P, Ferns GA. Effect of vitamin C on ambulatory blood pressure and plasma lipids in older persons. J Hypertens 2000;18:411–415. DOI: 10.1097/00004872-200018040-00009

[61] Block G, Mangels AR, Norkus EP, Patterson BH, Levander OA, Taylor PR. Ascorbic acid status and subsequent diastolic and systolic blood pressure. Hypertension 2001;37:261–267. DOI: 10.1161/01.hyp.37.2.261

[62] Ghosh SK, Ekpo EB, Shah IU, Girling AJ, Jenkins C, Sinclair AJ. A double-blind, placebo-controlled parallel trial of vitamin C treatment in elderly patients with hypertension. Gerontology 1994;40:268–272. DOI: 10.1159/000213595

[63] Galley HF, Thornton J, Howdle PD, Walber BE, Webster NR. Combination oral antioxidant supplementation reduces blood pressure. Clin Sci (Lond) 1997;92:361–365.

[64] Mullan BA, Young IS, Fee H, McCance DR. Ascorbic acid reduces blood pressure and arterial stiffness in type 2 diabetes. Hypertension 2002;40:804–809. DOI: 10.1161/01.hyp.0000039961.13718.00

[65] Padayatty SJ, Katz A, Wang Y, Eck P, Kwon O, Lee JH et al. Vitamin C as an antioxidant: evaluation of its role in disease prevention. J Am Coll Nutr 2003;22:18–35. DOI: 10.1080/07315724.2003.10719272

[66] Rapola JM, Virtamo J, Ripatti S, Huttunen JK, Albanes D, Taylor PR et al. Randomised trial of a-tocopherol and b-carotene supplements on incidence of major coronary events in men with previous myocardial infarction. Lancet 1997;349:1715–1720. DOI: 10.1016/s0140-6736(97)01234-8

[67] Dietary supplementation with n-3 polyunsaturated fatty acids and vitamin E after myocardial infarction: results of the GISSI-Prevenzione Trial. Lancet 1999;354:447–455. DOI: 10.1016/s0140-6736(99)07072-5

[68] Lonn E, Bosch J, Yusuf S, Sheridan P, Pogue J, Arnold JM et al. Effects of long-term vitamin E supplementation on cardiovascular events and cancer: a randomized controlled trial. JAMA 2005;293:1338–1347. DOI: 10.1001/jama.293.11.1338

[69] Lee IM, Cook NR, Gaziano JM, Gordon D, Ridker PM, Manson JE et al. Vitamin E in the primary prevention of cardiovascular disease and cancer: the Women's Health Study: a randomized controlled trial. JAMA 2005;294:56–65. DOI: 10.1001/jama.294.1.56

[70] Ward NC, Wu JH, Clarke MW, Puddey IB, Burke V, Croft KD et al. The effect of vitamin E on blood pressure in individuals with type 2 diabetes: a randomized, double-blind, placebo-controlled trial. J Hypertens 2007;25:227–234. DOI: 10.1097/01.hjh.0000254373.96111.43

[71] Münzel T, Keaney JF Jr. Are ACE inhibitors a "magic bullet" against oxidative stress? Circulation 2001;104:1571–1574. DOI: 10.1161/hc3801.095585

[72] Heller R, Werner-Felmayer G, Werner ER. Antioxidants and endothelial nitric oxide synthesis. Eur J Clin Pharmacol 2006;62:21–28. DOI: 10.1007/s00228-005-0009-7

[73] Heller R, Werner-Felmayer G, Werner ER. Alpha-tocopherol and endothelial nitric oxide synthesis. Ann N Y Acad Sci 2004;1031:74–85. DOI: 10.1196/annals.1331.007

[74] Bilodeau JF, Hubel CA. Current concepts in the use of antioxidants for the treatment of preeclampsia. J Obstet Gynaecol Can 2003;25:742–750.

[75] Plantinga Y, Ghiadoni L, Magagna A, Giannarelli C, Franzoni F, Taddei S et al. Supplementation with vitamins C and E improves arterial stiffness and endothelial function in essential hypertensive patients. Am J Hypertens 2007;20:392–397.

[76] Rodrigo R, Guichard C, Charles R. Clinical pharmacology and therapeutic use of antioxidant vitamins. Fundam Clin Pharmacol 2007;21:111–127. DOI: 10.1111/j.1472-8206.2006.00466.x

[77] Suzuki H, DeLano FA, Parks DA, Jamshidi N, Granger DN, Ishii H et al. Xanthine oxidase activity associated with arterial blood pressure in spontaneously hypertensive rats. Proc Natl Acad Sci USA 1998;95:4754–4759. DOI: 10.1073/pnas.95.8.4754

[78] DeLano FA, Parks DA, Ruedi JM, Babior BM, Schmid-Schönbein GW. Microvascular display of xanthine oxidase and NADPH oxidase in the spontaneously hypertensive rat. Microcirculation 2006;13:551–566. DOI: 10.1080/10739680600885152

[79] Feig DI, Soletsky B, Johnson RJ. Effect of allopurinol on blood pressure of adolescents with newly diagnosed essential hypertension: a randomized trial. JAMA 2008;300:924–932. DOI: 10.1001/jama.300.8.924]

[80] Mazzali M, Hughes J, Kim Y, Jefferson JA, Kang DK, Gordon KL et al. Elevated Uric Acid Increases Blood Pressure in the Rat by a Novel Crystal-Independent Mechanism. Hypertension 2001;38:1101–1106. DOI: 10.1161/hy1101.092839

[81] Goicoechea M, Vinuesa SG, Verdalles U, Ruiz-Caro C, Ampuero J, Rincón A et al. Effect of allopurinol in chronic kidney disease progression and cardiovascular risk. Clin J Am Soc Nephrol 2010;5:1388–1393. DOI: 10.2215/cjn.01580210

[82] George J, Struthers A. The role of urate and xanthine oxidase in vascular oxidative stress: future directions. Ther Clin Risk Manag 2009;5:799–803. DOI: 10.2147/tcrm.s5701

[83] Miller S, Walker SW, Arthur JR, Nicol F, Pickard K, Lewin MH et al. Selenite protects human endothelial cells from oxidative damage and induces thioredoxin reductase. Clin Sci (Lond) 2001;100:543–550. DOI: 10.1042/cs20000299

[84] Faure P, Ramon O, Favier A, Halimi S. Selenium supplementation decreases nuclear factor-kappa B activity in peripheral blood mononuclear cells from type 2 diabetic patients. Eur J Clin Invest 2004;34:475–481. DOI: 10.1111/j.1365-2362.2004.01362.x

[85] Kim IY, Stadtman TC. Inhibition of NF-kappaB DNA binding and nitric oxide induction in human T cells and lung adenocarcinoma cells by selenite treatment. Proc Natl Acad Sci 1997;94:12904–12907. DOI: 10.1073/pnas.94.24.12904

[86] Campbell L, Howie F, Arthur JR, Nicol F, Beckett G. Selenium and sulforaphane modify the expression of selenoenzymes in the human endothelial cell line EAhy926 and protect cells from oxidative damage. Nutrition 2007;23:138–144. DOI: 10.1016/j.nut.2006.10.006

[87] Takizawa M, Komori K, Tampo Y, Yonaha M. Paraquat-induced oxidative stress and dysfunction of cellular redox systems including antioxidative defense enzymes glutathione peroxidase and thioredoxin reductase. Toxicol In Vitro 2007;21:355–363. DOI: 10.1016/j.tiv.2006.09.003

[88] Faure P. Protective effects of antioxidant micronutrients (vitamin E, zinc and selenium) in type 2 diabetes mellitus. Clin Chem Lab Med 2003;41:995–998. DOI: 10.1515/cclm.2003.152

[89] Brigelius-Flohé R, Banning A, Schnurr K. Selenium-dependent enzymes in endothelial cell function. Antioxid Redox Signal 2003;5:205–215. DOI: 10.1089/152308603764816569]

[90] Ito Y, Fujita T. Trace elements and blood pressure regulation. Nippon Rinsho 1996;54:106–110.

[91] Zhou X, Ji WJ, Zhu Y, He B, Li H, Huang TG et al. Enhancement of endogenous defenses against ROS by supra-nutritional level of selenium is more safe and effective than antioxidant supplementation in reducing hypertensive target organ damage. Med Hypotheses 2007;68:952–956. DOI: 10.1016/j.mehy.2006.09.058]

[92] Lymbury RS, Marino MJ, Perkins AV. Effect of dietary selenium on the progression of heart failure in the ageing spontaneously hypertensive rat. Mol Nutr Food Res 2010;54:1436–1444. DOI: 10.1002/mnfr.201000012

[93] Mistry HD, Wilson V, Ramsay MM, Symonds ME, Broughton Pipkin F. Reduced selenium concentrations and glutathione peroxidase activity in preeclamptic pregnancies. Hypertension 2008;52:881–888. DOI: 10.1161/hypertensionaha.108.116103

[94] Nawrot TS, Staessen JA, Roels HA, Den Hond E, Thijs L, Fagard RH et al. Blood pressure and blood selenium: a cross-sectional and longitudinal population study. Eur Heart J 2007;28:628–633. DOI: 10.1093/eurheartj/ehl479

[95] Tian N, Rose RA, Jordan S, Dwyer TM, Hughson MD, Manning RD Jr. N-Acetylcysteine improves renal dysfunction, ameliorates kidney damage and decreases blood pressure in salt-sensitive hypertension. J Hypertens 2006;24:2263–2270. DOI: 10.1097/01.hjh.0000249705.42230.73

[96] Pechánová O, Zicha J, Kojsová S, Dobesová Z, Jendeková L, Kunes J. Effect of chronic N-acetylcysteine treatment on the development of spontaneous hypertension. Clin Sci (Lond) 2006;110:235–242. DOI: 10.1042/cs20050227

[97] Zembowicz A, Hatchett RJ, Radziszewski W, Gryglewski RJ. Inhibition of endothelial nitric oxide synthase by ebselen: Prevention by thiols suggests the inactivation by ebselen of a critical thiol essential for the catalytic activity of nitric oxide synthase. J Pharmacol Exp Ther 1993;267:1112–1118.

[98] De la Fuente M, Victor VM. Ascorbic acid and N-acetylcysteine improve in vitro the function of lymphocytes from mice with endotoxin-induced oxidative stress. Free Radic Res 2001;35:73–84. DOI: 10.1080/10715760100300611

[99] Penugonda S, Mare S, Goldstein G, Banks WA, Ercal N. Effects of N-acetylcysteine amide (NACA), a novel thiol antioxidant against glutamate-induced cytotoxicity in neuronal cell line PC12. Brain Res 2005;1056:132–138. DOI: 10.1016/j.brainres.2005.07.032

[100] Rodrigo R, Bosco C. Oxidative stress and protective effects of polyphenols: comparative studies in human and rodent kidney. A review. Comp Biochem Physiol C Toxicol Pharmacol 2006;142:317-327. DOI: 10.1016/j.cbpc.2005.11.002

[101] Pietta P, Simonetti P, Gardana C, Brusamolino A, Morazzoni P, Bombardelli E. Relationship between rate and extent of catechin absorption and plasma antioxidant status. Biochem Mol Biol Int 1998;46:895–903. DOI: 10.1080/15216549800204442

[102] Duarte J, Andriambeloson E, Diebolt M, Andriantsitohaina R. Wine polyphenols stimulate superoxide anion production to promote calcium signaling and endothelial-dependent vasodilatation. Physiol Res 2004;53:595–602.

[103] Zenebe W, Pechánová O, Andriantsitohaina R. Red wine polyphenols induce vasorelaxation by increased nitric oxide bioactivity. Physiol Res 2003;52:425–432.

[104] Pechánová O, Rezzani R, Babál P, Bernátová I, Andriantsitohaina R. Beneficial effects of Provinols: cardiovascular system and kidney. Physiol Res 2006;55:17–30.

[105] Rodrigo R, Gil D, Miranda-Merchak A, Kalantzidis G. Antihypertensive role of polyphenols. Adv Clin Chem 2012;58:225–254.

[106] Ward NC, Hodgson JM, Croft KD, Burke V, Beilin LJ, Puddey IB. The combination of vitamin C and grape-seed polyphenols increases blood pressure: a randomized, double-blind, placebo-controlled trial. J Hypertens 2005;23:427–434. DOI: 10.1097/00004872-200502000-00026

[107] Koh ET. Effect of vitamin C on blood parameters of hypertensive subjects. J Okla State Med Assoc 1984;77:177–182.

[108] Taddei S, Virdis A, Ghiadoni L, Magagna A, Salvetti A. Vitamin C improves endothelium-dependent vasodilation by restoring nitric oxide activity in essential hypertension. Circulation 1998;97:2222–2229. DOI: 10.1161/01.cir.97.22.2222

[109] Hajjar IM, George V, Sasse EA, Kochar MS. A randomized, double-blind, controlled trial of vitamin C in the management of hypertension and lipids. Am J Ther 2002;9:289–293. DOI: 10.1097/00045391-200207000-00005

[110] Sato K, Dohi Y, Kojima M, Miyagawa K, Takase H, Katada E et al. Effects of ascorbic acid on ambulatory blood pressure in elderly patients with refractory hypertension. Arzneimittelforschung 2006;56:535–540. DOI: 10.1055/s-0031-1296748

[111] Juraschek SP, Guallar E, Appel LJ, Miller ER. Effects of vitamin C supplementation on blood pressure: a meta-analysis of randomized controlled trials. Am J Clin Nutr 2012;95:1079–1088. DOI: 10.3945/ajcn.111.027995

[112] Rodrigo R, Prat H, Passalacqua W, Araya J, Bächler JP. Decrease in oxidative stress through supplementation of vitamins C and E is associated with a reduction in blood pressure in patients with essential hypertension. Clin Sci (Lond) 2008;114:625–634. DOI: 10.1042/cs20070343

[113] Barrios V, Calderón A, Navarro-Cid J, Lahera V, Ruilope LM. N-acetylcysteine potentiates the antihypertensive effect of ACE inhibitors in hypertensive patients. Blood Press 2002;11:235–239. DOI: 10.1080/08037050213760.

[114] Schneider MP, Delles C, Schmidt BM, Oehmer S, Schwarz TK, Schmieder RE et al. Superoxide scavenging effects of N-acetylcysteine and vitamin C in subjects with essential hypertension. Am J Hypertens 2005;18:1111–1117.

[115] Kim MK, Sasaki S, Sasazuki S, Okubo S, Hayashi M, Tsugane S. Lack of long-term effect of vitamin C supplementation on blood pressure. Hypertension 2002;40:797–803. DOI: 10.1161/01.hyp.0000038339.67450.60

Chapter 4

Omega-3 Polyunsaturated Fatty Acids in Blood Pressure Control and Essential Hypertension

GianLuca Colussi, Cristiana Catena,
Marileda Novello and Leonardo A. Sechi

Additional information is available at the end of the chapter

http://dx.doi.org/10.5772/63501

Abstract

Hypertension is a worldwide problem that affects up to 22% of adults and contributes to the global burden of disability due to cardiovascular disease. Several factors influence blood pressure and participate to the development of hypertension. Among these factors, polyunsaturated fatty acids of the omega-3 family (omega-3 PUFA) are effective hypotensive agents. Through their anti-inflammatory and antioxidant properties, omega-3 PUFA can improve cardiac hemodynamics and vascular function and potentially reduce arterial stiffness and atherosclerotic damage. However, despite this promising evidence many meta-analyses on the cardiovascular effect of omega-3 PUFA were inconclusive. The choice of the omega-3 PUFA sources, baseline tissue content of these fatty acids, and individual compliance to their intake can be reasons for such a discrepancy between studies. Basic and clinical research on these fatty acids documents interesting mechanisms through which these molecules could be useful in the treatment of hypertension and its related organ damage. The role of the maternal dietary habit during pregnancy and the quality of prenatal growth on the effect of omega-3 PUFA in cardiovascular system need further investigations. This chapter summarizes the literature of the past 30 years on the antihypertensive effects of this family of essential fatty acids.

Keywords: Omega-3 fatty acids, Cardiovascular disease, Atherosclerosis, Vascular function, Oxidative stress

1. Introduction

Worldwide, hypertension affects more than one billion people and about 22% of individuals older than 18 years suffer from this disease. Untreated hypertension increases the risk and mortality for myocardial infarction and stroke, as well as it is responsible for chronic invalidating disorders such as coronary and peripheral vascular diseases, heart and renal failure, and visual impairment, all problems that heavily impact the individual's quality of life [1]. Although a descending trend of blood pressure levels has been observed in the past decades [2], hypertension remains the most underdiagnosed, undertreated, and uncontrolled problem [3] among the noncommunicable diseases. For these reasons, the prevention of hypertension is one of the main goals of the global healthcare system.

Primary or essential hypertension is diagnosed when secondary causes of high blood pressure are excluded [4]. Therefore defined, essential hypertension is a modifiable cardiovascular risk factor often associated with several inappropriate conditions related to lifestyle habits, such as overweight/obesity, excess of alcohol consumption, and high salt intake. Lifestyle changes have proven to reduce blood pressure and are highly recommended as the first step to treat hypertensive disease in all affected patients [4]. Among these changes, dietary habits have a primary role because food quantity affects directly body weight and food quality can modulate some minerals and nutrients associated with blood pressure regulation. For example, low salt and low alcohol intake, and increased consumption of polyunsaturated fatty acids of the omega-3 family (omega-3 PUFA) have shown to reduce blood pressure levels and in some cases to reduce the cardiovascular risk [5]. In this chapter, we present evidence of the beneficial effects of omega-3 PUFA on blood pressure and hypertension-related organ complications.

2. Biochemistry and physiology of the omega-3 PUFA

Long-chain PUFA are present in all tissues of mammals; tough mammals cannot directly synthesize these fatty acids because they lack enzymes to make double bonds at some position in the fatty acid chain. Therefore, long-chain PUFA need to be consumed with diet and for that reason they are "essential" fatty acids. Essential PUFA are those of the omega-6 and omega-3 families, whereas nonessential are those of the omega-7 and omega-9. Nonessential PUFA families can be synthesized directly from endogenous saturated fatty acids. The "omega" letter indicates the last methyl carbon opposed to the carboxyl group of the acyl chain and the expression of "minus 6" or "minus 3" indicates the position of the first double bond from the last methyl group. Fatty acids are abbreviated with the C letter standing for "carbon" followed by the number of carbons in the molecule, the number of double bonds separated by colon, and the PUFA family name [6].

Linoleic acid (C18:2, LA) is the precursor of long-chain omega-6 PUFA that is abundant in vegetable oils such as those derived from soybean, corn, and rapeseed and in some species of insects. The omega-6 arachidonic acid (C20:4, AA) derives from LA through elongation and desaturation of the acyl chain (**Figure 1**) and it is involved in important cellular processes including eicosanoids and endocannabinoids production, inflammation, and hemostasis. The content of AA in vegetables is poor and its main source is animal-derived food. Alpha linolenic acid (C18:3, ALA), an analog of LA with one more double bond, is the precursor of long-chain omega-3 PUFA. By elongation and desaturation of its acyl chain, it is converted into the two principal long-chain omega-3 PUFA, the eicosapentaenoic acid (C20:5, EPA) and the docosahexaenoic acid (C22:6, DHA). ALA is from plant origin where it is abundant in seeds and vegetable oils, whereas EPA and DHA are mainly from marine source. In particular, fish directly synthesize EPA and DHA by ingesting phytoplankton enzymes. Since in humans the rate of conversion of ALA in EPA and DHA is relatively slow, the main source of omega-3 PUFA is seafood (**Table 1**). Enrichment in omega-3 PUFA content of cell membranes can be reached by omega-3 consumption for a relatively short time (days or weeks) [7].

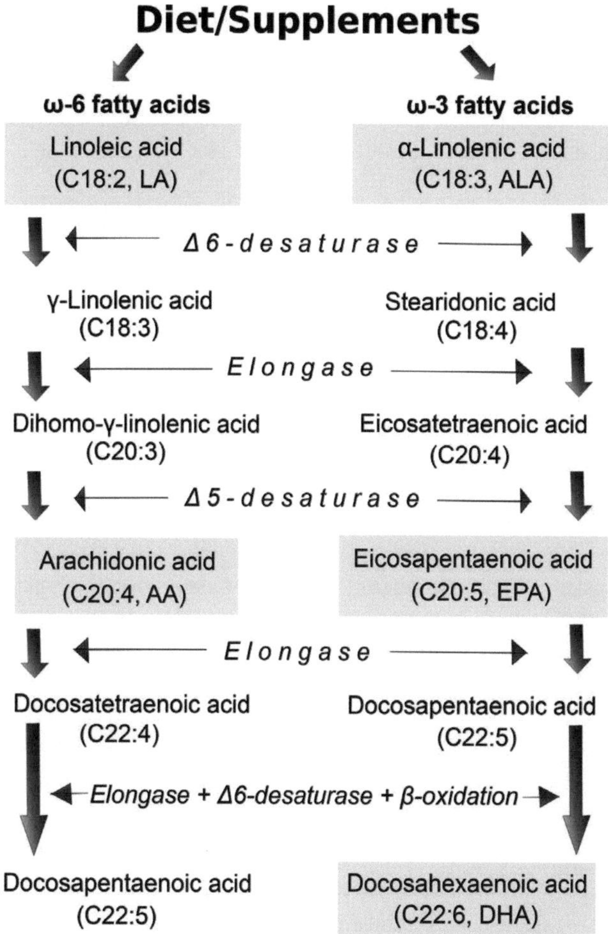

Figure 1. Biosynthesis of long-chain omega-6 and omega-3 polyunsaturated fatty acids from precursor essential fatty acids. The same elongase and desaturase enzymes act on linoleic and alpha-linolenic acids to produce omega-6 arachidonic acid and omega-3 eicosapentaenoic and docosahexaenoic acids, respectively. Only the last step of the biosynthetic pathway is located in peroxisomes where the beta-oxidation of 24-carbon long-chain fatty acids produce the final 22-carbon chains.

Source	Total PUFA (g/100g)	LA (g/100g)	AA (g/ 100g)	ALA (g/100g)	EPA (g/100g)	DHA (g/100g)	Amount (g) to provide about 1 g of omega-3 PUFA	Cholesterol (mg/100g)
Salmon oil	40.324	1.543	0.675	1.061	13.023	18.232	3	485
Menhaden oil	34.197	2.154	1.169	1.490	13.168	8.562	5	521
Sardine oil	31.867	2.014	1.756	1.327	10.137	10.656	5	710
Cod liver oil	22.541	0.935	0.935	0.935	6.898	10.968	6	570
Herring oil	15.604	1.149	0.289	0.763	6.273	4.206	7	766
Flaxseed oil	67.849	14.327	0	53.368	0	0	2	0
Mackerel, Atlantic, cooked, dry heat	4.300	0.147	0.051	0.113	0.504	0.699	83	75
Herring, Atlantic, cooked, dry heat	2.735	0.167	0.077	0.132	0.909	1.105	50	77
Salmon, Atlantic, farmed, cooked, dry heat	4.553	0.666	1.273	0.113	0.690	1.457	47	63
Tuna, fresh, bluefin, cooked, dry heat	1.844	0.068	0.055	-	0.363	1.141	66	49
Tuna, fresh, yellowfin, cooked, dry heat	0.175	0.023	0.018	0.002	0.015	0.105	833	47
Trout, mixed species, cooked, dry heat	1.922	0.224	0.242	0.199	0.259	0.677	107	63
Halibut, Atlantic and Pacific, cooked, dry heat	0.352	0.041	0.017	0.013	0.080	0.155	425	60
Cod, Atlantic, cooked, dry heat	0.292	0.006	0.028	0.001	0.004	0.154	633	55
Flaxseeds	28.730	5.903	0	22.813	0	0	4	0

Data from the National Nutrient Database for Standard Reference 28 (2015). United States Department of Agriculture.

PUFA, polyunsaturated fatty acids; LA, linolenic acid; AA, arachidonic acid; ALA, alpha-linolenic acid; EPA, eicosapentaenoic acid; and DHA, docosahexaenoic acid.

Table 1. Polyunsaturated fatty acids and cholesterol composition of the major edible sources of omega-3 polyunsaturated fatty acids.

Fatty acids are quickly incorporated in phospholipids of plasma, platelets, neutrophil, and red blood cells, whereas enrichment of other tissues takes longer time. Omega-3 PUFA accumulate especially in cerebral cortex, retina, testes, muscle, and liver; omega-6 are ubiquitous in all tissues. The process of elongation and desaturation of precursors of PUFA is competitive because the synthesis of omega-6 and omega-3 PUFA utilizes the same enzymatic pathway. Despite that, ALA is a more affine substrate for desaturases and conversion of ALA into long-chain omega-3 PUFA is more efficient than that of LA into AA. Therefore, increased ALA availability reduces AA formation and the balance between omega-6 and omega-3 PUFA content in cell membranes can be modulated by changing the dietary habit. Accordingly, it has been shown that populations that live in regions with higher seafood consumption have lower omega-6 to omega-3 PUFA ratio than populations that live in farming-prevalent regions with a lower omega-3 PUFA consumption. Interestingly, the former populations are those with the lowest risk for cardiovascular mortality [8].

Deficiency of PUFA is rare in humans, because normal diet contains an adequate amount of omega-6 and omega-3 PUFA. However, signs of severe PUFA deficiency have been documented in premature infants with limited lipid stores or when these infants were fed with low lipid formulas; such signs were severe skin rash, loss of hair, and irritability. Several clinical conditions may also be associated with PUFA deficiency [9]. Clinical manifestations associated with PUFA deficiency consist of dermatitis, increased skin-water permeability, susceptibility to infection, higher sensitivity to radiation damage, impaired wound healing, hematological abnormalities, and fatty liver disease. Biochemically, PUFA deficiency is associated with an increased eicosatrienoic acid (C20:3 omega-9) to AA ratio (Holman index) because mammals can use oleic acid (C18:1 omega-9) as a precursor of long-chain PUFA only in the absence of the other families [10].

3. Effects of omega-3 PUFA on blood pressure regulation

Arterial blood pressure is the product of cardiac output and peripheral vascular resistance to blood flow. Cardiac output results from the stroke volume times the heart rate, whereas the vascular resistance to blood flow depends on the vascular function. Regulation of arterial blood pressure derives from a complex interaction between cardiovascular cell components with autocrine, paracrine, and endocrine factors and the involvement of the nervous and immune systems. Many physiologic systems are involved in blood pressure regulation such as that of baroreceptor signals, natriuretic peptides, renin-angiotensin-aldosterone, kinin-kallikrein, and catecholamine. In addition, several genetic, anthropometric, and dietetic factors can influence blood pressure, such as family history, age, gender, body mass index, and consumption of salt. Classically, hypertension is a multifactorial complex disease mainly related to an initial abnormality in the kidney that leads to inappropriate tubular sodium retention, intravascular volume expansion, cardiac overload, vascular dysfunction, and sustained high blood pressure levels [11].

Arterial hypertension is defined in adults when systolic (SBP) and diastolic (DBP) blood pressure levels persist over 140 or 90 mm Hg, respectively [4]. In fact, over these thresholds lowering blood pressure is protective for the occurrence of organ damage and cardiovascular events. Reducing blood pressure by a few mm Hg in hypertensive patients can significantly decrease the incidence of stroke and coronary events [12] independently of the class of drug used [13]. Omega-3 PUFA intake has shown to reduce blood pressure especially in hypertensive patients by interacting with several mechanisms of blood pressure regulation (**Table 2**).

Mechanisms of blood pressure regulation

- Reduction of stroke volume and heart rate
- Improvement of left ventricle diastolic filling
- Reduction of peripheral vascular resistances
  - Improvement of endothelial-dependent and -independent vasodilation
    - Stimulation of nitric oxide production
    - Reduction of the asymmetric di-methyl-arginine (ADMA)
    - Reduction of endothelin-1
    - Relaxation of vascular smooth muscle cells
    - Metabolic effects on perivascular adipocytes
    - Endothelial regeneration

Mechanisms of hypertension-related organ damage protection

- Anti-inflammatory, antioxidant, and antithrombotic effects
- Reduction of arterial stiffness
- Experimental effects on left ventricular hypertrophy and abnormal gene expression
- Effects on atherosclerotic plaque progression and stability

Table 2. Mechanisms by which omega-3 polyunsaturated fatty acids can modulate blood pressure levels and protect from the hypertension-related organ damage.

3.1. Effects of omega-3 PUFA on cardiac function and hemodynamics

Omega-3 PUFA can influence blood pressure by acting on the cardiac hemodynamics. In particular, the influence of omega-3 PUFA on the electrophysiological properties of cardiomyocytes can account for the reduced heart rate and the antiarrhythmic effect of these molecules [14]. Mozaffarian et al. [15] published a meta-analysis on the effects of omega-3 PUFA on resting heart rate demonstrating that fish oil treatment can reduce the heart rate by few beats per minute with respect to placebo. Omega-3 PUFA have shown also to improve heart rate variability, heart rate response during exercise, and heart rate post-exercise recovery by modulating the vagal tone [16, 17].

Influences of omega-3 PUFA on heart rate and peripheral vascular resistance may explain the effects of these fatty acids on the left ventricular function. Studies on nonhuman primates firstly showed that fish oil consumption can enhance left ventricular diastolic filling by improving left ventricular diastolic volume, stroke volume, and myocardial efficiency [18, 19]. In addition, other experimental studies demonstrated that omega-3 PUFA can blunt the hypertrophic response of the left ventricle to the pressure overload and prevent the abnormal gene expression of cardiomyocytes [20, 21]. Evidence for hemodynamic effects of omega-3 PUFA in humans was also reported. In a parallel double-blind randomized controlled trial (RCT) in 224 young-adult and middle-aged healthy men, 4 g/day of ethyl ester DHA reduced the heart rate of 2.2 bpm with respect to placebo without affecting blood pressure levels. In another study, a small group of about 50 men taking omega-3 PUFA improved left ventricular diastolic filling assessed by echocardiography when compared to controls [22]. In a cross-sectional study, an increased intake of non-fried fish (tuna or other broiled or backed fish) was associated with lower blood pressure, lower heart rate, lower systemic vascular resistances, greater stroke volume, and better ventricular diastolic function. Conversely, fried fish intake was associated with worse cardiac function [23].

3.2. Effects of omega-3 PUFA on vascular function

Vascular function results from a complex interaction between neurohormonal signaling, circulating cells, immune system, and different components of the vascular wall. These components consist of endothelial cells, vascular smooth muscle cells, extracellular matrix, and perivascular adipocytes. There is a clear relationship between inflammation, oxidation, thrombosis, and endothelial dysfunction, conditions continuously interacting in a vicious circle that promote high blood pressure and the atherosclerotic process. Omega-3 PUFA have shown to modulate vascular resistance and blood pressure by acting on several determinants of the vascular function.

3.2.1. Omega-3 PUFA in inflammation and thrombosis

Omega-3 PUFA affect several mechanisms of the inflammatory process [24]. The intake of omega-3 PUFA increases these fatty acids in phospholipids of cells involved in inflammation at the expenses of omega-6 PUFA. Since AA is the precursor of the pro-inflammatory and pro-thrombotic eicosanoids (prostaglandins, leukotrienes, and thromboxanes), the reduction of AA by increasing omega-3 PUFA decreases the amount of AA-derived eicosanoids. In addition, EPA competes with AA for cyclooxygenase and lipoxygenase enzymes generating eicosanoid derivatives that are less pro-inflammatory and pro-thrombotic than those derived from AA.

Omega-3 PUFA are involved in the production of "specialized pro-resolving mediators" (SPMs) from EPA and DHA through the activity of cyclooxygenase and lipoxygenase enzymes. These molecules include resolvins (E- and D-series), protectins, and maresins. Their amount increases in plasma of subjects with a high intake of omega-3 PUFA and can be found in human milk during the first month of lactation. These molecules are actively involved in the termination (resolution) of an acute inflammatory process by activating local resolution programs that include inhibition of trans-endothelial neutrophil migration, reduced pro-inflammatory cytokines production, limitation of leukocyte recruitment, enhancement of macrophage uptake of debris, bacteria and apoptotic cells, and tissue repair [25].

Omega-3 PUFA exert their anti-inflammatory properties also by inhibiting other pro-inflammatory mediators (platelet-activating factor, PAF; interleukin (IL)-1, -2, -6, and -8; tumor necrosis factor alpha) and several pro-inflammatory transcription factors (activator protein-1, AP-1; nuclear factor kappa-light-chain-enhancer of activated B cells, nuclear factor (NF)-κB) [26, 27]. EPA and DHA can disrupt the small heterogeneous membrane microdomains (lipid raft) of inflammatory cells by changing their lipid composition. In these microdomains, several important processes for the cell take place, especially the activation of the pro-inflammatory NF-κB [28].

In addition, omega-3 PUFA can modulate the activity of inflammasomes. Inflammasomes are a group of sensor and receptor proteins of the innate immunity assembled in an intracytoplasmic complex in response to harmful stimuli [29]. These stimuli consist of exogenous product such as bacterial or endogenous advanced glycation end products (AGEs), cholesterol crystals in atherosclerotic lesions, and oxidized low-density lipoproteins (ox-LDL) [30]. EPA and DHA can inhibit the inflammasome activation through the G-protein receptor (GPR)120/beta-arrestin2-dependent pathway by suppressing the nuclear translocation of the NF-κB [31] and by stimulating inflammasome autophagy [32].

3.2.2. Omega-3 PUFA in mechanisms of endothelial dysfunction

Several experimental and human studies have demonstrated that omega-3 PUFA can improve endothelial function in both normal and damaged endothelium. In endothelial cells, the incubation with EPA stimulates the production of nitric oxide (NO) through the activation and translocation of the endothelial nitric oxide synthase (eNOS) from caveolae (a special type of cell membrane lipid raft) to the cytoplasm [33]. In experimental studies, NO produced via eNOS after EPA stimulation induced endothelial-dependent vasodilation of arteries [33, 34]. Omega-3 PUFA enhance endothelial-dependent vasodilation also in arteries with a damaged endothelium [35], by reducing plasma levels of the asymmetric dimethylarginine (ADMA), a potent endogenous inhibitor of the eNOS activity [36].

Other mechanisms by which omega-3 PUFA can improve endothelial dysfunction are antioxidation [37], reduction of the vasoconstrictive endothelin-1 (ET-1) [38], and the generation of omega-3 PUFA-derived epoxides from the metabolic pathway of the cytochrome P450 epoxygenases [39]. Recently, Hoshi et al. elucidated with an elegant work that DHA can directly induce relaxation of the vascular smooth muscle cells (VSMCs) and acutely reduce blood pressure in anesthetized mice. This effect was mediated by a direct hyperpolarization of the VSMC induced by DHA through the stimulation of the large-conductance calcium- and voltage-activated potassium channels (BK channels) [40]. The activation of BK channels by DHA depends from the activity of cytochrome P450 epoxygenase, since its selective inhibition abolishes the effect [41].

Omega-3 PUFA can modulate endothelial function also by regulating the endocrine activity of the perivascular adipose cells. Experimentally, ALA stimulates the release of adiponectine, an anti-inflammatory, insulin sensitizer, and vasodilating adipokine, from mature adipocytes by inhibiting calcium current through the calcium-permeable nonselective cationic channels [42]. Other metabolic important effects of omega-3 PUFA on the adipose cells are increased sensitivity to insulin through PPAR-gamma and GPR120 stimulation [28, 43] and increased production of anti-inflammatory endocannabinoids [44].

Omega-3 PUFA demonstrate an important endothelium protective and reparative effect. The treatment with EPA partially repairs endothelial damage induced by hyperlipidemia in rabbits [45]. Reparative effects of omega-3 PUFA can be mediated by their capacity to stimulate endothelial progenitor cells availability and by promoting endothelial regeneration and neo-angiogenesis in damaged vessels. These effects have been observed in experimental model of diabetic retinopathy [46] and cerebrovascular ischemia [47], and also in healthy individuals [48]. Recently, an endothelial regenerative effect of omega-3 PUFA has been demonstrated in low cardiovascular risk patients. In these patients, omega-3 PUFA promoted the production of endothelial progenitor cells and reduced the presence of endothelial cell-damaged micro-particles [49].

3.2.3. *Omega-3 PUFA in endothelial dysfunction in human studies*

Endothelial cell function can be indirectly assessed *in vivo* in humans by stimulating endothelial NO production with pharmacological or mechanical stimuli (endothelial-dependent vasodilation) and comparing the induced vasodilatory response with that induced by an exogenous nitrate-donor compounds (endothelial-independent vasodilation) [50]. The difference between endothelial-dependent and -independent vasodilation is proportional to the extent of endothelial dysfunction [51]. Endothelial dysfunction assessed with these techniques is an independent predictor of cardiovascular events and mortality [52]. Omega-3 PUFA have shown to improve endothelial-dependent vasodilation in several RCTs. The results of these studies were summarized in two recent systematic reviews and meta-analyses [53, 54]. In the first were included 16 RCTs involving 901 participants who took a dose of omega-3 PUFA ranging from 0.45 to 4.5 g/day for a mean of 56 days. Omega-3 PUFA slightly improved the flow-mediated vasodilation (FMD) of the brachial artery in treated patients. The effect was present especially in patients affected by a pathological condition respect to healthy subjects and was greater with a higher dose of omega-3 PUFA [53]. In the second meta-analysis were included 23 studied with 1385 participants. The source of omega-3 PUFA was fish oil with a dose ranging from 0.45 to 4.53 g/day and a treatment duration from 2 to 52 weeks. Again, the FMD response of the brachial artery was slightly better in treated patients. However, an inverse association between study quality and the improvement of FMD due to fish oil supplementation was observed and when authors considered only high-quality RCTs (19 studies) no overall effect was observed anymore [54]. Recently, many RCTs of different quality on the effect of omega-3 PUFA on endothelial-dependent vasodilation have been published. However, results of these studies are conflicting and again a final conclusion cannot be drawn [55–59].

4. Effects of omega-3 PUFA on hypertension and hypertensive-related organ damage

The first evidence of the hypotensive effect of omega-3 PUFA was observed more than 30 years ago and was summarized in two seminal systematic reviews and meta-analyses about 10 years later. The first meta-analysis selected 17 controlled clinical trials including 728 normotensive healthy individuals and 291 untreated hypertensive patients without any other comorbidity. The analysis showed a significant blood pressure reduction for SBP and DBP only in hypertensive patients. The omega-3 PUFA-lowering effect was directly related to the baseline levels of blood pressure [60]. The second meta-analysis included 31 controlled clinical trials with 1356 participants who were healthy or at risk for cardiovascular disease. The mean dose of omega-3 PUFA used was of 4.8 g/day as fish or fish oil for 3–24 weeks of treatment. Again, omega-3 PUFA reduced SBP and DBP only in hypertensive patients. Importantly, there was a total dose-response effect of −0.66/−0.35 mm Hg/g assumed of omega-3 PUFA [61]. Thereafter, many meta-analyses on the effect of omega-3 PUFA on blood pressure have been published [62–66] and are summarized in **Table 3**. All these meta-analyses confirmed a significant although small hypotensive effect of these fatty acids especially in hypertensive patients who are not taking any antihypertensive drugs. Evidence from observational prospective studies suggests also that baseline omega-3 PUFA intake can be associated with the occurrence of future development of hypertension [67].

First author, publication year [Ref.]	Included studies (individuals)	Populations	EPA+DHA (median, g/day)	Duration (median, weeks)	Effect on SBP (mm Hg, 95% CI)	Effect on DBP (mm Hg, 95% CI)
Apple, 1993 [60]	11 (728)	Healthy subjects	3.35	5	−1.0 (−2.0 to 0.0)	−0.5 (−1.2 to 0.2)
	6 (291)	Untreated hypertensive patients	5	8	−5.5 (−8.1 to −2.9)	−3.5 (−5.0 to −2.1)
Morris, 1993 [61]	8 (569)	Healthy subjects	4.3	6	−0.4 (−1.6 to 0.8)	−0.7 (−1.5 to 0.1)
	9 (415)	Hypertensive patients	4.75	6	−3.4 (−5.9 to −0.9)	−2.0 (−3.3 to −0.7)
Geleijnse*, 2002 [62]	27 (1354)	Without hypertension	–	–	−1.03 (−2.40 to 0.14)	−1.17 (−1.91 to −0.43)
	23 (760)	With hypertension	–	–	−3.97 (−5.66 to −2.15)	−2.46 (−3.44 to −1.47)
Dickinson, 2006 [63]	8 (375)	Hypertensive patients	4.5	11	−2.3 (−4.3 to −0.2)	−2.2 (−4.0 to −0.4)
Campbell, 2013 [64]	9 (1049)	Normotensive subjects	2.55	12	−0.50 (−1.44 to 0.45)	−0.53 (−1.24 to 0.19)
	8 (475)	Hypertensive patients	3.4	11	−2.56 (−4.53 to −0.58)	−1.47 (−2.53 to −0.41)

First author, publication year [Ref.]	Included studies (individuals)	Populations	EPA+DHA (median, g/day)	Duration (median, weeks)	Effect on SBP (mm Hg, 95% CI)	Effect on DBP (mm Hg, 95% CI)
Miller, 2014 [66]	56 (3533)	Normotensive subjects	2.6	6.5	−1.25 (−2.05 to −0.46)	−0.62 (−1.22 to −0.02)
	16 (942)	Untreated hypertensive patients	3	6	−4.51 (−6.12 to −2.83)	−3.05 (−4.35 to −1.74)

PUFA, polyunsaturated fatty acids; EPA, eicosapentaenoic acid; DHA, docosahexaenoic acid; CI, confidence intervals.

* Studies included in subgroup analysis were not specified; therefore, no median dose and treatment duration can be calculated.

Table 3. Principal meta-analytical studies on the effects of omega-3 polyunsaturated fatty acids on blood pressure levels in healthy subjects and hypertensive patients.

Another source of omega-3 PUFA, flaxseeds or flaxseed-derived oil, showed anti-inflammatory, antioxidant, and blood pressure-lowering effects in animals and cardiovascular risk patients. Flaxseed is the seed of *Linum usitatissimum*, the richest source of ALA. A recent meta-analysis by Khalesi et al. [68] on 14 trials demonstrated a significant lowering effect on SBP (1.77 mm Hg; 95% confidence interval (CI): −3.45 to −0.09, $P = 0.04$) and DBP (1.58 mm Hg; 95% CI: −2.64 to −0.52, $P = 0.003$) of flaxseeds or flaxseed oil intake. An interesting mechanism suggested for blood pressure reduction of flaxseed was the inhibition of the epoxide hydrolase by ALA that reduced the production of vasoconstrictive oxylipins [69].

4.1. Studies with ambulatory blood pressure monitoring

Ambulatory blood pressure monitoring (ABPM) evaluates blood pressure levels over 24 h giving information on daytime and nighttime blood pressure profiles and their circadian variations. ABPM is a useful tool for the diagnosis of hypertension and for definition of the full-day efficacy of antihypertensive treatments. Several observational and interventional studies have evaluated the effect of omega-3 PUFA on ABPM, though with inconsistent results [70, 71]. We followed up a group of uncomplicated hypertensive patients who were advised to take a diet rich of PUFA by assuming a fish meal three times a week for 6 months. ABPM parameters and omega-3 PUFA enrichment of red blood cell plasma membranes were evaluated at baseline and at the end of the study. Twenty-four-hour and nighttime SBP/DBP were reduced only in patients that increased omega-3 PUFA in cell membranes and the effect was more pronounced in patients with a lower baseline omega-3 PUFA content [72]. Our findings underline the importance of the baseline omega-3 PUFA status in cell membranes as a determinant of the hypotensive effect of these fatty acids. Also, our observation might explain the discrepancy observed among previous studies that did not assess the compliance to dietary prescriptions.

The different effect of EPA and DHA on blood pressure was evaluated by Mori et al. in a small RCT of overweight mild hyperlipidemic men. Specifically, at the end of the follow-up only DHA treatment reduced 24 h and daytime ambulatory SBP/DBP with respect to placebo

(5.8/3.3 and 3.5/2.0 mm Hg, respectively). Also, DHA treatment was effective to reduce 24-h, daytime, and nighttime heart rate [73].

4.2. Arterial stiffness

Arterial stiffening is caused by the loss of vascular elasticity due to factors such as aging and atherosclerosis. It depends from the structural properties of the arterial wall that affect the manner in which pressure, blood flow, and arterial diameter change within each heartbeat. Arterial stiffness depends from the balance between extracellular proteins and their distribution along the arterial wall. An increased arterial stiffness is associated with hypertension and it is an independent direct predictor of cardiovascular events. The measurement of velocity of the pulse-wave propagation (pulse-wave velocity, PWV) between two vascular points is an accepted method to assess arterial stiffness [74]. Pase et al. summarized in a systematic review the effect of omega-3 PUFA supplementation on PWV and other indexes of arterial stiffness. Ten trials met the inclusion criteria with 550 participants randomized to take a dose of omega-3 PUFA ranging from 0.64 to 3.00 g/day or placebo for a period of 6–105 weeks. Studies involved healthy subjects and patients with overweight, diabetes, hypertension, and dyslipidemia. The treatment with omega-3 PUFA improved arterial stiffness and the effect was independent of changes in blood pressure, heart rate, or body mass index. Neither significant heterogeneity nor publication bias was detected [75]. The same author showed recently in a new larger RCT on healthy subjects that a high dose of fish oil (6 g/day) but not a low dose (3 g/day) could reduce aortic pulse pressure and aortic augmentation pressure, two indirect measures of central blood pressure and arterial stiffness, respectively [76].

The reasons for improvement of arterial stiffness with the use of omega-3 PUFA can be related to the hypotensive, anti-inflammatory, and antioxidative effects of these fatty acids, as well as to their ability to improve endothelial cell function. A low maternal habit in fish consumption during pregnancy is an independent predictor of arterial stiffness later in the childhood life but not of elevated blood pressure [77]. The inverse association between maternal omega-3 PUFA intake and arterial stiffness persists with child aging and it is independent of the individual's fish consumption [77, 78]. Additional evidence of the beneficial effect of omega-3 PUFA on the vascular structure comes from the inverse association between omega-3 PUFA intake and the cross-sectional diameter of arteries. It was demonstrated that a larger brachial artery diameter is a significant independent predictor of future cardiovascular events [79, 80]. Accordingly, we and other authors have reported an inverse association between the brachial artery cross-sectional diameter and the consumption of fish or the concentration of circulatory omega-3 PUFA [81, 82]. We reported also that the membrane content of omega-3 PUFA is directly associated with the extent of the vasodilatory response to sublingual nitrate administration, supporting the evidence of a beneficial effect of these fatty acids on the vascular wall [82].

Since aging is another important determinant of arterial stiffening and hypertension, it is interesting to note that blood levels of omega-3 PUFA are inversely related with telomere shortening, a marker of cell senescence, in patients with coronary heart disease [83]. Telomere shortening reflects the generation of oxidative stress and inflammation that characterizes cellular ageing, and omega-3 PUFA might protect cells and slow this process. In a group of overweight patients, supplemental intake of omega-3 PUFA for 4 months increased omega-3 to omega-6 ratio in plasma phospholipids and this ratio was associated with telomeres length of leukocytes. In this study, omega-3 PUFA reduced also the proportion of plasma F2-isoprostanes, a marker of lipid peroxidation and oxidative stress [84]. Similar results were reported in elderly individuals with mild cognitive impairment [85].

4.3. Atherosclerotic lesions

Omega-3 PUFA have shown to modulate atherosclerotic plaque formation and stability. The carotid intima-media thickness (cIMT) is an early marker of atherosclerotic damage that precedes plaque formation and is easily assessed in humans by ultrasonography. We have recently demonstrated that a diet rich of fish for 1 year can reduce cIMT of patients with uncomplicated hypertension. This effect was observed only in those patients who were compliant with dietary prescription [86]. Similar findings on early atherosclerotic lesions were reported in other studies with different populations [87–89], but not in all those that have investigated this problem [90]. Interesting observation by Skilton and coworkers might help to explain these discrepancies. These authors demonstrated that a factor, which significantly affects the benefit of PUFA supplementation to slow cIMT progression, is the presence of an impaired prenatal growth [91]. As a consequence, dietary omega-3 PUFA supplementation in children with a history of impaired prenatal growth is protective from subsequent carotid wall thickening [92].

In addition to their preventive effect on the formation of atherosclerotic plaques, omega-3 PUFA could stabilize existing plaques. In patients with carotid stenosis, fish oil supplementation increases omega-3 PUFA content of plaques. This was associated with a thickening fibrous cup and reduction of intra-plaque inflammation and macrophage infiltration [93]. Similar results were obtained in another group of patients awaiting endarterectomy in which omega-3 PUFA supplementation reduced the intra-plaque content of foam cells and T-lymphocytes and lowered the expression of metalloproteinases, interleukins, and intracellular adhesion molecules [94]. Omega-3 PUFA supplementation can act favorably also on less critical plaques, as those not responsible for an acute coronary syndrome (non-culprit lesions) [95]. Although the beneficial effects of omega-3 PUFA on atherosclerotic plaques are mainly attributed to their anti-inflammatory and antioxidant properties, it was shown that these fatty acids increase the amount of cholesterol of high-density lipoprotein (HDL) [96–98] and reduce plasma levels of lipoprotein(a) [99, 100]. Finally, some studies have shown that omega-3 PUFA intake can enhance the beneficial effects of cardio-protective drugs such as statins and the acetylsalicylic acid [101–104].

Despite the evidence of many effects of omega-3 PUFA in opposing the atherosclerotic process, meta-analytical studies on their use in primary and secondary cardiovascular prevention provided inconclusive results [5].

5. Conclusions

This chapter has analyzed the effects of omega-3 PUFA on blood pressure and their potential benefit for the treatment of hypertension and its related organ damage. Substantial evidence supports the existence of a small hypotensive effect of these fatty acids in hypertensive patients that appears more related to the use of DHA and dietary compliance. Evidence in support of a protective effect of omega-3 PUFA on hypertension-related organ damage is much weaker. Lack of a clear benefit from marine food or other sources of these fatty acids in cardiovascular prevention has limited their use in the clinical practice. Nonetheless, a regular fish intake remains recommended by international guidelines.

Research on omega-3 PUFA has provided many interesting results in the cardiovascular field, but new areas need to be explored. Although effective in hypertensive patients, no studies have evaluated the effects of omega-3 PUFA on specific types of hypertension-related organ damage such as left ventricular hypertrophy, nephroangiosclerosis, and retinopathy. The role of omega-3 PUFA during pre-natal development and potential effects on post-natal cardio-vascular outcomes will also need further investigation.

Author details

GianLuca Colussi*, Cristiana Catena, Marileda Novello and Leonardo A. Sechi

*Address all correspondence to: gianluca.colussi@uniud.it

Division of Internal Medicine, Department of Experimental and Clinical Medical Sciences, University of Udine, Udine, Italy

References

[1] Lim SS, Vos T, Flaxman AD, et al. A comparative risk assessment of burden of disease and injury attributable to 67 risk factors and risk factor clusters in 21 regions, 1990-2010: a systematic analysis for the Global Burden of Disease Study 2010. *Lancet* 2012; 380: 2224–2260.

[2] Hopstock LA, Bønaa KH, Eggen AE, et al. Longitudinal and secular trends in blood pressure among women and men in birth cohorts born between 1905 and 1977: The Tromsø Study 1979 to 2008. *Hypertension* 2015; 66: 496–501.

[3] Ikeda N, Sapienza D, Guerrero R, et al. Control of hypertension with medication: a comparative analysis of national surveys in 20 countries. *Bull World Health Organ* 2014; 92: 10–19C.

http://dx.doi.org/10.5772/63501

[4] Mancia G, Fagard R, Narkiewicz K, et al. 2013 ESH/ESC Guidelines for the management of arterial hypertension. *Eur Heart J* 2013; 31: 1281–1357.

[5] Colussi G, Catena C, Sechi LA. ω-3 polyunsaturated fatty acids effects on the cardiometabolic syndrome and their role in cardiovascular disease prevention: an update from the recent literature. *Recent Adv Cardiovasc Drug Discov* 2015; 9: 78–96.

[6] Colussi G, Catena C, Baroselli S, et al. Omega-3 fatty acids: from biochemistry to their clinical use in the prevention of cardiovascular disease. *Recent Patents Cardiovasc Drug Discov* 2007; 2: 13–21.

[7] Sprecher H. Metabolism of highly unsaturated n-3 and n-6 fatty acids. *Biochim Biophys Acta* 2000; 1486: 219–231.

[8] Bjerregaard P, Dyerberg J. Mortality from ischaemic heart disease and cerebrovascular disease in Greenland. *Int J Epidemiol* 1988; 17: 514–519.

[9] Jeppesen PB, Christensen MS, Høy CE, et al. Essential fatty acid deficiency in patients with severe fat malabsorption. *Am J Clin Nutr* 1997; 65: 837–843.

[10] Holman RT, Johnson S. Changes in essential fatty acid profile of serum phospholipids in human disease. *Prog Lipid Res* 1981; 20: 67–73.

[11] Androulakis ES, Tousoulis D, Papageorgiou N, et al. Essential hypertension: is there a role for inflammatory mechanisms? *Cardiol Rev* 2009; 17: 216–221.

[12] MacMahon S, Peto R, Cutler J, et al. Blood pressure, stroke, and coronary heart disease. Part 1, Prolonged differences in blood pressure: prospective observational studies corrected for the regression dilution bias. *Lancet* 1990; 335: 765–774.

[13] Law MR, Morris JK, Wald NJ. Use of blood pressure lowering drugs in the prevention of cardiovascular disease: meta-analysis of 147 randomised trials in the context of expectations from prospective epidemiological studies. *BMJ* 2009; 338: b1665.

[14] Kang JX. Reduction of heart rate by omega-3 fatty acids and the potential underlying mechanisms. *Front Physiol* 2012; 3: 416.

[15] Mozaffarian D, Geelen A, Brouwer IA, et al. Effect of fish oil on heart rate in humans a meta-analysis of randomized controlled trials. *Circulation* 2005; 112: 1945–1952.

[16] Ninio DM, Hill AM, Howe PR, et al. Docosahexaenoic acid-rich fish oil improves heart rate variability and heart rate responses to exercise in overweight adults. *Br J Nutr* 2008; 100: 1097–1103.

[17] Macartney MJ, Hingley L, Brown MA, et al. Intrinsic heart rate recovery after dynamic exercise is improved with an increased omega-3 index in healthy males. *Br J Nutr* 2014; 112: 1984–1992.

[18] McLennan PL, Barnden LR, Bridle TM, et al. Dietary fat modulation of left ventricular ejection fraction in the marmoset due to enhanced filling. *Cardiovasc Res* 1992; 26: 871–877.

[19] Charnock JS, McLennan PL, Abeywardena MY. Dietary modulation of lipid metabolism and mechanical performance of the heart. *Mol Cell Biochem* 1992; 116: 19–25.

[20] Duda MK, O'Shea KM, Lei B, et al. Dietary supplementation with omega-3 PUFA increases adiponectin and attenuates ventricular remodeling and dysfunction with pressure overload. *Cardiovasc Res* 2007; 76: 303–310.

[21] Shah KB, Duda MK, O'Shea KM, et al. The cardioprotective effects of fish oil during pressure overload are blocked by high fat intake: role of cardiac phospholipid remodeling. *Hypertension* 2009; 54: 605–611.

[22] Grimsgaard S, Bønaa KH, Hansen JB, et al. Effects of highly purified eicosapentaenoic acid and docosahexaenoic acid on hemodynamics in humans. *Am J Clin Nutr* 1998; 68: 52–59.

[23] Mozaffarian D, Gottdiener JS, Siscovick DS. Intake of tuna or other broiled or baked fish versus fried fish and cardiac structure, function, and hemodynamics. *Am J Cardiol* 2006; 97: 216–222.

[24] Calder PC. Marine omega-3 fatty acids and inflammatory processes: Effects, mechanisms and clinical relevance. *Biochim Biophys Acta* 2015; 1851: 469–484.

[25] Serhan CN. Pro-resolving lipid mediators are leads for resolution physiology. *Nature* 2014; 510: 92–101.

[26] Meydani SN, Endres S, Woods MM, et al. Oral (n-3) fatty acid supplementation suppresses cytokine production and lymphocyte proliferation: comparison between young and older women. *J Nutr* 1991; 121: 547–555.

[27] Zhao Y, Chen LH. Eicosapentaenoic acid prevents lipopolysaccharide-stimulated DNA binding of activator protein-1 and c-Jun N-terminal kinase activity. *J Nutr Biochem* 2005; 16: 78–84.

[28] Oh DY, Talukdar S, Bae EJ, et al. GPR120 is an omega-3 fatty acid receptor mediating potent anti-inflammatory and insulin-sensitizing effects. *Cell* 2010; 142: 687–698.

[29] Guo H, Callaway JB, Ting JP-Y. Inflammasomes: mechanism of action, role in disease, and therapeutics. *Nat Med* 2015; 21: 677–687.

[30] Witztum JL, Lichtman AH. The influence of innate and adaptive immune responses on atherosclerosis. *Annu Rev Pathol* 2014; 9: 73–102.

[31] Yan Y, Jiang W, Spinetti T, et al. Omega-3 fatty acids prevent inflammation and metabolic disorder through inhibition of NLRP3 inflammasome activation. *Immunity* 2013; 38: 1154–1163.

[32] Williams-Bey Y, Boularan C, Vural A, et al. Omega-3 free fatty acids suppress macrophage inflammasome activation by inhibiting NF-κB activation and enhancing autophagy. *PloS One* 2014; 9: e97957.

[33] Omura M, Kobayashi S, Mizukami Y, et al. Eicosapentaenoic acid (EPA) induces Ca(2+)-independent activation and translocation of endothelial nitric oxide synthase and endothelium-dependent vasorelaxation. *FEBS Lett* 2001; 487: 361–366.

[34] Lawson DL, Mehta JL, Saldeen K, et al. Omega-3 polyunsaturated fatty acids augment endothelium-dependent vasorelaxation by enhanced release of EDRF and vasodilator prostaglandins. *Eicosanoids* 1991; 4: 217–223.

[35] Engler MB, Engler MM, Ursell PC. Vasorelaxant properties of n-3 polyunsaturated fatty acids in aortas from spontaneously hypertensive and normotensive rats. *J Cardiovasc Risk* 1994; 1: 75–80.

[36] Raimondi L, Lodovici M, Visioli F, et al. n-3 polyunsaturated fatty acids supplementation decreases asymmetric dimethyl arginine and arachidonate accumulation in aging spontaneously hypertensive rats. *Eur J Nutr* 2005; 44: 327–333.

[37] Wang H-H, Hung T-M, Wei J, et al. Fish oil increases antioxidant enzyme activities in macrophages and reduces atherosclerotic lesions in apoE-knockout mice. *Cardiovasc Res* 2004; 61: 169–176.

[38] Chisaki K, Okuda Y, Suzuki S, et al. Eicosapentaenoic acid suppresses basal and insulin-stimulated endothelin-1 production in human endothelial cells. *Hypertens Res* 2003; 26: 655–661.

[39] Frömel T, Fleming I. Whatever happened to the epoxyeicosatrienoic Acid-like endothelium-derived hyperpolarizing factor? The identification of novel classes of lipid mediators and their role in vascular homeostasis. *Antioxid Redox Signal* 2015; 22: 1273–1292.

[40] Hoshi T, Wissuwa B, Tian Y, et al. Omega-3 fatty acids lower blood pressure by directly activating large-conductance Ca2+-dependent K+ channels. *Proc Natl Acad Sci U S A* 2013; 110: 4816–4821.

[41] Wang R, Chai Q, Lu T, et al. Activation of vascular BK channels by docosahexaenoic acid is dependent on cytochrome P450 epoxygenase activity. *Cardiovasc Res* 2011; 90: 344–352.

[42] Sukumar P, Sedo A, Li J, et al. Constitutively active TRPC channels of adipocytes confer a mechanism for sensing dietary fatty acids and regulating adiponectin. *Circ Res* 2012; 111: 191–200.

[43] Neschen S, Morino K, Rossbacher JC, et al. Fish oil regulates adiponectin secretion by a peroxisome proliferator-activated receptor-gamma-dependent mechanism in mice. *Diabetes* 2006; 55: 924–928.

[44] Meijerink J, Plastina P, Vincken J-P, et al. The ethanolamide metabolite of DHA, docosahexaenoylethanolamine, shows immunomodulating effects in mouse peritoneal and RAW264.7 macrophages: evidence for a new link between fish oil and inflammation. *Br J Nutr* 2011; 105: 1798–1807.

[45] Cayli S, Sati L, Seval-Celik Y, et al. The effects of eicosapentaenoic acid on the endothelium of the carotid artery of rabbits on a high-cholesterol diet. *Histol Histopathol* 2010; 25: 141–151.

[46] Tikhonenko M, Lydic TA, Opreanu M, et al. N-3 polyunsaturated fatty acids prevent diabetic retinopathy by inhibition of retinal vascular damage and enhanced endothelial progenitor cell reparative function. *PloS One* 2013; 8: e55177.

[47] Wang J, Shi Y, Zhang L, et al. Omega-3 polyunsaturated fatty acids enhance cerebral angiogenesis and provide long-term protection after stroke. *Neurobiol Dis* 2014; 68: 91–103.

[48] Spigoni V, Lombardi C, Cito M, et al. N-3 PUFA increase bioavailability and function of endothelial progenitor cells. *Food Funct* 2014; 5: 1881–1890.

[49] Wu S-Y, Mayneris-Perxachs J, Lovegrove JA, et al. Fish-oil supplementation alters numbers of circulating endothelial progenitor cells and microparticles independently of eNOS genotype. *Am J Clin Nutr* 2014; 100: 1232–1243.

[50] Deanfield JE, Halcox JP, Rabelink TJ. Endothelial function and dysfunction: testing and clinical relevance. *Circulation* 2007; 115: 1285–1295.

[51] Ludmer PL, Selwyn AP, Shook TL, et al. Paradoxical vasoconstriction induced by acetylcholine in atherosclerotic coronary arteries. *N Engl J Med* 1986; 315: 1046–1051.

[52] Inaba Y, Chen JA, Bergmann SR. Prediction of future cardiovascular outcomes by flow-mediated vasodilatation of brachial artery: a meta-analysis. *Int J Cardiovasc Imaging* 2010; 26: 631–640.

[53] Wang Q, Liang X, Wang L, et al. Effect of omega-3 fatty acids supplementation on endothelial function: a meta-analysis of randomized controlled trials. *Atherosclerosis* 2012; 221: 536–543.

[54] Xin W, Wei W, Li X. Effect of fish oil supplementation on fasting vascular endothelial function in humans: a meta-analysis of randomized controlled trials. *PLoS One* 2012; 7: e46028.

[55] Grenon SM, Owens CD, Nosova EV, et al. Short-term, high-dose fish oil supplementation increases the production of omega-3 fatty acid-derived mediators in patients with peripheral artery disease (the OMEGA-PAD I Trial). *J Am Heart Assoc* 2015; 4: e002034.

http://dx.doi.org/10.5772/63501

[56] Singhal A, Lanigan J, Storry C, et al. Docosahexaenoic acid supplementation, vascular function and risk factors for cardiovascular disease: a randomized controlled trial in young adults. *J Am Heart Assoc* 2013; 2: e000283.

[57] Siasos G, Tousoulis D, Oikonomou E, et al. Effects of Ω-3 fatty acids on endothelial function, arterial wall properties, inflammatory and fibrinolytic status in smokers: a cross over study. *Int J Cardiol* 2013; 166: 340–346.

[58] Oh PC, Koh KK, Sakuma I, et al. Omega-3 fatty acid therapy dose-dependently and significantly decreased triglycerides and improved flow-mediated dilation, however, did not significantly improve insulin sensitivity in patients with hypertriglyceridemia. *Int J Cardiol* 2014; 176: 696–702.

[59] Tousoulis D, Plastiras A, Siasos G, et al. Omega-3 PUFAs improved endothelial function and arterial stiffness with a parallel antiinflammatory effect in adults with metabolic syndrome. *Atherosclerosis* 2014; 232: 10–16.

[60] Appel LJ, Miller ER, Seidler AJ, et al. Does supplementation of diet with 'fish oil' reduce blood pressure? A meta-analysis of controlled clinical trials. *Arch Intern Med* 1993; 153: 1429–1438.

[61] Morris MC, Sacks F, Rosner B. Does fish oil lower blood pressure? A meta-analysis of controlled trials. *Circulation* 1993; 88: 523–533.

[62] Geleijnse JM, Giltay EJ, Grobbee DE, et al. Blood pressure response to fish oil supplementation: metaregression analysis of randomized trials. *J Hypertens* 2002; 20: 1493–1499.

[63] Dickinson HO, Mason JM, Nicolson DJ, et al. Lifestyle interventions to reduce raised blood pressure: a systematic review of randomized controlled trials. *J Hypertens* 2006; 24: 215–233.

[64] Campbell F, Dickinson HO, Critchley JA, et al. A systematic review of fish-oil supplements for the prevention and treatment of hypertension. *Eur J Prev Cardiol* 2013; 20: 107–120.

[65] Hartweg J, Farmer AJ, Holman RR, et al. Meta-analysis of the effects of n-3 polyunsaturated fatty acids on haematological and thrombogenic factors in type 2 diabetes. *Diabetologia* 2007; 50: 250–258.

[66] Miller PE, Van Elswyk M, Alexander DD. Long-chain omega-3 fatty acids eicosapentaenoic acid and docosahexaenoic acid and blood pressure: a meta-analysis of randomized controlled trials. *Am J Hypertens* 2014; 27: 885–896.

[67] Yang B, Shi M-Q, Li Z-H, et al. Fish, long-chain n-3 PUFA and incidence of elevated blood pressure: a meta-analysis of prospective cohort studies. *Nutrients* 2016; 8: 58.

[68] Khalesi S, Irwin C, Schubert M. Flaxseed consumption may reduce blood pressure: a systematic review and meta-analysis of controlled trials. *J Nutr* 2015; 145: 758–765.

[69] Caligiuri SPB, Aukema HM, Ravandi A, et al. Flaxseed consumption reduces blood pressure in patients with hypertension by altering circulating oxylipins via an α-linolenic acid–induced inhibition of soluble epoxide hydrolase. *Hypertension* 2014; 64: 53–59.

[70] Prisco D, Paniccia R, Bandinelli B, et al. Effect of medium-term supplementation with a moderate dose of n-3 polyunsaturated fatty acids on blood pressure in mild hypertensive patients. *Thromb Res* 1998; 91: 105–112.

[71] Russo C, Olivieri O, Girelli D, et al. Omega-3 polyunsaturated fatty acid supplements and ambulatory blood pressure monitoring parameters in patients with mild essential hypertension. *J Hypertens* 1995; 13: 1823–1826.

[72] Colussi G, Catena C, Dialti V, et al. Fish meal supplementation and ambulatory blood pressure in patients with hypertension: relevance of baseline membrane fatty acid composition. *Am J Hypertens* 2014; 27: 471–481.

[73] Mori TA, Bao DQ, Burke V, et al. Docosahexaenoic acid but not eicosapentaenoic acid lowers ambulatory blood pressure and heart rate in humans. *Hypertension* 1999; 34: 253–260.

[74] Townsend RR, Wilkinson IB, Schiffrin EL, et al. Recommendations for improving and standardizing vascular research on arterial stiffness: a scientific statement from the American heart association. *Hypertension* 2015; 66: 698–722.

[75] Pase MP, Grima NA, Sarris J. Do long-chain n-3 fatty acids reduce arterial stiffness? A meta-analysis of randomised controlled trials. *Br J Nutr* 2011; 106: 974–980.

[76] Pase MP, Grima N, Cockerell R, et al. The effects of long-chain omega-3 fish oils and multivitamins on cognitive and cardiovascular function: a randomized, controlled clinical trial. *J Am Coll Nutr* 2015; 34: 21–31.

[77] Bryant J, Hanson M, Peebles C, et al. Higher oily fish consumption in late pregnancy is associated with reduced aortic stiffness in the child at age 9 Years. *Circ Res* 2015; 116: 1202–1205.

[78] Reinders I, Murphy RA, Song X, et al. Higher plasma phospholipid n-3 PUFAs, but lower n-6 PUFAs, are associated with lower pulse wave velocity among older adults. *J Nutr* 2015; 145: 2317–2324.

[79] Yeboah J, Crouse JR, Hsu F-C, et al. Brachial flow-mediated dilation predicts incident cardiovascular events in older adults: the Cardiovascular Health Study. *Circulation* 2007; 115: 2390–2397.

[80] Yeboah J, Folsom AR, Burke GL, et al. Predictive value of brachial flow-mediated dilation for incident cardiovascular events in a population-based study: the multi-ethnic study of atherosclerosis. *Circulation* 2009; 120: 502–509.

[81] Anderson JS, Nettleton JA, Herrington DM, et al. Relation of omega-3 fatty acid and dietary fish intake with brachial artery flow-mediated vasodilation in the Multi-Ethnic Study of Atherosclerosis. *Am J Clin Nutr* 2010; 92: 1204–1213.

[82] Colussi G, Catena C, Dialti V, et al. The vascular response to vasodilators is related to the membrane content of polyunsaturated fatty acids in hypertensive patients. *J Hypertens* 2015; 33: 993–1000.

[83] Farzaneh-Far R, Lin J, Epel ES, et al. Association of marine omega-3 fatty acid levels with telomeric aging in patients with coronary heart disease. *JAMA* 2010; 303: 250–257.

[84] Kiecolt-Glaser JK, Epel ES, Belury MA, et al. Omega-3 fatty acids, oxidative stress, and leukocyte telomere length: A randomized controlled trial. *Brain Behav Immun* 2013; 28: 16–24.

[85] O'Callaghan N, Parletta N, Milte CM, et al. Telomere shortening in elderly individuals with mild cognitive impairment may be attenuated with ω-3 fatty acid supplementation: a randomized controlled pilot study. *Nutrition* 2014; 30: 489–491.

[86] Colussi G, Catena C, Dialti V, et al. Effects of the consumption of fish meals on the carotid IntimaMedia thickness in patients with hypertension: a prospective study. *J Atheroscler Thromb* 2014; 21: 941–956.

[87] He K, Liu K, Daviglus ML, et al. Intakes of long-chain n-3 polyunsaturated fatty acids and fish in relation to measurements of subclinical atherosclerosis. *Am J Clin Nutr* 2008; 88: 1111–1118.

[88] Dai X, Zhang B, Wang P, et al. Erythrocyte membrane n-3 fatty acid levels and carotid atherosclerosis in Chinese men and women. *Atherosclerosis* 2014; 232: 79–85.

[89] Hjerkinn EM, Abdelnoor M, Breivik L, et al. Effect of diet or very long chain omega-3 fatty acids on progression of atherosclerosis, evaluated by carotid plaques, intima-media thickness and by pulse wave propagation in elderly men with hypercholesterolaemia. *Eur J Cardiovasc Prev Rehabil* 2006; 13: 325–333.

[90] Angerer P, Kothny W, Störk S, et al. Effect of dietary supplementation with omega-3 fatty acids on progression of atherosclerosis in carotid arteries. *Cardiovasc Res* 2002; 54: 183–190.

[91] Skilton MR, Mikkilä V, Würtz P, et al. Fetal growth, omega-3 (n-3) fatty acids, and progression of subclinical atherosclerosis: preventing fetal origins of disease? The Cardiovascular Risk in Young Finns Study. *Am J Clin Nutr* 2013; 97: 58–65.

[92] Skilton MR, Ayer JG, Harmer JA, et al. Impaired Fetal Growth and Arterial Wall Thickening: A Randomized Trial of Omega-3 Supplementation. *Pediatrics* 2012; 129: e698–e703.

[93] Thies F, Garry JMC, Yaqoob P, et al. Association of n-3 polyunsaturated fatty acids with stability of atherosclerotic plaques: a randomised controlled trial. *Lancet* 2003; 361: 477–485.

[94] Cawood AL, Ding R, Napper FL, et al. Eicosapentaenoic acid (EPA) from highly concentrated n–3 fatty acid ethyl esters is incorporated into advanced atherosclerotic plaques and higher plaque EPA is associated with decreased plaque inflammation and increased stability. *Atherosclerosis* 2010; 212: 252–259.

[95] Yamano T, Kubo T, Shiono Y, et al. Impact of eicosapentaenoic acid treatment on the fibrous cap thickness in patients with coronary atherosclerotic plaque: an optical coherence tomography study. *J Atheroscler Thromb* 2015; 22: 52–61.

[96] Colussi G, Catena C, Mos L, et al. The metabolic syndrome and the membrane content of polyunsaturated fatty acids in hypertensive patients. *Metab Syndr Relat Disord* 2015; 13: 343–351.

[97] Venturini D, Simão ANC, Urbano MR, et al. Effects of extra virgin olive oil and fish oil on lipid profile and oxidative stress in patients with metabolic syndrome. *Nutrition* 2015; 31: 834–840.

[98] Jones PJH, Senanayake VK, Pu S, et al. DHA-enriched high-oleic acid canola oil improves lipid profile and lowers predicted cardiovascular disease risk in the canola oil multicenter randomized controlled trial. *Am J Clin Nutr* 2014; 100: 88–97.

[99] Shinozaki K, Kambayashi J, Kawasaki T, et al. The long-term effect of eicosapentaenoic acid on serum levels of lipoprotein (a) and lipids in patients with vascular disease. *J Atheroscler Thromb* 1996; 2: 107–109.

[100] Colussi GL, Baroselli S, Sechi L. Omega-3 polyunsaturated fatty acids decrease plasma lipoprotein(a) levels in hypertensive subjects. *Clin Nutr* 2004; 23: 1246–1247.

[101] Nishio R, Shinke T, Otake H, et al. Stabilizing effect of combined eicosapentaenoic acid and statin therapy on coronary thin-cap fibroatheroma. *Atherosclerosis* 2014; 234: 114–119.

[102] Block RC, Abdolahi A, Tu X, et al. The effects of aspirin on platelet function and lysophosphatidic acids depend on plasma concentrations of EPA and DHA. *Prostaglandins Leukot Essent Fatty Acids* 2015; 96: 17–24.

[103] Block RC, Kakinami L, Jonovich M, et al. The combination of EPA+DHA and low-dose aspirin ingestion reduces platelet function acutely whereas each alone may not in healthy humans. *Prostaglandins Leukot Essent Fatty Acids* 2012; 87: 143–151.

[104] Toyama K, Nishioka T, Isshiki A, et al. Eicosapentaenoic Acid combined with optimal statin therapy improves endothelial dysfunction in patients with coronary artery disease. *Cardiovasc Drugs Ther* 2014; 28: 53–59.

Chapter 5

Psychiatric Comorbidity in Essential Hypertension

(Pattern, Prevalence of Psychiatric Comorbidity and Quality of Life in Subjects with Essential Hypertension)

Aborlo Kennedy Nkporbu and
Princewill Chukwuemeka Stanley

Additional information is available at the end of the chapter

http://dx.doi.org/10.5772/64104

Abstract

The prevalence of essential hypertension has continued to increase worldwide, and its consequences have remained a growing concern. A number of sociodemographic and clinical variables may however serve as key determinants of the extent to which it is associated with psychiatric comorbidity as well as impairment of quality of life. The aim of this study, therefore, was to determine the sociodemographic and clinical factors that may influence the level of psychiatric comorbidity and quality of life associated with persons with essential hypertension attending the general outpatient clinic of the University of Port Harcourt Teaching Hospital (UPTH). Following ethical approval and informed consent from the participants, 360 subjects making up the study group were recruited based on the study's inclusion and exclusion criteria. A pilot study was carried out. Subjects were further administered with the study's instruments including the socio-demographic/clinical questionnaire, GHQ-12, WHO Composite International Diagnostic Interview (WHOCIDI) and the WHOQOL-Bref. The data were analysed using the Statistical Package for Social Sciences version 16 statistical package. Confidence interval was set at 95%, while p-value of less than 0.05 was considered statistically significant. The study found a prevalence of psychiatric comorbidity of 64.4% among the hypertensives. Among the study group, there was no significant relationship between the presence of psychiatric comorbidity and age class (p = 0.350), gender (p = 0.22), level of education (p = 043), income class (p = 0.81) and occupation. Persons who were married were significantly more likely to have a psychiatric comorbidity (p = 0.001). There was also no significant relationships between age of onset of illness (p = 0.60), duration of illness (p = 0.73), duration of treatment (p = 0.82) and self-stigma (p = 0.15). The findings of this study support the impression that essential hypertension is a chronic debilitating illness, associated with psychiatric comorbidity and reduced quality of life, that is largely significantly influenced by a number of sociodemographic and clinical factors. The results support the call that the management of patients with essential hypertension should include attention to the mental health status of the sufferers.

Keywords: pattern and prevalence, essential hypertension, psychiatric comorbidity, QOL, UPTH

1. Introduction

There is a growing population of persons with essential hypertension (HT) worldwide despite all efforts at increasing education and awareness about it [1–19]. World Health Organization (WHO) estimates that non-communicable diseases like hypertension and other heart diseases, stroke, depression and cancers will increase by 60% by 2020 and are likely to triple in Nigeria and other sub-Saharan African countries in the next 50 years. According to the World Health Report, non-communicable diseases including diabetes mellitus, arthritis and cardiovascular diseases make up to about 22% of all deaths in the region in the year 2000; cardiovascular diseases alone accounted for 9.2% of the total deaths [20]. Indeed, it has already been projected that up to three quarters of the world's hypertensive population will be in economically developing countries by the year 2025 [7]. With increased prevalence rates and the resultant greater economic and health burden [8–10], nations like China and Nigeria will feel the impact mostly due to their population size.

Hypertension constitutes a greater percentage of all the referrals from other nonpsychiatric units seeking for psychiatric evaluation in the University of Port Harcourt Teaching Hospital (UPTH) [21]. Essential hypertension runs the features of chronicity, with subsequent need for long-term medications, adverse effects on the central nervous system (CNS), high rate of mortality and morbidity [10, 22, 23] and impact on emotion [24, 25] (the component that is often neglected). In addition, patients with hypertension need extensive education, attitudinal change, coping and healthy lifestyle, including diet and exercise. The need for these adjustments is imperative considering the immediate changes that usually accompany the diagnosis of the condition. They include burden of the diseases, regular hospital visits, complications arising from the primary illness and job adjustment. For these reasons, together with their direct effects on the central nervous system (CNS), no doubt, the patients commonly present with varying degrees of psychopathology [26–30]. Psychopathology is the inward or outward manifestation of a disordered psychic system.

Essential hypertension is a severe, chronic systemic disease and is becoming increasingly associated with psychiatric comorbidity, as high as 30–60% at present [31–36]. It carries enormous burden on both the patients and the caregivers [37, 8–10]. Unfortunately, there appears to be a general under-recognition or late recognition of, and in some cases poor attention to, the psychiatric component by clinicians [38–42] particularly in this environment [43]. This is often accompanied by increased severity and clinical deterioration of these illnesses, poor management and prognosis with eventual high mortality rates. Late recognition of mental disorders in hypertensive patients is related, among others, with diminished coping capacity at diagnosis, failure at primary prevention, poor antihypertensive adherence [44–47], impairment in quality of life (QOL) [48–56], greater social burden, overall increases in healthcare costs [57–59], and also higher mortality [8]. Also, psychological distress and lifestyle variables among patients with hypertension are equally associated with noncompliance.

To further compound the problem is the co-existence of other medical conditions like diabetes and obesity, with hypertension. Their presence further worsens the clinical outlook, complicates treatment and causes noncompliance [60]. Hypertension can, either singly or in association with other adverse psychosocial and clinical factors, predispose to psychiatric disorders. Furthermore, some of the medications employed in the management of these conditions have been associated with inherent neuropsychiatric complications [61, 62] either as direct side effects, from drug interactions with psychoactive substances, from multiple drug therapy or with other concomitantly administered drugs for other comorbid conditions.

Apart from the above aetiological links, a common pathway—sympathetic pathway [63–66] —seems to mediate both essential hypertension and most anxiety disorders. It is equally important to note that baseline adverse psychosocial factors, psychological distress or clearly identified psychiatric conditions have been implicated as predictors of hypertension [67–72]. In light of the foregoing, there appears to be a bidirectional relationship between associated psychiatric disorders and hypertension. This propensity to be associated with emotional disturbances, with tendency to either predispose to or comorbid with psychiatric disorders, has further increased the degree to which they affect the psychological well-being and quality of life of the sufferers [73–80]. The focus of medical practice has always tended towards relieving physical symptoms, in this case hypertension, which often neglects the huge impact on the psychological well-being, psychiatric comorbidity and the overall quality of life of the sufferers, often occasioning monumental health consequences [81, 82].

A prompt multidisciplinary approach involving evaluation, counselling and treatment of mental disorders in hypertensive patients is becoming more important [83]. Therefore, the determination of the nature and magnitude of psychiatric comorbidity, the additive effects on psychological well-being and quality of life and emphasis on the need for mental health component in the management of essential hypertension and other chronic medical conditions form the areas of concern of this study.

2. Overview of hypertension

Hypertension is defined as a persistent elevation in blood pressure (BP) over an acceptable upper limit of normal values of systolic and diastolic blood pressures [84]. Objectively, hypertension is blood pressure persistently equal to or greater than 140/90 mmHg [85]. The systolic pressure is the pressure at the peak of the heart's contraction, while diastolic blood pressure is the pressure when the heart relaxes. Blood pressure varies from moment to moment and has a diurnal variation, being highest at 10 am and lowest at 3 am [86]. Hypertension may be of unknown cause called essential hypertension or hyperpiesia [87] or may have an underlying cause when it is known as secondary hypertension. Hypertension has been classified by the World Health Organization/International Society of Hypertension into mild, moderate, severe and high normal [83].

Hypertension is a non-communicable chronic disease, often requiring long-term treatment. The incidence may be on the increase as a result of increasing urbanisation and changing lifestyles in the world [88–92]. Hypertension is regarded a major public health problem [29], and it is an important threat to the health of adults in sub-Saharan Africa [93, 94].

Secondary hypertension indicates that the high blood pressure (HBP) is a result of another underlying condition, such as kidney disease or tumours (adrenal adenoma or phaeochromocytoma). The pathogenesis of essential hypertension is not clearly understood [95, 96]. However, different investigators have proposed the kidney, peripheral resistance vessels and the sympathetic nervous system as the seat of the primary abnormality [97]. In reality, the problem is probably multifactorial. On the other hand, most mechanisms leading to secondary hypertension are well understood [97]. Some studies have tried to implicate genetic and environmental aetiologies to hypertension [98–101]. Disorder of the autonomic system, as in the case of sympathetic nervous system overactivity and others include imbalance in the renin-angiotensin-aldosterone system, chronic exposure to stress, chronic use of alcohol and other associated medical diseases like diabetes.

3. Epidemiology of hypertension

The prevalence of hypertension is probably on the increase in developing countries, including Nigeria, where adoption of western lifestyles and the stress of urbanisation, both of which are expected to increase the morbidity associated with unhealthy lifestyles, are not on the decline [102, 103]. The prevalence of hypertension depends on both racial composition of the population of the study and the criteria for defining the condition [104]. In Nigeria, it is the commonest non-communicable disease; over 4.3 million Nigerians above the age of 15 years are classified as being hypertensives [105, 106].

Risk factors have equally become important in the aetiology of hypertension. A study found that as high as 62% of the total population of hypertensive lived with at least two risk factors, mainly diabetes mellitus and alcohol use. Several other studies both in Nigeria and elsewhere have also implicated diabetes, calcium salt and fat intake from consumption of processed food [91], participating in jobs with minimal activities, obesity [92], consumption of caffeine [89, 108, 109] and alcohol [107], smoking and hypercholesterolemia [110, 111]. A proportion of the diabetic population (20%) suffered from isolated systolic hypertension [106]. In a meta-analysis of nine studies carried out in Nigeria with similar methodology, the authors [93, 112–115] summarised the prevalence of hypertension in population of Nigeria for a 20-year period (1990–2009), in which two reviewers, independently, were used during the selection process, so as to reduce bias as much as possible.

In spite of the peculiarities found in studies on hypertension in different parts of the world, it is important to note that in all areas, hypertension (HT) or high blood pressure (HBP) is a heterogeneous set of disorders. Social and cultural factors have a direct aetiologic effect on hypertension, and these factors are responsible for most of the differences in disease prevalence in different parts of the world. High blood pressure is a mass phenomenon responsible for high morbidity and mortality affecting millions of people the world over [30], and with the notable exception of a few non–salt-eating primitive societies, it occurs everywhere. Diseases of the cardiovascular system are among the most important causes of morbidity in the industrialised world [30, 116, 117], accounting for over one-third of all deaths in the United States [118, 119]. A study [7] estimates a worldwide prevalence of between 10 and 15% of adult populations to have high blood pressure which also agrees with findings in Africa [120]. However, other studies have reported a worldwide prevalence of 15–30% in adults [121]. Studies from the Western world identified five factors associated with hypertension: increasing age, obesity, elevated pressure in blood relative, environment and race [116].

4. Hypertension and psychopathology

The relationship between hypertension and emotional disturbance or psychiatric morbidity could be described as bidirectional, or better still, as taking the form of a vicious cycle. Apart from the genetic components, persistent environmental stressors are well-known triggers for hypertension [25, 31, 122]. They reset and over amplify the sympathetic outflow [62–65, 123]. The neurotransmitter that fuels the sympathetic pathway, noradrenaline, is consequently overelaborated and becomes hyperactive. This causes both hypertension and anxiety disorders including generalised anxiety disorder (GAD), panic disorder, acute stress disorder and PTSD. On the other hand, the presence of anxiety alone can cause hypertension in predisposed individuals [49, 50]. The chronicity of hypertension, persistent and recurrent symptoms, impairment in functioning capacity, other adverse and enduring environmental psychosocial burdens and even the thought of these can also in turn cause anxiety and may also quickly drive the patient into depression, suicidal ideation or attempt and ultimately suicide. Long-standing untreated depression in hypertensive patients can be complicated with psychosis [23]. Also, hypertension can be complicated with cerebrovascular accident (CVA), with its attendant neuropsychiatric sequelae including depression, anxiety, mild-to-severe cognitive impairment, personality changes, vascular dementia and psychosis.

Lishman identified the interest of psychiatry in hypertension, besides the obvious consequences of its central nervous system effects and noted:

1. The intriguing possibility of psychological factors as a part causation of essential hypertension.

2. Symptoms of hypertension like headache, fatigue, etc. appear to arise secondarily from knowledge of the disorder than increased blood pressure per se.

3. Iatrogenic psychiatric effects can figure prominently in the use of antihypertensive drugs.

He suggested possible explanations including drugs taken, feeling ill and attendance to hospital per se and possibly more pre-morbidly neurotic individuals becoming hypertensive patients. Other various writers have also looked in depth at purely psychological attributes in hypertensive subjects either causally or effectually [106, 124]. Fundamental advances in the understanding of hypertension from then have coincided with theories of anxiety states and affective disorders suggesting catecholamines as mediators. These find common ground in suggested mechanisms for producing increased arterial pressure [62–65, 123].

Studies have shown that stress-related situations, issue of job loss and unemployment [24], prolonged difficulties, being under stress and people at war front were shown to have elevated blood pressures [25, 31, 122]. It has been found that stress increases the level of cortisol which causes increased deposition of arteriosclerotic deposits in the intima of blood vessels. These depositions gradually narrow the lumen of the vessels, which in turn increases arterial pressure resulting into hypertension. The same elevated cortisol has been implicated in depression and also explains the high rate of depression associated with disorders that primarily involve cortisol-like Cushing's syndrome [125, 126]. It has also been suggested that hypertensive individuals exhibit more aggressive traits than others and that these may be hidden or suppressed, becoming manifest by abnormal elevation of blood pressure [127].

Psychosocial stressors, especially job-related stressors, predicted hypertension more strongly in men than in women in these data as in those of other investigators [50]. Other potential hypertension risk factors included social alienation and low level of education and ethnicity, which are independent predictors of hypertension. Indicators of subjective distress and low educational status, on the other hand, appeared more predictive of hypertension in women than in men. The excess impact of psychosocial stress on the development of hypertension in men compared with women may be related to sex differences in reactions to cardiovascular stress reactivity [127].

Some other studies that have examined the association of hypertension with psychological distress, such as anxiety and depressive symptoms, have produced mixed findings. Several studies have reported positive associations [128, 129], whereas others have observed weak or no associations. Other numerous studies have produced evidence that patients with depression have an increased risk of developing cardiovascular disease [48]. Also, depression in untreated hypertension might increase risk of developing cardiovascular disease. There is even some evidence to suggest lower blood pressure (BP) in participants with depressive or anxiety disorders. These areas of uncertainty call for further research (longitudinal) to evaluate the true associations between mental disorders and hypertension.

The findings of other studies that depressive disorder was associated with lower systolic blood pressure (SBP), although the use of tricyclic antidepressants was associated with greater risk of hypertension, may simply correspond with increased risk of weight gain associated with these agents [130]. Similar findings have been made with psychotropic medications. These studies are limited by their cross-sectional design, which made it difficult to infer causality or determine the direction of the observed relationship between hypertension and psychological distress. A related issue is the effect of labelling patients as hypertensive. Several studies have suggested that individuals 'labelled' as hypertensive might adopt a sick role that can negatively affect quality of life [74–79]. For this reason, the association between hypertension and psychological distress may be because of a direct effect of the BP itself, adverse effects of treatment or the consequences of labelling.

Another study also found that health-related quality of life, including physical functioning, vitality, mental health and pain thresholds, was better in unaware compared with aware hypertensive participants [78]. Several mechanisms have been postulated to explain the effects of labelling. Some evidence suggests that the act of labelling somebody as hypertensive can cause increases in sympathetic activity during mental stress [123], which might partly explain the reason for the poor mental health of patients with hypertension. In a study of 214 normotensive and mildly hypertensive participants, the perception of being hypertensive was associated with greater anxiety during clinic BP measurement and may be due to the white coat effect [131].

Another study also observed direct associations between the use of alcohol (daily >14 g intake of ethanol) and kola nut consumption in men and isolated systolic hypertension [124]. The survey showed that over 10% of the population taking kola nuts (at least one in 2 days) and/or alcohol is hypertensive. Caffeine has been identified as a significant cause of hypertension [79]. The authors [79] therefore concluded that programmes to improve treatment of hypertension should not only focus on lifestyle variables like smoking and alcohol, but they should also include the identification and treatment of substance abuse and dependence disorders.

Besides anxiety and depression, a range of other psychiatric problems may occur following cerebrovascular accident resulting from hypertension. They include cognitive disorders and personality changes [127], especially with the involvement of the right hemisphere. In fact, untreated hypertension can equally cause cognitive impairment, which is commonly seen in organic psychiatry [97]. A study done in two communities in Ibadan metropolis, Nigeria, by Ogunniyi and Baiyewu found a high rate of incident (vascular) dementia with psychological and behavioural components as complications of hypertension [43]. Studies have also found out the association between hypertension and erectile dysfunction in men. A study noted 1% of psychogenic impotence and 1% secondary to the effect of some antihypertensive drugs like methyldopa and reserpine [29].

This study was therefore designed to evaluate the sociodemographic and clinical correlates of psychiatric comorbidity in hypertensive patients. This, no doubt, would be of immense relevance to the practice of consultation liaison psychiatry in the West African subregion and contribute to the corpus of knowledge on chronic medical conditions and aid care/service providers to plan better management strategies that will also accord premium to the psychological component and well-being of these patients. Impairments, disabilities and handicaps from chronic conditions may thus be limited and patients' dignity and functional capacity enhanced.

5. Aim

The study was to determine the pattern and prevalence of psychiatric comorbidity and quality of life in subjects with essential hypertension.

6. Methodology

In this cross-sectional study, following ethical approval from the hospital and informed consent from the participants, 360 subjects making up the study group were recruited based on the study's inclusion and exclusion criteria, after a pilot study for both groups. In addition, the hypertensives were screened for human immunodeficiency virus (HIV) infection. Subjects were further administered with the study's instruments including the sociodemographic questionnaire, General Health Questionnaire, version 12 (GHQ-12), World Health Organization Composite International Diagnostic Interview (WHOCIDI) and the brief version of the WHO Quality of Life (WHOQOL-Bref) instrument. Severity of hypertension was determined using the modern classification by the WHO/International Society of Hypertension into mild, moderate and severe. Those considered suitable for the study were patients who had been seen and diagnosed as having essential hypertension by the consultant family physicians and internists.

The hypertensive patients have all had basic investigations: i.e. full blood count, blood urea and electrolytes estimation and urinalysis, in most cases. In addition, some had electrocardiograms (ECG), chest X-rays, serum cholesterol, uric acid, creatinine and creatinine clearance estimations. Investigation results were all recorded in the case notes. Hypertensive patients with primary myocardial or valvular disease, cardiac failure or renal failure or who had a stroke or coronary heart disease, diabetes, asthma or other chronic illnesses or those found to be acutely ill were excluded. Patients were required to have been diagnosed for at least the past 1 year and have had at least 6 months of treatments. The data were analysed using the Statistical Package for Social Sciences version 16 statistical package. Confidence interval was set at 95%, while p-value of less than 0.05 was considered statistically significant.

7. Study instruments

The following instruments were used in this study:

- Sociodemographic/clinical questionnaire
- General Health Questionnaire, version 12 (GHQ-12)
- World Health Organization Composite International Diagnostic Interview (WHOCIDI)

8. Results

8.1. Sociodemographic and clinical correlates of psychiatric morbidity in study group

Out of the 360 subjects with essential hypertension who fulfilled the inclusion criteria, 141 (39.2%) were males and 219 (60.8%) females. The mean age for the study group (hypertensives)

http://dx.doi.org/10.5772/64104

was 45.57 years. More than half of all the subjects 257 (71.4%) were married. The majority (78.0%) had attained at least a secondary level of education.

Variables	Essential hypertensive			
	Total	Psychiatric diagnosis	No psychiatric diagnosis	Statistical analysis
Age				$X^2 = 3.27$
<20	0	0 (0.0%)	0 (0.0%)	df = 4
20–29	16	9 (3.8%)	7 (5.6%)	p = 0.35
30–39	77	49 (20.8%)	28 (22.6%)	
40–49	132	82 (34.7%)	50 (40.3%)	
≥50	135	96 (40.7%)	39 (31.5%)	
	360	236 (65.6%)	124 (34.43%)	
Sex				$X^2 = 1.52$
Male	141	87 (36.9%)	54 (43.5%)	df = 1
Female	219	149 (63.1%)	70 (56.5%)	p = 0.22
Marital status				$X^2 = 20.94$
Married	257	153 (64.8%)	104 (83.9%)	df = 4
Single	38	25 (10.6)	13 (105.5%)	p < 0.001
Divorced	3	8 (1.30%)	0 (0.0%)	
Separated	8	8 (3.4%)	0 (0.0%)	
Widowed	54	47 (19.9%)	7 (5.6%)	
Education				$X^2 = 2.78$
None	17	10 (4.2%)	7 (5.6%)	df = 3
Primary	76	55 (23.3%)	21 (16.9%)	p = 0.43
Secondary	128	85 (36.0%)	43 (34.7%)	
Tertiary	139	86 (36.4)	53 (42.7%)	
Tribe				$X^2 = 0.43$
Hausa	7	3 (1%)	4 (1.1%)	df = 2
Ibo	75	41 (11.4%)	34 (9.4%)	p = 0.81
Yoruba	20	10 (2.8%)	10 (2.8%)	
Ijaw	83	52 (14.4%)	31 (8.6%)	
Ogoni	62	29 (8.1%)	33 (9.2%)	
Ikwerre	79	48 (13.3%)	31 (8.6%)	
Others	24	16 (4.4%)	8 (2.2%)	

Variables	Essential hypertensive			
	Total	Psychiatric diagnosis	No psychiatric diagnosis	Statistical analysis
Average monthly income				$X^2 = 23.86$
Low	83	54 (24.8%)	29 (24.2%)	df = 3
Average	159	104 (47.7%)	54 (45.0)	$p < 0.001$
High	97	60 (27.5%)	37(30.8)	
Reaction to diagnosis				$X^2 = 14.41$
Normal	38	18 (7.6%)	20 (16.1%)	df = 10
Sad	175	101 (42.8%)	74 (59.7%)	$p = 0.16$
Very sad	146	116 (49.2%)	30 (24.2%)	
Wish to die	1	1 (0.4%)	0 (0.0%)	
Mode of getting drugs				$X^2 = 13.09$
From the government	106	42 (11.7%)	64 (17.8%)	df = 3
Self-purchase	202	146 (40.6%)	56 (15.6%)	$p = 0.57$
Both	52	35 (9.7%)	17 (4.7%)	
Source of support				$X^2 = 15.06$
Charity organisation	14	9 (2.5%)	5 (1.4%)	df = 3
Fiends	36	27 (7.5%)	9 (2.5%)	$p = 0.33$
Relatives	92	60 (16.7%)	32 (8.9%)	
None	218	143 (39.8%)	75 (20.8%)	
Domestic situation				$X^2 = 12.41$
Partner	37	22 (6.1%)	15 (4.2%)	df = 3
Family	307	213 (59.2%)	94 (26.1%)	$p = 0.51$
Friends	7	3 (0.8%)	4 (1.1%)	
None	9	5 (1.4%)	4 (1.1%)	
Blood pressure				$X^2 = 16.40$
BP within normal range	0	0 (0%)	0 (0%)	df = 3
Mild hypertension	119	49 (13.7%)	70 (19.4%)	$p = 0.001$
Moderate hypertension	161	114 (31.7%)	47 (13.1%)	
Severe hypertension	80	73 (20.3%)	7 (1.9%)	
Occupation				$X^2 = 17.63$
Managers	5	3 (1.3%)	2 (1.6%)	df = 10
Professionals	15	5 (2.0%)	10 (2.8%)	$p = 0.82$

Variables	Essential hypertensive			
	Total	Psychiatric diagnosis	No psychiatric diagnosis	Statistical analysis
Technicians and associate professionals	30	23 (7.7%)	7 (5.6%)	
Clerical support workers	46	32 (13.6%)	14 (11.3%)	
Service and sales workers	29	18 (7.6%)	11 (8.9%)	
Skilled agricultural forestry and fishery workers	30	23 (9.7%)	7 (5.6%)	
Craft and related trade workers	54	33 (13.6%)	22 (17.27%)	
Plant and machine operators and assemblers	47	31 (13.1%)	16 (12.9%)	
Elementary occupation	72	50 (21.2%)	22 (21.8%)	
Armed forces occupation	3	1 (0.4%)	2 (1.6%)	
Unemployed	22	17 (7.2%)	5 (4.0%)	
Age of onset of disease				$X^2 = 1.89$
20–29	27	18 (7.6%)	9 (7.3%)	df =3
30–39	102	62 (26.3%)	40 (32.3%)	p = 0.60
40–49	169	112 (47.5%)	57 (46.0%)	
>50	62	44 (18.6%)	18 (14.5%)	
Duration of illness				$X^2 = 0.63$
1–5	316	208 (88.1%)	108 (87.1%)	df = 2
6–10	30	18 (7.6%)	12 (9.7%)	p = 0.73
11 and above	14	10 (4.2%)	4 (3.2%)	
Duration of treatment				$X^2 = 0.91$
<1	74	46 (19.5%)	28 (22.6%)	df = 3
1–5	242	162 (68.6%)	80 (64.5%)	p = 0.82
6–10	31	19 (8.1%)	12 (9.7%)	
>10	13	9 (3.8%)	4 (3.2%)	
Missed treatment				$X^2 = 1.89$
Yes	73	61 (16.9%)	12 (3.3%)	df = 3
No	287	171 (47.5%)	116 (32.2%)	p = 0.003
STIGMA				$X^2 =2.13$
Yes	4	4 (1.7%)	0 (0.0%)	df = 1
No	356	232 (98.3%)	124 (100.0%)	p = 0.15

Table 1. Sociodemographic variables and psychiatric comorbidity among hypertensives.

More than one quarter of all the subjects, 241 (66.9%), were within low to average income range of less than 10,000–30,000 naira monthly. The majority, 169 (46.9%), had their onset of illness at the age range of 40–49 years. Persons who were married were significantly more likely to have a psychiatric comorbidity ($p < 0.001$). Also, those who reacted with either 'very sad' or a 'wish to die' when they received the diagnosis of the medical conditions were more likely to have psychiatric comorbidity ($p = 0.001$). See **Table 1.**

8.2. Pattern and prevalence of psychiatry morbidity in subjects with essential hypertension

A total of 232 (64.4%) subjects had associated psychiatric comorbidity, while 128 (35.5%) had no psychiatric diagnosis. Out of the total number with psychiatric comorbidity, 106 (29.4%) had a depressive illness, generalised anxiety disorder (GAD) was diagnosed in 58 (16.2%) patients, 32 (9.3%) patients had sexual dysfunction out of which 27 (7.5%) had male erectile dysfunction, while 5 (1.4%) had hyposexual dysfunction and was diagnosed all in females (see **Figure 1**).

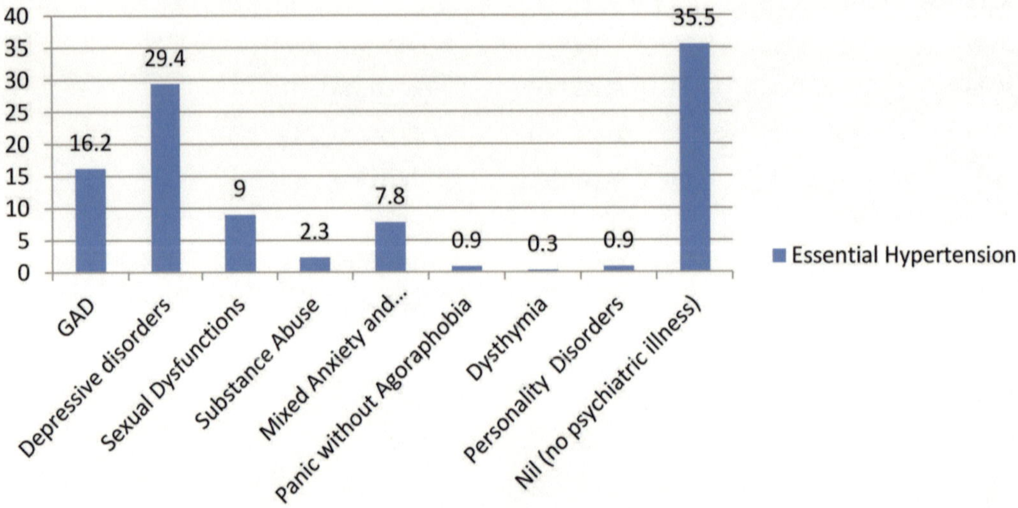

Figure 1. Bar chart showing the pattern and prevalence of psychiatric morbidity among persons with essential hypertension.

It is important to note that 20 (5.6%) patients were diagnosed with more than one condition. Erectile dysfunction and substance abuse were diagnosed in one patient; one respondent had GAD, substance abuse and erectile dysfunction; five respondents had GAD and hyposexual dysfunction; six had GAD and male erectile dysfunction, two had mixed anxiety and depression and male erectile dysfunction; and five had depressive illness and male erectile dysfunction. This accounted for the excess above 590 patients if the total diagnoses are summed up (see **Table 2**).

S/N	Diagnosis	Essential hypertension		
		Freq.	Male	Female
1	Substance abuse/male erectile dysfunction	1 (0.3%)	1 (1.7%)	0 (0.0%)
2	Generalise anxiety disorder/substance abuse/male erectile dysfunction	1 (0.3)	1 (1.7%)	0 (0.0%)
3	Generalised anxiety disorder	36 (10.0%)	17 (11.8%)	19 (8.8%)
4	Generalised anxiety disorder with somatic features	10 (2.8%)	4 (6.8%)	6 (2.8%)
5	Generalised anxiety disorder	5 (1.4%)	0 (0.0%)	5 (2.3%)
6	Generalised anxiety disorder/male erectile dysfunction	6 (1.7%)	6 (4.2%)	0 (0.0%)
7	Mixed anxiety and depression/male erectile dysfunction	2 (0.6%)	2 (3.4%)	0 (0.0%)
8	Moderate depression/male erectile dysfunction	4 (1.1%)	4 (6.8%)	0 (0.0%)
9	Mild depression/male erectile dysfunction	1 (0.3%)	1 (1.7%)	0 (0.0%)
10	Male erectile dysfunction	12 (3.3%)	12 (7.3%)	0 (0.0%)
11	Mild depressive disorders	35 (9.7%)	5 (3.5%)	30 (13.9%)
12	Dysthymia	1 (0.3%)	0 (0.0%)	1 (0.5%)
13	Mild depression with anxiety features	10 (2.8%)	2 (3.4%)	8 (3.7%)
14	Mild depression with somatic features	7 (1.9%)	1 (1.7%)	6 (2.8%)
15	Mixed anxiety and depressive disorders	21 (5.8%)	5 (3.5%)	16 (7.4%)
16	Moderate depressive disorders	36 (10.0%)	8 (3.6%)	28 (3.0%)
17	Panic disorder without agoraphobia	4 (1.1%)	2 (3.4%)	2 (1.0%)
18	Severe depression with psychotic features	8 (2.2%)	2 (3.4%)	6 (2.8%)
19	Personality disorders	5 (1.4%)	4 (6.8%)	1 (0.5%)
20	Substance abuse	6 (1.7%)	5 (3.5%)	1 (0.5%)
21	Nil (no diagnosis)	128 (35.5%)	57 (15.8%)	71 (19.7%)
	Total	**360 (100%)**	**144 (39.5)**	**216 (32.9%)**

Table 2. Pattern and prevalence of psychiatry morbidity in subjects with essential hypertension.

9. Association of psychiatric comorbidity with quality of life in persons with essential hypertension

From the study, psychiatric comorbidity was negatively statistically significantly associated with QOL in all domains except in General Health Facet in both medical conditions. Among the hypertensives patients, those with psychiatric comorbidity performed better on psychological and social domains (see **Table 3**).

Domains of QOL	Quality of life in persons with essential hypertension			
	Quality of life of all hypertensive patients	Psychiatric comorbidity	No psychiatric comorbidity	Statistical analysis
Physical domain	50.97 ± 14.671	45.98 ± 13.064	60.46 ± 12.788	t = −10.07 df = 358 p < 0.001
Psychological domain	54.20 ± 22.186	56.60 ± 24.914	61.05 ± 13.362	t = −4.35 df = 358 p < 0.001
Social domain	54.51 ± 26.13	48.06 ± 26.114	66.80 ± 21.378	t = − 6.87 df = 358 p < 0.001
Environment domain	50.01 ± 16.91	44.95 ± 14.831	59.62 ± 16.503	t = −8.57 df = 358 p < 0.001
General health facet	49.34 ± 22.44	47.98 ± 21.896	51.91 ± 23.319	t = −1.58 df = 358 p < 0.001

Table 3. Association of psychiatric morbidity with quality of life in persons with essential hypertension.

10. Discussion

The study on the psychiatric comorbidities associated with essential hypertension was conceptualised mainly from the observation of the relatively high frequency with which requests for psychiatric consultation were being received over time from other clinical departments in UPTH, particularly internal medicine. The observation was later confirmed by a study [43]. The study was, thus, started with the main objectives of determining the pattern and prevalence of psychiatric morbidity among persons with essential hypertension attending the outpatients clinic of UPTH. A cross-sectional design was adopted, with a sequential use of four study instruments, followed by analysis of data using the various statistical methods.

From the study, the prevalence of essential hypertension was noted to be increasing with age and was about twice higher, in the age groups 40–49 and 50 and above, compared to age group of 30–39, and about six times higher compared with age group 20–29. This result is consistent with earlier studies which reported that about 4.3 million Nigerians above the age of 15 years are classified as being hypertensive. Furthermore, the prevalence has been said to be related to age, particularly in females, with a substantial increase occurring after the age of 50 [36].

Though essential hypertension commonly starts in middle age, the illness may progressively become worse with attendant incapacitating symptoms that may infringe on the functional capacity of the individual and thereby lowering the quality of life. Africans usually seek medical attention mostly when illness has worsened with disabling symptoms, and in most cases late, in spite of awareness of the diagnosis. This is particularly more so for essential hypertension. Moreover, cultural factors, poverty and inaccessibility to healthcare facilities often contribute to this delay. This could also explain the over-representation of the older age group in the hypertensive patients in this study, who are more superstitious, poor and with low-income capacity and hence unable to seek health care, particularly timely. Furthermore, essential hypertension is a chronic disease, and most of the respondents diagnosed over 5–10 years ago are still on maintenance antihypertensive therapy.

On the other hand, the rising prevalence of hypertension with age could be a reflection of exposure to enduring stressors, poor dietary habit, lack of exercise and other culturally permissible hazardous lifestyle [36].

The most prevalent age of onset of hypertension was ages 40–49, with 169 respondents or 46.9%. This was in agreement with other studies, which had established that the illness is commonest after 40 years. It is interesting to note that the number of patients steadily increased with increasing age of onset of illness with a sharp decrease after the age of 50. Hypertension beginning after the age of 50 years is most likely to be secondary hypertension [23]. This result is therefore in consonant with the methodology adopted in this study, where all those with any other concurrent medical illnesses were excluded in other not to introduce bias. However, it was difficult for most of the respondents to know exactly the age of onset of disease since majority only became aware of the diagnosis during their first or routine hospital visits.

Females predominated in the study with 60.8%, and although essential hypertension is more common in males, females may have been over-represented in this study due to two reasons. First, African females tend to have lower blood pressure than males early in life with a reversal of the trend after the ages 45–50 years [35, 36]. This may be due to hormonal changes associated with the preparation for or actual menopause occurring in this age group, coupled with the increasing family and domestic (stressors) responsibilities shouldered by married females in this age group. Interestingly, in this study, there was high prevalence of the married females in both groups. Another probable reason for the predominance of females in this study is that females are more willing and likely to volunteer their symptoms easier than males and consequently tend to have better health-seeking behaviours.

The married group was over-represented in the study (71.4%). This preponderance might be due to low rates of divorce and separation, which may reflect a dominance of Christianity in the study environment. Furthermore, widows constituted a significant percentage (15%) among the hypertensives, next to the married group. Widowhood, no doubt, hurts and often results in severe emotional trauma, particularly when it is sudden and early in life. More than half of the subjects who were single (10.6%) were above the age of 30 years, many of whom were unemployed. In Africa, due to sociocultural values, a female not yet married at the age of 30 years and above calls for concern not only to her but also to her family members. Majority of the separated group were females. Although lower rates of psychiatric comorbidities were found among these categories, both separation and divorce are capable of impacting enormous psychological trauma in affected individuals.

Also from the study, it was found that more of each of the categories—married, separated and widowed—had more psychiatric comorbidity among patients with hypertension. A possible explanation could be that in hypertension, marital difficulties, separation and even widowhood may serve as baseline psychosocial factors that may act either singly or in synergy with the medical stressor (hypertension) to cause psychiatric comorbidity. The presence of these psychosocial stressors alone can equally predispose to hypertension. Thus, in hypertension, psychological stressors are both causal and effectual.

Most of the subjects in this study had attained various levels of formal education especially secondary and tertiary. Perhaps the influence of westernisation and urbanisation in Rivers State, Niger Delta and Nigeria might have played an important role. Furthermore, the cosmopolitan nature of Port Harcourt, domiciling majority of ethnic groups in Nigeria, with over 50% of Nigeria's oil and gas business, makes education a priority. A good number (39%) of the subjects with hypertension had tertiary education. The fact that they were educated may have increased their chances of employment and possibly ability to seek quality health care and timely, too. It is equally important to note that perhaps the older one becomes, and probably with more education, the more his or her socioeconomic and family responsibilities, with their accompanying stressors.

A number of studies have implicated environmental stressors as important aetiological factors in high blood pressure, particularly in already genetically predisposed individuals [82]. Occupational environments in Nigeria had remained stressful due to lack of job security and poor wages and remunerations, confronting countless demands from members of the family in a poverty-ravaged economy such as ours. This is supported by the fact that the percentage of females with tertiary education was significantly less compared to other educational levels. The incidence of psychiatric comorbidity was lowest among those with tertiary education. Hence, education tended to have some protective influence on the psyche of the study subjects. Expectedly, those with higher level of education were more likely to secure better employment, earn better income and have better access to quality health care. Thus, in this study, results showed that being employed correlated positively, while unemployment correlated negatively with occurrence of psychiatric comorbidity.

From the study, essential hypertension was associated more with low income. Stable income, no doubt, is an important stabilising factor for any chronic illness. In this study, income level negatively correlated with psychiatric comorbidity in hypertension. The higher the income level, the lower the prevalence of psychiatric illness in hypertension. Among the hypertensives, there was preponderance of older adults; however, as it has to do with income level, it appears to be a combined effect of both income and age in the study.

African extended family may also be contributory. Sharing the burden of disease by relatives in the African extended family system may be an advantage to the outcome of chronic illnesses like hypertension, as it tends to distribute responsibility from such patients to other family members. This was evident from this study where 85% of hypertensives live with their supportive family members. Adequate social support has been identified as a key factor in relieving or decreasing psychosocial burden associated with chronic medical conditions.

Expectedly, the longer the duration of these illnesses, the more likelihood of developing psychopathology. Interestingly, however, the reverse was observed in this study, as psychiatric comorbidity steadily decreased with increasing duration of illness. This might suggest that with the passage of time, one tended to absorb the initial shock of diagnosis and had adequately readjusted to the medical condition. Secondly, they might have stabilised on medications. The high rate of psychiatric illnesses among those in treatment between 1 and 5 years could probably reflect an over-representation of subjects in this category ab initio. Also, the effect of advancing age might have played a role as many would have died from complications of the illness. This was reflected in this study as subjects in the category of duration of treatment greater than 10 years were fewer. Mortality rates in this medical condition have remained high [93].

The reduced rate of psychiatric comorbidity among the category that has had treatment for 6 years and above could suggest that most of the medications being used in these clinics in the treatment of patients with essential hypertension even though they potentially may be associated with neuropsychiatric side effects [82] were cautiously used and properly monitored. This might have resulted into minimal rate of psychiatric side effects even with prolonged use.

From the results of this present study, the prevalence of psychiatric morbidity in the hypertensives was 64.4%. This was slightly higher than results from previous studies [62]. Ohene, in his study in Benin City, found a prevalence of 35% psychiatric morbidity among persons with essential hypertension [62]. Although these results seem to be far apart, the difference might reflect the increasing environmental stressors and economic hardship, increasing spate of insecurity in Nigeria and particularly in the Niger Delta, which has significantly worsened over the last 10 years.

Hypertension alone can present with psychiatric morbidity, and this may be aggravated by adverse environmental factors. Adverse environmental factors can in turn predispose to essential hypertension and mental illness. Indeed, this relationship describes a sustained vicious circle. Another possible reason for the observed difference was that in the study by Ohene [62], GHQ-30 was used which is a less-sensitive version when compared with GHQ-12 (used in this study). Thirdly, the sample size was smaller, i.e. 40 patients compared with 360 hypertensives used in this study. The higher the sample size, the higher the likelihood of diagnosis of psychiatric morbidity. Furthermore, several studies have suggested that hospital-based treatment of hypertensives tends to be associated with higher neuroticism and levels of psychiatric morbidity than their counterparts on community-based treatment. Another plausible reason could be the use of some antihypertensive particularly calcium channel blockers and α-methyldopa, implicated recently in psychiatry comorbidity among patients on treatment for hypertension.

Out of the total number with psychiatric illness, 232 (64.4%), depression was significantly the commonest with 29.4% as against 16% in Ohene's study [62]. Depression was mostly the mild and moderate types with few cases presenting with psychotic features which were mostly mood congruent. This might also be due to reasons earlier given for overall psychiatric disorders. Hypertension presents with very disabling symptoms, which could impair the functional capability of the sufferer. This, coupled with other adverse depressogenic environmental factors, might predispose the patient to depressive illness. There was significant predominance of females with depression. This finding, which is consistent with the gender distribution of depression, may equally reflect the willingness of the female gender to volunteer information on their health, hence, better health-seeking behaviour. Hypertensive disease, which carries the risk of both physical and emotional burden, is likely to affect the mood-regulating centre of the brain, i.e. the limbic system.

The prevalence of generalised anxiety disorder was 16.1% in this study. Previous study had found 12%. This could possibly be more frequent. The effect of propranolol and benzodiazepines (bromazepam and diazepam), which are commonly used medications in the General Outpatient Department, may have been responsible for the relatively low prevalence. Males were 48.2% and females 51.8%. Again, the observed gender bias is in line with existing literature. Earlier studies have suggested that hypertensives were more neurotic, more insecure, more conservative and more tense.

Hypertension and generalised anxiety disorder are somewhat similar illnesses, sharing common pathway—the sympathetic pathway. It is for this reason that medications like beta blockers such as propranolol and some benzodiazepine that act by dampening the activity of the sympathetic pathway have comparable usefulness in both disease conditions. Another reason to 'drive home' the relationship between hypertension and anxiety is that fundamental advances in the understanding of hypertension have coincided with the theories of anxiety states and affective disorders, suggesting catecholamines—particularly known here is noradrenaline [11].

This finds common ground in suggested mechanism for producing increased arterial pressure and neurotic states [11]. This is also consistent with the study by Kidson [94], who argued that higher neurotic scores of his hypertensive outpatients were due to a 'reactive state' occurring in them contrary to other study [113], which reported the absence of neuroticism among newly hypertensives and suggested that drug treatment could cause the observed neurosis. However, in this study, the inclusion criteria of 1 year duration of illness stand to disprove this, and it also appears that most of the hypertensives with diagnosis of anxiety were not due to their medication, and most were having one psychosocial stressor or the other that may either be responsible for or worsen the hypertension, anxiety or even both.

Panic disorder was diagnosed in 1.1% of hypertensive patients in this study. Many workers have consistently established that most of the major deleterious effects of high blood pressure are in the heart, blood vessels, kidneys and brain [11]. Therefore, with the strong connection between the heart and cardiovascular system, hypertension and the psyche, diagnosis of panic disorder in hypertensive subjects might not be a surprising finding. In fact, other names that have been given to anxiety neurosis (now obsolete) include cardiac neurosis, irritable heart syndrome, soldier's heart, nervous tachycardia, vasomotor neurosis, vasoregulatory asthenia and disordered action of heart, among others. Strikingly, these names mainly further imply the close and strong association between the heart or cardiovascular system and anxiety states.

Considering the fact that psychiatric morbidity was most prevalent in the unemployed, elementary and low-income workers, separated and divorced, all baseline psychosocial factors, capable of causing depressive illness, anxiety disorders and other mental illnesses, hypertension is commonly associated with stressful conditions. This is in line with findings from other studies which also showed that some common aetiological factors like stress-related situations, issues of job loss and unemployment, prolonged difficulties and people at war front were shown to have hypertension and anxiety [100]. It has been found that stress, which potentially causes anxiety, also increases the level of cortisol which in turn causes increased deposition of arteriosclerotic deposits in the intima of blood vessels [11]. These deposits gradually narrow the lumen of the vessels. This in turn increases arterial pressure resulting in hypertension [11].

Sexual dysfunction was diagnosed in 9.0% of hypertensive patients. Of this, 84% had male erectile dysfunction, while 16% who were all females had hyposexual dysfunction. Hyposexual desire disorder (HSDD) is sexual dysfunction with decreased libido, lack of sexual motivation and decreased sexual fantasies. Some studies have found associations between hypertension and erectile dysfunction in men, while others have implicated effects of some antihypertensive drugs like methyldopa and reserpine [50, 62], in addition to psychogenic impotence. However, in this study no patient was being treated with reserpine, and of the 27 males with erectile dysfunction, only negligible three subjects were on methyldopa.

Another diagnosis that was made among eight of the hypertensives was substance abuse. More than 80% of them had alcohol-related disorder with the male-to-female ratio of 7:1. Although the gender gap was wide, substance abuse generally is commoner among males than females. There is a bidirectional relationship between substance abuse and hypertension, i.e. substance abuse particularly alcohol can cause hypertension while hypertension, on the other hand, can precipitate substance abuse due to frustration [70, 71]. People with hypertension tend to abuse substance mainly to self-medicate their depression or to abate the many anxiety or anxiety-like symptoms that characterised hypertension, hence the use of propranolol and diazepam which have anxiolytic effects.

Personality disorder was seen in 5% of the hypertensive subjects. The concept of type A behaviour pattern (TABP), also referred to as type A personality, which appears fairly well established as a strong correlate of coronary heart disease (CHD), strongly supports a relationship between hypertension and personality disorder [93]. High blood pressure (HBP) is identified as major risk factor to CHD, which is reported to be on the increase in Nigeria. However, the present study found a low rate of personality disorder.

Hypertensive subjects with more than one psychiatric morbidity were seen in this study. Twelve percent had both GAD and sexual dysfunction, while 8% had both major depression and sexual dysfunction. This equally agrees with the multifactorial aetiological basis of essential hypertensive with environmental stressors playing as much significant role as genetic factors.

For quality of life among patients with hypertension, studies in western countries have shown inconsistent findings. There are no local studies to compare with the present study where both psychiatric comorbidity and QOL were studied together. However, a study that compared QOL of epileptics, schizophrenics and hypertensives found that the last fared poorly on all domains except on overall quality of life where they all faired equally. Some authors have opined that quality of life will be poor in the developing countries like Nigeria where factors of finances, social relationships, health and personal safety are considered to be poor. Hypertension in adults has a high impact on the economy and with consequent low quality of life of individuals. The results in this study are consistent with many studies elsewhere [27]. It also agrees with a population-based study, which found a lower health status in the hypertensives compared with individuals free from hypertension. This finding varied a little from previous studies where all domains of QOL except domain 4 (environment) and health satisfaction were affected by psychiatric comorbidity.

11. Conclusion/recommendations

The findings of this study support the impression that essential hypertension is a chronic debilitating illness, associated with psychiatric comorbidity. In both groups, being divorced was associated with lower QOL in some domains. The results support the call that the management of patients with hypertension should include attention to their mental health status and subjective quality of life in order to enhance the quality of care.

Author details

Aborlo Kennedy Nkporbu* and Princewill Chukwuemeka Stanley

*Address all correspondence to: nakpigi2008@yahoo.com

Department of Neuropsychiatry, University of Port Harcourt Teaching Hospital, Port Harcourt, Nigeria

References

[1] Oviasu VO. The pattern and prevalence of heart disease in Benin, Nigeria. Niger Med J. 1989;8:83–85.

[2] Wokoma FS, Alasia DD. Blood pressure pattern in Barako: a rural community in Rivers State, Nigeria. Niger J. 2011;11:813.

[3] Akpa MR, Alasia DD, Emmen-Chioma PC. An appraisal of hospital based blood pressure control in Port Harcourt, Nigeria. Niger Health J. 2008;8:27–30.

[4] UnachukwuCN, Agomoh DI, Alasia DD. Pattern of non-communicable diseases among medical admissions in Port Harcourt, Nig. Nig. J Clin Pract. 2008;11(1):14–17.

[5] Adefuye BO, Adefuye PO, Oladepo TO, Familoni OB, Olurunga TO. Prevalence of hypertension and other cardiovascular risk factors in an African Urban, sub-urban religious community. Niger Med Pract. 2009;55(1–2):4–8.

[6] Cooper R, Rotimi C, Ataman S, McGee D, Osotimehin B, Kadiri S, et al. The prevalence of hypertension in seven populations of west African origin. Am Public Health. 1997;87(2):160–168

[7] Kearney PM, Whelton M, Renoids K, Muntner, P Whenton KP. Global burden of hypertension: analysis of worldwide data. Lancet 2005;365:217–223

[8] Murray CJ, Lopez AD. Mortality by cause for eight regions of the world. Global burden of disease. Lancet, 1997;349:1269–1276.

[9] OgbagbonEK, Okesina AB, Biliaminu SA. Prevalence of hypertension and associated variables in paid workers in Ilorin, Nigeria. Niger J. Clin. Pract. 2008;11(4):342–346.

[10] Lawes CM, Vander Hoorn S, Law MR Eliot P, McMahon S, Rodgers A. Blood pressure and the global burden of disease 2000. Part II: estimate of attributable burden. J Hypertens. 2006;24:423–430.

[11] Cappuccio FP, Cook DG, Atkinson RW and Strazzullo P. Prevalence, detection, and management of cardiovascular risk factors in different ethnic groups in south London. Heart. 1997;78(6):555–563

[12] Cooper R, Rotimi C, Ataman S, McGee D, Osotimehin B, Kadiri S, et al. The prevalence of hypertension in seven populations of West African origin. Am Public Health. 1997;87(2):160–168

[13] Adedoyin RA, Mbada CE, Balogun MO, Martins T, Adabayo RA, Akintomide A. Prevalence and pattern of hypertension in a semi-urban community in Nigeria. Eur J Cardiovasc Prev Rehabil. 2008;15(6):683.687.

[14] Cappuccio FP, Micah FB, Emmeth L, Kerry SM. Prevalence, detection, management and control of hypertension in Ashanti, West Africa. Hypertens. 2004;43:10–17.

[15] Cappuccio FP, Cook DG, Atkinson RW, Stuzzullo P. Prevalence, detection, management of cardiovascular risk factors in different ethnic groups in South Africa. J Health, 1997;78:555–563

[16] Lawoyin TO, Azuzu MC, Kaufman J, Rotimi C, Oweaje E, Johnson L, Cooper R. Prevalence of cardiovascular risk factors in an African, urban inner city community. West Afr Med. 2002;21:208–211.

[17] Chamontin B, Poggi L, Lang T, Menard J, Chevalier H, Gallois H, Cremier O. Prevalence, treatment and control of hypertension in the French population: data from a survey on high blood pressure in general practice, 1994. Am J Hypertens. 1998;11:759–62.

[18] Wolf-Maier K, Cooper RS, Banegas JR, Giampaoli S, Hense HW, Joffres NM, Kastarinen M, Poulter N, Primatesta P, Rodriguez-Artalejo F, Steg-mayr B, Thamm M, Tuomilehto J, Vanuzzo D, Vescio F. Hypertension, prevalence and blood pressure levels in 6 European countries, Canada, and the United States. JAMA. 2003;89:2363–9.

[19] Hajjar I, Kotchen TA. Trends in prevalence, awareness, treatment, and control of hypertension in the United States, 1988–2000. JAMA. 2003; 290:199–206.

[20] Health Reform Foundation of Nigeria (HERFON) (2009, August) 'Impact challenges and long-term, implications of antiretroviral therapy programme in Nigeria'

[21] Nkporbu AK, Ugbomah L, Stanley PC. Pattern and prevalence of psychiatric consultations in other non-psychiatric facilities in the University of Port Harcourt Teaching Hospital: a 5-year review. Niger Health J. 2014;14;1, 13–20.

[22] Ogbagbon EK, Okesina AB, Biliaminu SA. Prevalence of hypertension and associated variables in paid workers in Ilorin, Nigeria. Niger J Clin Pract. 2008;11(4):342–346.

[23] Oviasu VO. High blood pressure: a silent mysterious killer, a primary preventive approach. Inaugural Lecture. Ambik Press, Benin City, 1988;89.

[24] Lown B, De Silva RA, Reich P, Murawsk BJ. Psychological factors in sudden cardiac death. Am J Psychiatry. 1980;137:1325–1335.

[25] Kearney PM, Whelton M, Renoids K, Muntner P, Whenton KP. Global burden of hypertension: analysis of worldwide data Lancet 2005;365:217–223

[26] Cotlington EM, Brook BM, House IS, Hawthorne VM. Psychosocial factors and blood pressure in the Michigan Statewide Blood Pressure Survey. Am J Epidemiol. 1985;121:515–529.

[27] Nyklicek I, Vingerhoets JJ, Van Heck GL. Hypertension and objective and self-reported stressor exposure: a review. J Psychosom Res. 1996;40:585–601.

[28] Carroll D, Phillips AC, Gale CR, Batty GD. Generalized anxiety and major depressive disorders, their comorbidity and hypertension in middle-aged men. Psychosom Med. 2010;72:16–19.

[29] Landsbergis PA, Sctnrmll FL, Warren K, Pickering IC, Schwartz 28.Association between ambulatory blood pressure and alternative formulations of job strain. Stand Work Environ Health. 1994;20:349–363.

[30] Roberts RE, Kaplan GA, Camacha TO. Psychological distress and mortality: evidence from the Alameda County Study. Soc Sci Med 1990; 31:527–530.

[31] Arodime EB,Ike SO,Nwokedinke SC.Case fatality among hypertensive-related admission in Enugu, Nigeria. Niger J Clin Pract, 2009:12(2):153–156.

[32] Goldney RD, Phillips PJ, Fisher LJ, Wilson DH. Diabetes, depression, and quality of life – a population study. Diabetes Care. 2004;27:1066–1070.

[33] Spiegel D, Giese-Davis J. Depression and cancer: mechanisms and disease progression. Biol Psychiatry. 2003;54:269–282.

[34] Chobanian AV, Bakris GL, Black HR, Cushman WC, Green LA, Izzo JL Jr, Jones DW, Materson BJ, Oparil S, Wright JT Jr, Roccella EJ. Seventhresport of the Joint National

committee on Prevention, Detection, Evaluation, and Treatment of High Blood Pressure. Hypertension. 2003;42:1206–1252.

[35] Norbert S, Wolfganf T, Johannrs K. Mental disorders and hypertension: factors associated with awareness and treatment of hypertension in the general population of Germany. Psychosom Med. 2006;68:246–252.

[36] Erhun WO, Olayiwola, G, Agbani EO, and Omotoso NS. Prevalence of hypertension in a University Community in South Western Nigeria. Afr J Biomed Res Ibadan Biomed Commun Group. 2005;8:15–19.

[37] Gwatkin D, Guillot M, Heuveline P. The burden of disease among the global poor. Lancet, 2000;354:586–589.

[38] Wenzel U, Roben T, Schwietzer G, Stahl RAK. The treatment of arterial hypertension: a questionnaire survey among doctors in general practice. Deut Med Wochenschr. 2001;126:1454–1459.

[39] Hartley RM, Velez R, Morris RW, Dsouza MF, Heller RF. Confirming the diagnosis of mild hypertension. BMJ 1983;286:287–289.

[40] Gupta K. Undertreatment of hypertension: a dozen reasons. Arch Intern Med 2002;162:2246–2247.

[41] Oliveria SA, Lapuerta P, McCarthy BD, L'Italien GJ, Berlowitz DR, Asch SM. Physician-related barriers to the effective management of uncontrolled hypertension. Arch Intern Med 2002;162:413–420.

[42] Hyman DJ, Pavlik VN. Poor hypertension control: let's stop blaming the patients. Cleve Clin J Med 2002:69(10):793–799.

[43] Ogunniyi O, Lane KA, BAiyewu O, Gao S, Gureje O, Unversagt FW, Murrell JR, Smith-Gamble V, Hall KS, Hendrie HC. Hypertension and incident dementia in community-dwelling elderly Yoruba Nigerians. Acta Neurol Scand. 2011.

[44] Hyman DJ, Pavlik VN. Characteristics of patients with uncontrolled hypertension in the United States. N Engl J Med. 2001;345:479–86.

[45] DiMatteo MR. Social support and patient adherence to medical treatment: a meta-analysis. Health Psychol. 2004;23:207–18.

[46] DiMatteo MR, Lepper HS, Croghan TW. Depression is a risk factor for noncompliance with medical treatment—meta-analysis of the effects of anxiety and depression on patient adherence. Arch Intern Med. 2000;160:2101–7.

[47] Schmitz N, Kruse J. The relationship between mental disorders and medical service utilization in a representative community sample. Soc Psychiatry Psychiatr Epidemiol. 2002;37:380–6.

[48] Anderson RB, Testa MA. Symptom distress checklists as a component of quality-of-life measurement comparing prompted reports by patient and physician with concurrent adverse event reports via the physician. Drug Inf. J. 1994;28:89–14.

[49] Testa MA, Simonson DC. Measuring quality of life in hypertensive patients with diabetes. Postgrad Med J. 1988;64:(Suppl 3):50–58.

[50] Testa MA, Hollenberg Anderson RA, Williams GH. Assessment of quality of life by patient and spouse during antihypertensive therapy with atenolol and nifedipine gastrointestinal therapeutic system. Am J Hypertens. 1991;4:363–373.

[51] Olusina AK, Ohaeri JU. Subjective quality of life of recently discharged Nigerian Psychiatric patients. Soc Psychiatry Epidemiol. 2003;38(12):707–704.

[52] Concepts of Health-Related Quality of Life. In: Patrick DL, Erickson P. Health Status and Health Policy: Quality of Life in Health Care Evaluation and Resource Allocation. New York: Oxford University Press, 1993;76–112.

[53] Wenzel U, Roben T, Schwietzer G, Stahl RAK. The treatment of arterial hypertension: a questionnaire survey among doctors in general practice. Deut Med Wochenschr. 2001;126:1454–1459.

[54] Croog SH, Levine S, Tests MA, et al. The effects of antihypertensive therapy on the quality of life. N Engl J Med. 1986;314:157–164.

[55] Testa MA. Interpreting quality-of-life clinical trial: data for use in the clinical practice of antihypertensive therapy. J Hypertens Suppl. 1987;5:S9-S13.

[56] Ii W, Liu L, Purnte JG, Li Y, Jiang X, Jin S, Ma. H, Kong L, Ma L, He X, Ma S, Chen C. Hypertension and health related quality of life: an epidemiological study in patients attending hospital clinic in China. J Hypertens. 2005;23(9):1667–1676.

[57] Rice D, Kelman S, Miller L. The economic burden of mental illness. Hosp Community Psychiatry. 1992;43:1227–1232.

[58] DuPont R, Rice D, Miller L, Shiraki S, Rowland C, Hanwood H. Economic costs of anxiety. J Anxiety. 1996;2:167–172.

[59] French M, Mauskopf J, League J, Roland E. Estimating the dollar value of health outcomes from drug abuse Interventions. Med Care. 1996;34:890–910.

[60] Briganti EM, Shaw JE, Chadban SJ, Zimmet PZ, Welborn TA, McNeil JJ, Atkins RC. Untreated hypertension among Australian adults: the 1999–2000 Australian Diabetes, Obesity and Lifestyle Study. Med J Aust. 2003;179:135–139.

[61] Testa MA, Anderson RB, Nackley JF, Hollenberg NK. Quality of life and antihypertensive therapy in men: a comparison of Captopril with Enalapril. N Engl J Med. 1993;328:907–913.

[62] Ohene S. Psychiatric Morbidity among Patients with Essential Hypertension Attending Out-Patient Clinics in University of Benin Teaching Hospital. Dissert. WACP, 2003.

[63] Somers VK, Anderson EA, Mark AL. "Sympathetic neural mechanisms in human hypertension". Curr Opin Nephrol Hypertens 1993;2(1):96–105.

[64] Takahashi H. "[Sympathetic hyperactivity in hypertension]" (in Japanese). Nippon Rinsho. 2008;66(8):1495–1502.

[65] Esler M. "The sympathetic system and hypertension". Am J Hypertens. 13(6 Pt 2):99S–105S.

[66] Mark AL. "The sympathetic nervous system in hypertension: a potential long-term regulator of arterial pressure". J Hypertens Suppl. 1996;14(5):S159–S165.

[67] Fauvel JP, Quelin P, Ducher M, Rakotomalala H, Laville M. Perceived job stress but not individual cardiovascular reactivity to stress is related to higher blood pressure at work. Hypertension. 2001;38(1):71–75.

[68] Gwatkin D, Guillot M, Heuveline P. The burden of disease among the global poor. Lancet, 2000;354:586–589.

[69] Rutledge T, Hogan BE. A quantitative review of prospective evidence linking psychological factors with hypertension development. Psychosom Med. 1999;64(5):758–766.

[70] Jee SH, He J, Whelton PK, et al. The effect of chronic coffee drinking on blood pressure: a meta-analysis of controlled clinical trials. Hypertension. 1999;33:647–652.

[71] Lane JD, Pieper CF, Phillips-Bute BG, Bryant JE, Kuhn CM. Caffeine affects cardiovascular and neuroendocrine activation at work and home. Psychosom Med. 2002;64(4): 595. 603.

[72] Mathews JD. Alcohol use, hypertension and coronary heart disease. Clin Sci Mol Med. 1976;3:66 IS663S.

[73] Mena-Martin FJ, Martin-Escudero JC, Simal-Blanco F, Carretero-Ares JL, Arzua-Mouronte D, Herreros-Fernandez V. Health-related quality of life of subjects with known and unknown hypertension: results from the population-based Hortega study. J Hypertens. 2003;21:1283–1289.

[74] Wittchen HU, Carter RM, Pfister H, Montgomery SA, Kessler RC. Disabilities and quality of life in pure and comorbid generalized anxiety disorder and major depression in a national survey. Int Clin Psychopharmacol 2000;15:319–328.

[75] Anderson RB, Testa MA. Symptom distress checklists as a component of quality-of-life measurement comparing prompted reports by patient and physician with concurrent adverse event reports via the physician. Drug Inf J. 1994;28:89–14.

[76] Testa MA, Simonson DC. Measuring quality of life in hypertensive patients with diabetes. Postgrad Med J. 1988;64:(Suppl 3):50–58.

[77] Lenderking WR, Gelber RD, Cotton DL, et al. Evaluation of the quality of life associated with Zidovudine treatment in asymptomatic human immunodeficiency virus Infection. N Engl J Med. 1994;330:738–743.

[78] Olusina AK, Ohaeri JU, Subjective quality of life of recently discharged Nigerian Psychiatric patients. Soc Psychiatry Epidemiol. 2003;38(12):707–704.

[79] Concepts of Health-Related Quality of Life. In: Patrick DL, Erickson P. Health Status and Health Policy: Quality of Life in Health Care Evaluation and Resource Allocation. New York: Oxford University Press, 1993;76–112.

[80] Testa MA, Lenderking WR. Interpreting pharmacoeconomic and quality-of –life clinical trial data for use in therapeutics. Pharmacoeonomics. 1992;2:107–117.

[81] Wells K, Golding J, Burman M. Psychiatric disorder in a sample of the general population with and without chronic medical conditions. Am J Psychiatry. 1988;145:976–981

[82] Evans D, Charney D. Mood disorders and medical illness a major public health problem. Blot Psychiatry. 2003;64:177–180.

[83] Guidelines Subcommittee. World Health Organization – International Society of Hypertension Guideline for the management of hypertension. J Hypertens. 1999;17:151–183.

[84] Davidson's principles and practice of internal medicine. Text book of Internal Medicine, 10th ed. Edinburgh, United Kingdom.

[85] Falase AO, Akinkugbe OO. A Compendium of Clinical Medicine. Spectrum Books Limited, Ibadan, 1999;2: 55–128.

[86] Millar-Craig MW, Bishop CN, Baftery EB. Circadian variation of blood pressure. Lancet 1978:795–797.

[87] Carretero OA, Opani S. Essential hypertension. Part I: 2000.

[88] Jee SH, He J, Whelton PK, et al. The effect of chronic coffee drinking on blood pressure: a meta-analysis of controlled clinical trials. Hypertension. 1999;33:647–652.

[89] Lane JD, Pieper CF, Phillips-Bute BG, Bryant JE, Kuhn CM. Caffeine affects cardiovascular and neuroendocrine activation at work and home. Psychosom Med. 2002;64(4): 595. 603.

[90] Mathews JD. Alcohol use, hypertension and coronary heart disease. Clin Sci Mol Med. 1976;3:66 IS663S.

[91] Cutler JA, Brittain E. Calcium and blood and pressure: an epidemiologic perspective. Am J Hypertens. 1990;3:137S 146S

[92] David M, Deyu P, Nilgoon K, Debesh D, Keith N. The relationship between body, weight and the prevalence of isolated systolic hypertension in older subjects. J Clin Hypertens. 2000;2(4):248–252.

[93] Cooper R, Rotimi C, Ataman S, McGee D, Osotimehin B, Kadiri S, et al. The prevalence of hypertension in seven populations of West African origin. Am Public Health. 1997;87(2):160–168

[94] Cappuccio FP, Micah FB, Emmeth L, Kerry SM. Prevalence, detection, management and control of hypertension in Ashanti, West Africa. Hypertens. 2004;43:10–17.

[95] Amoah AGB. Hypertension in Ghana: a cross-sectional community prevalence study in Greater Accra. Ethn Dis. 2003;13:310–315. Medline.

[96] Akinkugbe OO. The Nigerian hypertension programme. J Hum Hypertens. 1996;10:S43–S46.

[97] Oparil S, Zaman MA, Calhoun DA. "Pathogenesis of hypertension". Ann Intern Med. 2003;139(9):761–76.

[98] Corvol P, Persu A, Gimenez-Roqueplo AP, Jeunemaitre X. "Seven lessons from two candidate genes in human essential hypertension: angiotensinogen and epithelial sodium channel". Hypertension 1999;33(6):1324–1323.

[99] Feinleib M, Garrison RJ, Fabsi.tz R, et al. "The NHLBI twin study of cardiovascular disease risk factors: methodology and summary of results". Am J Epidemiol. 1977;106(4):284–285

[100] Biron P, Mongeau JG, Bertrand D. "Familial aggregation of blood pressure in 558 adopted children". Can Med Assoc J. 1976;115(8):773–774.

[101] Lifton RP, Gharavi AG, Geller DS. "Molecular mechanisms of human hypertension". 2001;104(4):545–556.

[102] Castelli WP. Epidemiology of coronary heart disease. The Framingham Study. Am J Med. 1984;76:4–12.

[103] Chhabra MK, Lal A, Sharma KK. Status of "lifestyle" modification in hypertension. J. Indian Med Assoc. 2001;99(9):504–508

[104] Gordon HW. Hypertensive vascular disease. Harrison's principles of internal medicine. McGraw-Hill companies, Inc. 2001;15;246:1414–1430.

[105] Robinson S, Young T, Roos 1. Estimating the burden of disease. Comparing administrative data and self-reports. Med Cure. l997;35(9):932–947.

[106] Erhun WO, Olayiwola G, Agbani EO, Omotoso NS. Prevalence of hypertension in a University Community in South Western Nigeria. Afr J Biomed Res Ibadan Biomed Commun Group. 2005;8:15–19.

[107] Susan L, Margot WS, George AK. Psychosocial predictors of hypertension in men and women.

[108] Hyman DJ, Pavlik VN. Poor hypertension control: let's stop blaming the patients. Cleve Clin J Med. 2002:69(10):793–799.

[109] Klang MJ, Wang NY, Meoni LA, Brancati FL, Cooper LA, Liang KY, Young JH, Ford DE. Coffee intake and risk of hypertension: the Jo1 Hopkins precursors study. Arch Intern Med. 2003;63(3):370–371.

[110] Oparinde DP,Opadijo OG, Akande AA, Ogunro PS, Akinwusi PO, Okesina AB, Oyelele AO. High risk coronary heart disease, lipid fractions and transferring saturation among hypertensive Nigerians. J Hypertens. 2005;5:211–213.

[111] Opadijo OG, Akande AA, Jimoh AK. Prevalence of coronary heart disease risk factors in Nigeria with systemic hypertension. J Hypertens. 2004;23:85–90.

[112] Ogbagbon EK, Okesina AB, Biliaminu SA. Prevalence of hypertension and associated variables in paid workers in Ilorin, Nigeria. Niger J Clin Pract 2008;11(4):342–346.

[113] Adedoyin RA, Mbada CE, Balogun MO, Martins T, Adabayo RA, Akintomide A. Prevalence and pattern of hypertension in a semi-urban community in Nigeria. Eur J Cardiovasco Prev Rehabil. 2008;15(6):683–687.

[114] Kadiri S, Walker O, Salako BL, Akinkugbe O. Blood pressure, hypertension and correlates in urbanized workers in Ibadan. Nigeria: a revisit J Hum Hypertens. 1999;13:23–27.

[115] WHO/ISH. World Health Organization (WHO)/international society of hypertension (ISH) statement on management of hypertension. J Hypertens. 2003;21:1983–1992.

[116] Mosterd A, O'Agostirro RB, Silbersfiatz H, et al. Trends in the prevalence of hypertension, antihypertensive therapy, and left ventricular hypertrophy from 1950 to 1989. Engl J Med. 1999;340;1221–1227.

[117] Burt VL, Whulton F, Itoccella EJ, et al. Prevalence of hypertension in the US adult population results from the Third National Health and Nutrition Examination Survey, 1988-1991. Hypertension. 1995;25:305–313.

[118] Kannel WB. Framingham study insights into hypertensive risk of cardiovascular disease. Hypertens Res. 1995;18:181–196.

[119] Kannel WB. Hypertension as a risk factor for cardiac events—epidemiologic results of longterm studies. J Cardiovasc Pharmacol. 1993;21:S27–S37.

[120] Melander O, Orho M, Fagerudd J, et al. "Mutations and variants of the epithelial sodium channel gene in Liddle's syndrome and primary hypertension". Hypertension. 1998;31(5):11, 18–24.

[121] Van de Sande MAB, Bailey R, Faal H, Banya WA, Dolin P, Nyan OA, Ceesay SM, Walraven GE, Johnson GJ, McAdam KP. Nationwide prevalence study of hypertension and related non-communicable diseases. Trop Med Int Health. 1997;2:1039–1048.CrossRefMedline.

[122] Aro S. Occupational stress, health-related behavior, and blood pressure: a 5-year follow-up. Prey Med. 1994;13:333–348.

[123] Rostrup M, Kjeldsen SE, EideIK. Awareness of hypertension increases blood pressure and sympathetic responses to cold pressor test. Am J Hypertens. 1990;3:912–917.

[124] Norbert S, Wolfganf T, Johannrs K. Mental disorders and hypertension: factors associated with awareness and treatment of hypertension in the general population of Germany. Psychosom Med. 2006; 68:246–252.

[125] Hall J, Guyton E, Arthur C. Textbook of Medical Physiology. St. Louis, MO: Elsevier Saunders. 2006; pp. 228. ISBN 0-7216-0240-1.

[126] Saddocks BI, Saddocks V. Comprehensive Textbook of Psychiatry, vol. 1. 2005: 426–448.

[127] Spiro A, Aldwiri CM, Ward KB, Mroczek DK. Personality and the incidence of hypertension among older men: longitudinal findings from the Normative Aging Study. Health Psychol. 1995;14:563–569.

[128] Jonas ES, Franks P, Ingram DO. Are symptoms of anxiety and depression risk factors for hypertension? Longitudinal evidence from the National Health and Nutrition Examination Survey I Epidemiologic Follow-up Study. Arch Fam Med. 1997;6:43–49.

[129] Markovitz JH, Matthews KA, Kannel WB, Cobb JL, O'Agostino RB. Psychological predictors of hypertension in the Framingham Study. JAMA. 1993;270:2439–2443.

[130] Aronne IJ, Segal KR. Weight gain in the treatment of mood disorders. J Clin Psychiatry. 2003;64:22–29(suppl).

[131] Spruill TM, Pickering TG, Schwartz JE, Mostofsky E, Ogedegbe G, Clemow L, Gerin W. The impact of perceived hypertension status on anxiety and the white coat effect. Ann Behav Med. 2007;34:1–9.

Section 2

Hypertension Highlights

Chapter 6

Ambient Particulate Matter Air Pollution Exposure and Hypertension

Wen-Wen Bao and Guang-Hui Dong

Additional information is available at the end of the chapter

http://dx.doi.org/10.5772/63923

Abstract

The relationship between exposure to ambient particulate matter (PM) and hypertension in humans is controversial. The aim of the present meta-analysis was to quantify the predictability of ambient PM on the risk of incident hypertension in humans. The selection criteria included the studies that could provide quantitative estimates of the change in hypertension prevalence linked with exposure to either indicator of PM. The health outcome of "hypertension" was defined as systolic blood pressure (SBP) of 140 mmHg and greater and/or diastolic blood pressure (DBP) of 90 mmHg or greater and/or taking antihypertensive drugs or diagnosis by a physician or self-reported hypertension. A total of 647 studies were initially identified through online database searches, and finally five studies met the inclusion criteria. The combined results of reported relative risk from the five included studies revealed that ambient PM was positively associated with hypertension (OR = 1.03; 95% CI: 0.99–1.06), but this was not statistically significant. When stratified by the PM size, the results showed that the odds ratio for hypertension increased by 1.03 (95% CI: 0.93–1.14) per 10 μg/m^3 increase in $PM_{2.5}$, 1.04 (95% CI: 0.98–1.10) in PM_{10}, and 0.99 (95% CI: 0.92–1.07) in $PM_{2.5-10}$. In conclusion, to get more information about the associations between PM and hypertension, many studies need to be undertaken further to clarify these relationships.

Keywords: ambient particulate matter, hypertension, $PM_{2.5}$, PM_{10}, human

1. Introduction

Hypertension is the major risk factor for cardiovascular disease and other vascular diseases [1, 2] and renal disease [3, 4]. It has been considered as the most important cause of disability, and high blood pressure (BP; SBP > 110–115 mmHg) increased from the fourth-ranked risk factor for burden of disease in 1990 to the leading risk factor in 2010 [5]. Previous studies have concluded that high BP and hypertension are associated with genetic factor, diet and lifestyle [6], and environmental factors which include ambient air pollution as a potential risk factor as well [7].

Ambient air pollution is a complex mixture containing particulate matter (PM). In academia, PM can be divided into four fractions on the basis of aerodynamic diameter of PM, including thoracic particles (<10μm, PM_{10}), coarse particles (2.5–10μm, $PM_{2.5-10}$), fine particles (<2.5μm, $PM_{2.5}$), and ultrafine particles (<0.1μm) [8]. There are mounting evidences, especially relating PM_{10} and $PM_{2.5}$, which suggest that those kinds of particles of different aerodynamic diameter have been linked with elevated BP [9–11]. And several studies have reported ambient PM and risk of hypertension [12–19], but until now, there are no comprehensive evidences about outdoor PM exposure and risk of hypertension.

The aim of this study was to provide synthesized evidence of the hypertension risk associated with exposure to PM in ambient air, specifically $PM_{2.5}$ and PM_{10} and DPM, through conducted meta-analysis.

2. Methods

2.1. Literature search

We developed search terms to identify associated papers by using the medical headings (MeSH) in PubMed. Meanwhile, studies were also identified through Web of Science (WOS) and Scopus using relevant search terms, which include terms related to the exposure (air pollution, PM, inhalable particle, fine particle, $PM_{2.5}$, PM_{10}) and the outcome (hypertension/high BP). The reference lists of the papers were searched for possible relevant articles. We conducted literature search at PubMed, Web of Science (WOS), and Scopus on 6 November 2015, 1 January 2016, and 11 January 2016, respectively. The limitation of language is English. Through this process, a total of 662 potentially relevant papers were searched.

2.2. Study selection

Studies were included in the current meta-analysis to know if they provided quantitative estimates of residential exposure to $PM_{2.5}$ and/or PM_{10} and other PM. Further, studies were required to provide quantitative estimates of the change in hypertension prevalence linked with exposure to either indicator of PM; this could be reported as the change in risk per microgram per cubic meter or per quantile of exposure. Studies that reported results for the association of hypertension with other air pollutants or exposure to traffic but did not provide quantitative estimates for PM were not included in the meta-analysis. The health outcome of "Hypertension" was defined as systolic blood pressure (SBP) of 140 mmHg and greater and/or diastolic blood pressure (DBP) of 90 mmHg or greater and/or taking anti-hypertensive drugs or diagnosis by a physician or self-reported hypertension.

http://dx.doi.org/10.5772/63923

Though multiple publications included overlapping study populations, we included the publication that considered the largest number of cases and/or that evaluated results based on the longest follow-up. In addition, we did not place any restrictions based on whether or not a study adjusted for specific confounders. All risk estimates were abstracted by one of the authors and double checked for accuracy by a second author.

2.3. Data synthesis and analysis

All study estimates were converted to represent the change in hypertension risk per 10 μg/m^3 unit increase in exposure to $PM_{2.5}$, PM_{10}, or other PM. If we could not reliably convert the values in a particular study to the aforementioned units, we contacted the authors of the original study for further information. If information necessary to convert estimates could not be obtained, the study was excluded from consideration.

Estimates from the studies were combined using a random-effects model, which allowed between-study heterogeneity to contribute to the variance [20]. I^2 values are reported, representing the estimated percent of the total variance that is explained by between-study heterogeneity [21]. We also conducted chi-square tests of homogeneity to compare meta-estimates divided into subgroups by pollutants ($PM_{2.5}$, $PM_{2.5\text{–}10}$, PM_{10}, DPM). Finally, forest and funnel plots were created to provide a visual summary of the distribution of study-specific effect estimates. Instead of statistical tests of funnel plot asymmetry, we conducted trim and fill analyses. All analyses were conducted using STATA (v12.1; StataCorp, College Station, TX, USA). Noted $P < 0.05$ (two-tailed) was considered statistically significant except for the heterogeneity test, for which $P < 0.10$ (one-tailed) was used.

3. Results

3.1. Literature search and study characteristics

The detailed steps of our literature search are shown in **Figure 1**. A total of 647 citations were screened during the primary search. According to the title and abstract of every citation and included and excluded criteria, we identified 11 papers. After a detailed evaluation, two papers [18, 22] were excluded due to lack of data and two papers [17, 23] were excluded since the target population of the two studies comprises black women in the USA. Finally, the remaining five studies [12, 13, 15, 16, 19] published between 2009 and 2015 were included in the present meta-analysis. Of these, five cross-sectional studies were included. Two studies were conducted in the USA [15, 19], two in China [13, 16], and one in Germany [12].

3.2. Combined estimates of ambient particulate matter and the risk of hypertension

The effect estimates of individual studies and the combined effect estimates for hypertensive associated with PM, including $PM_{2.5}$, $PM_{2.5\text{–}10}$, PM_{10} and DPM, are presented in **Figure 2**. Hypertension among study population was not statistically significantly associated with a 10 μg/m^3 increment in PM (OR = 1.03; 95% CI: 0.99–1.06).

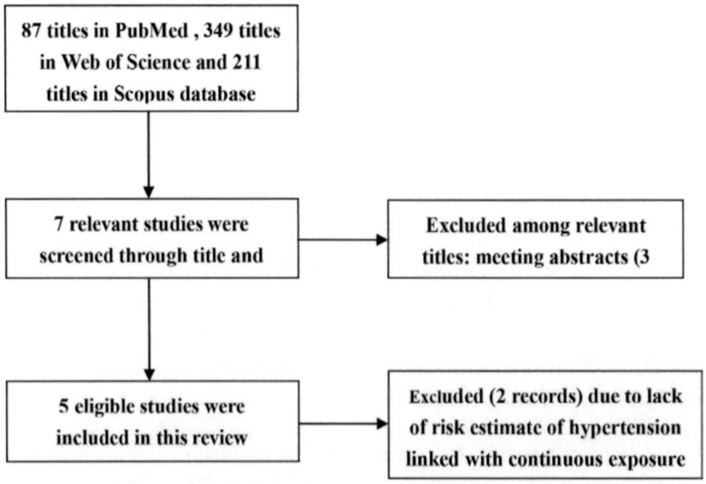

Figure 1. Flow diagram of screened, included and excluded publications.

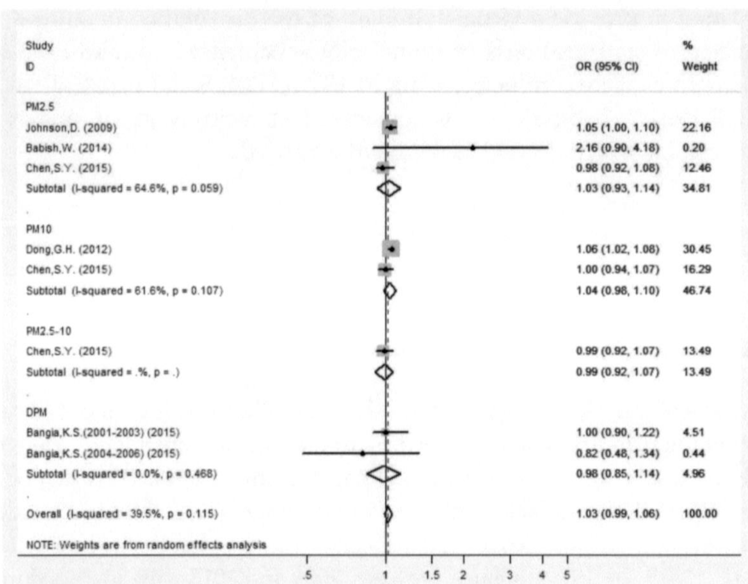

Figure 2. Estimates of hypertension risk associated with a 10 μg/m³ change in exposure to PM overall and by pollutant, including $PM_{2.5}$, $PM_{2.5–10}$, PM_{10}, DPM.

3.3. Subgroup analyses and publication bias

The results of our subgroup analyses showed that our pooled OR for the prevalence was 1.03 (95% CI, 0.93–1.14) with I^2 of 64.6% in $PM_{2.5}$ and 1.04 (95% CI, 0.98–1.10) with I^2 of 61.6% heterogeneity in PM_{10} and 0.98 (95% CI, 0.85–1.14) with no heterogeneity.

Funnel plots for each pollutant exhibited a notable asymmetry, reflecting no publication bias from vision (**Figure 3**). Introducing "trim and fill method", the results suggested no existed publication bias exist. For all exposures, the *P* values of Egger tests were statistically non-significant ($P = 0.496$). To sum up, the possibility of publication bias is small.

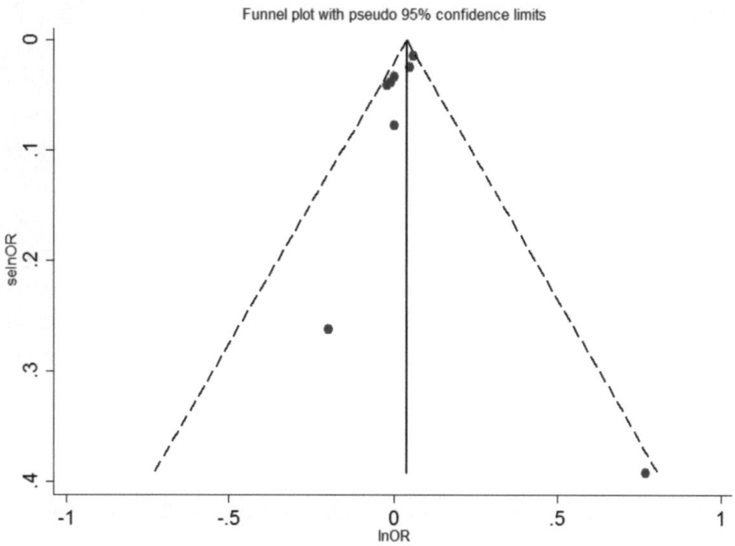

Figure 3. Funnel plot with pseudo 95% confidence limits.

4. Discussion

To our knowledge, this is the first systematic review and meta-analysis to pooled estimates linked with ambient PM and hypertension among general population. We selected and reviewed five large population-based cross-sectional studies, including a total of >200,000 general population. The pooled estimator of our meta-analysis showed that ambient PM was marginally associated, but not statistically significant, with hypertension among general population.

There are an increasing number of studies which have reported the association between PM and BP. Some studies showed that BP increased with short-term exposure to $PM_{2.5}$ of 10 μg/m³ [SBP 0.81 (95% CI: 0.19, 1.43) mmHg and DBP 0.63 (95% CI: 0.17, 1.10) mmHg] [24] and for each 10 μg/m³ increase of PM_{10}, pulse pressure and SBP increased by 0.583 (95% CI: 0.296–0.870) mmHg and 0.490 (95% CI: 0.056–0.925) mmHg, respectively in Geneva, and 0.183 (95% CI: 0.017–0.348) mmHg and 0.036 (95% CI: 0.042–0.561) mmHg, respectively in Lausanne [25]. Meanwhile, several studies also assessed the association between long-term exposure to particulate air pollution and BP. Fuks et al. reported that an interquartile increase in $PM_{2.5}$ (2.4 μg/m³) was associated with an estimated increase in mean SBP and DBP of 1.4 (95% CI: 0.5–

2.3) mmHg and 0.9 (95% CI: 0.4, 1.4) mmHg, respectively [18]. Also, Dong et al. found that the estimated increases in mean SBP and DBP were 0.87 (95% CI: 0.48–1.27) mmHg and 0.32 (95% CI: 0.08–0.56) mmHg per 19 μg/m^3 interquartile increase in PM_{10}, respectively [13].

Till now, only three epidemiology studies [14, 17, 26] have explored the effect of air pollution on the incidence of hypertension, and the results have been varied. A cohort study of 35,303 non-hypertensive adults from Ontario, Canada, with follow-up from 1996 to 2005, reported that the adjusted hazard ratio of incident (IRR) hypertension was 1.13 (95% CI: 1.05–1.22) for incident hypertension among individuals who were exposed to per 10 μg/m^3 increase of $PM_{2.5}$ [14]. Coogan et al. reported that in a cohort of black women living in Los Angeles, with exposure to $PM_{2.5}$ and nitrogen oxides, over follow-up from 1995 to 2005, the incidence rate ratio (IRR) for hypertension for a 10 μg/m^3 increase in $PM_{2.5}$ was 1.48 (95% CI: 0.95–2.31), and the IRR for the interquartile range (12.4 parts per billion) of nitrogen oxides was 1.14 (95% CI: 1.03–1.25) [17]. The third cohort of 33,275 participants was enrolled in this population-based cohort study. The IRR of self-reported incident hypertension among individuals who were exposed to nitrogen oxides (NOx) in the 95th quantile (>26.6 parts per billion), contrasted with those in the 5th quantile (<16.1 parts per billion), is 1.06 (95% CI: 0.92–1.23) after a mean follow-up of 5.3 years [26].

The strength of this study is mainly related to the large number of residents. In addition, none of the previous meta-analyses focused on investigating the relationship between ambient PM and hypertension. Compared with the cohort study of Canada [14], the existing problem of this meta-analysis is the study design. The evidence strength of the cohort study is higher than the cross-sectional study. Because of this, we need think about seriously the combined effects of this meta-analysis. And researchers should pay more attention to PM and hypertension.

4.1. Biological mechanisms associated with PM and hypertension

A potential mechanism relating exposure to $PM_{2.5}$ to hypertension may be its indirect effects mediated through systemic proinflammatory and oxidative responses, which may lead to increased sympathetic tone and potentially cause arterial remodeling. Oxidative stress may also increase the circulation of activated immune cells and inflammatory cytokines, which may subsequently induce endothelial dysfunction, leading to an imbalance in vascular homeostatic responses. If this happens repeatedly, it could result in an increased total peripheral resistance and a fixation of elevated BP [18]. Other mechanisms by which $PM_{2.5}$ may elevate BP include autonomic nervous system imbalance and direct vasoconstriction [17, 27]. Finally, PM exposure can reduce daytime sodium excretion and blunt the normal nocturnal reduction in BP. Over time, impaired renal handling of excess sodium may be partly responsible for elevated BP [27].

5. Limitations

There are some limitations of this meta-analysis which should be noted. First, only five screened papers were selected in this study due to the low number of studies associated with

http://dx.doi.org/10.5772/63923

ambient PM and hypertension among general population till now. And these five studies examined the relationship between PM and hypertension among general population using cross-sectional epidemiological study design, which precludes a causal interpretation of the complex relationship between outdoor PM and hypertension. Second, the exposure assessment of ambient PM is not consistent, so the risk of misclassification of different-level concentration might be amplified. Third, the degree of control for potential confounders is different. Covariates in common are included for all studies, including gender, age, body mass index, education, smoking status in most, but not all studies. And some reports indicated that diabetes mellitus and COPD (chronic obstructive pulmonary disease) are often associated with increased risk for hypertension [28, 29], but no studies had information on COPD and diabetes mellitus. Finally, not only do ambient PM concentrations and toxicity of major components vary largely over space [30] but also possibly other parameter such as season may be a potential confounder because seasonal variation in air pollution is well known [31].

6. Conclusion

The present meta-analysis of cross-sectional studies suggests that ambient PM may not contribute to the prevalence of hypertension from statistical perspective, but the evidence for a relationship between ambient particulate matter exposure and hypertension is still inconclusive because of limitations in study populations, study design, exposure characterization, and adjustment for important confounders and need researchers to pay more attention to PM and hypertension.

Author details

Wen-Wen Bao and Guang-Hui Dong*

*Address all correspondence to: donggh5@mail.sysu.edu.cn; donggh512@hotmail.com

Guangzhou Key Laboratory of Environmental Pollution and Health Risk Assessment, Department of Preventive Medicine, School of Public Health, Sun Yat-sen University, Yuexiu District, Guangzhou, PR China

References

[1] Poulter, N.R., D. Prabhakaran, and M. Caulfield, *Hypertension.* Lancet, 2015. 386(9995): pp. 801–12.

[2] Wong, N.D., et al., *Global cardiovascular risk associated with hypertension and extent of treatment and control according to risk group.* Am J Hypertens, 2012. 25(5): pp. 561–7.

[3] Klag, M.J., et al., *Blood pressure and end-stage renal disease in men.* N Engl J Med, 1996. 334(1): pp. 13–8.

[4] Hsu, C.Y., et al., *Elevated blood pressure and risk of end-stage renal disease in subjects without baseline kidney disease.* Arch Intern Med, 2005. 165(8): pp. 923–8.

[5] Lim, S.S., et al., *A comparative risk assessment of burden of disease and injury attributable to 67 risk factors and risk factor clusters in 21 regions, 1990–2010: A systematic analysis for the Global Burden of Disease Study 2010.* Lancet, 2012. 380(9859): pp. 2224–2260.

[6] Rahimi, K., C.A. Emdin, and S. MacMahon, *The epidemiology of blood pressure and its worldwide management*. Circ Res, 2015. 116(6): pp. 925–36.

[7] Hansson, G.K., *Inflammation, atherosclerosis, and coronary artery disease.* N Engl J Med, 2005. 352(16): pp. 1685–95.

[8] Brook, R.D., *Why physicians who treat hypertension should know more about air pollution.* J Clin Hypertens (Greenwich), 2007. 9(8): pp. 629–35.

[9] Hicken, M.T., et al., *Fine particulate matter air pollution and blood pressure: the modifying role of psychosocial stress.* Environ Res, 2014. 133: pp. 195–203.

[10] Brook, R.D., et al., *Hemodynamic, autonomic, and vascular effects of exposure to coarse particulate matter air pollution from a rural location.* Environ Health Perspect, 2014. 122(6): pp. 624–30.

[11] Bellavia, A., et al., *DNA hypomethylation, ambient particulate matter, and increased blood pressure: findings from controlled human exposure experiments.* J Am Heart Assoc, 2013. 2(3): p. e000212.

[12] Babisch, W., et al., *Associations between Traffic Noise, Particulate Air Pollution, Hypertension, and Isolated Systolic Hypertension in Adults: The KORA Study.* Environ Health Perspect, 2014. 122(5): pp. 492–8.

[13] Dong, G.H., et al., *Association between long-term air pollution and increased blood pressure and hypertension in China.* Hypertension, 2013. 61(3): pp. 578–84.

[14] Chen, H., et al., *Spatial association between ambient fine particulate matter and incident hypertension.* Circulation, 2014. 129(5): pp. 562–9.

[15] Johnson, D. and J.D. Parker, *Air pollution exposure and self-reported cardiovascular disease.* Environ Res, 2009. 109(5): p. 582–9.

[16] Chen, S.Y., et al., *Associations between long-term air pollutant exposures and blood pressure in elderly residents of Taipei city: A cross-sectional study.* Environ Health Perspect, 2015. 123(8): p. 779–784.

[17] Coogan, P.F., et al., *Air pollution and incidence of hypertension and diabetes mellitus in black women living in Los Angeles.* Circulation, 2012. 125(6): p. 767–72.

[18] Fuks, K., et al., *Long-term urban particulate air pollution, traffic noise, and arterial blood pressure.* Environ Health Perspect, 2011. 119(12): pp. 1706–11.

[19] Bangia, K.S., et al., *A cross-sectional analysis of polycyclic aromatic hydrocarbons and diesel particulate matter exposures and hypertension among individuals of Mexican origin.* Environ Health, 2015. 14:51.

[20] DerSimonian, R. and N. Laird, *Meta-analysis in clinical trials.* Control Clin Trials, 1986. 7(3): pp. 177–88.

[21] Higgins, J.P., et al., *Measuring inconsistency in meta-analyses.* Br Med J, 2003. 327(7414): pp. 557–60.

[22] Orru, H., et al., *Chronic traffic-induced PM exposure and self-reported respiratory and cardiovascular health in the RHINE Tartu Cohort.* Int J Environ Res Public Health, 2009. 6(11): pp. 2740–51.

[23] Basile, J.N. and M.J. Bloch, *Exposure to air pollution increases the incidence of hypertension and diabetes in black women living in Los Angeles.* J Clin Hypertens, 2012. 14(11): pp. 819–20.

[24] Chang, L.T., et al., *Short-term exposure to noise, fine particulate matter and nitrogen oxides on ambulatory blood pressure: A repeated-measure study.* Environmental Research, 2015. 140: pp. 634–40.

[25] Tsai, D.H., et al., *Short-term effects of particulate matters on pulse pressure in two general population studies.* J Hypertens, 2015. 33(6): pp. 1144–52.

[26] Sorensen, M., et al., *Long-term exposure to traffic-related air pollution associated with blood pressure and self-reported hypertension in a Danish Cohort.* Environ Health Perspect, 2012. 120(3): pp. 418–24.

[27] Tsai, D.H., et al., *Short-term increase in particulate matter blunts nocturnal blood pressure dipping and daytime urinary sodium excretion.* Hypertension, 2012. 60(4): pp. 1061–9.

[28] Mannino, D.M., et al., *Prevalence and outcomes of diabetes, hypertension and cardiovascular disease in COPD.* Eur Respir J, 2008. 32(4): pp. 962–9.

[29] Stone, I.S., N.C. Barnes, and S.E. Petersen, *Chronic obstructive pulmonary disease: a modifiable risk factor for cardiovascular disease?* Heart, 2012. 98(14): pp. 1055–62.

[30] Lelieveld, J., et al., *The contribution of outdoor air pollution sources to premature mortality on a global scale.* Nature, 2015. 525(7569): pp. 367–71.

[31] Liang, C.S., et al., *Review on recent progress in observations, source identifications and countermeasures of PM2.5.* Environ Int, 2016. 86: pp. 150–70.

Chapter 7

ACE I/D (Rs1799752), MTHFR C677T (Rs1801133), and CCR5 D32 (Rs333) Genes and their Association with Hypertension and Diabetic Nephropathy in Urban Areas of Costa Rica, Nicaragua, and Mexico

Lizbeth Salazar-Sanchez,
Juan Jose Madrigal-Sanchez,
Pedro Gonzalez-Martinez, Edel Paredes,
Ligia Vera-Gamboa, Norma Pavia Ruz and
Nina Valadez-Gonzalez

Additional information is available at the end of the chapter

http://dx.doi.org/10.5772/64548

Abstract

Aim: Type 2 diabetes mellitus (T2DM) is a procoagulant state because it is associated with increased risk of atherosclerosis. The purpose of this study was to investigate the prevalence in thrombotic markers that lead to hypercoagulability and its association with hypertension and diabetic nephropathy (DN).

Objective: To determine the association of molecular markers: (insertion/deletion) of the ACE gene Rs1799752, CCR5 D32 Rs333, and MTHFR C677T Rs1801133 with hypertension and DN in T2DM patients of urban areas in Costa Rica, Nicaragua, and Mexico.

Materials and methods: A total of 521 samples of diabetic patients were collected: 132 from Costa Rica, 192 from Nicaragua, and 197 from Mexico.

Results: A high prevalence of ACE genotype D/D ($p < 0.001$) and CCR5 ($p < 0.001$) in T2DM patients from the three different countries was found. The CCR5 D32/D32 genotype was seen in the population of Costa Rica. The prevalence of hypertension was 57.7% and nephropathy was 34% in overall T2DM patients. A statistical association was found; ACE polymorphism has significance with cardiovascular disease (CVD) $p = 0.02$, CCR5 D32 with dyslipidemia ($p = 0.008$), and hypertension ($p = 0.022$).

Conclusion: It is important to know the role of ACE and CCR5 molecular markers and their possible association with the development of microvascular complications in our populations.

Keywords: diabetes mellitus, diabetic nephropathy, urban areas, I/D ACE, C677TMTHFR, CCR5 D32, hypertension

1. Introduction

Diabetes is a disease of high human, economic, and social cost whose incidence has increased considerably. An estimation of seven million people develop the disease each year, which is equivalent to a person acquiring the disease every 5 s worldwide [1]. Clearly, diabetes is a disease in remarkable growth and is expected that by 2025 about 350 million people will have the disease, equivalent to 7.1% of the world population [2, 3]. The United Nations General Assembly adopted a resolution which recognizes diabetes as a threat and global epidemic due to its a chronic, debilitating, and costly nature associated with severe complications, which poses severe risks for families, member states, and the world [4].

Diabetes mellitus (DM) is one of the most common causes of morbidity and medical consultation in Mexico, Costa Rica, and Nicaragua [5]. DM patients, in Costa Rica, consume an enormous amount of medical resources, and their cost occupies the first place in all public hospitals and clinics [5, 6] due to its chronic complications such as lower extremity amputations, blindness, nephropathy, and heart disease, which in turn have devastating and irreversible effects on the health of people. All this has a major economic impact on people and the Health Social Security System [6, 7]. Therefore, with increasing number of diabetic patients, there is an increased demand for services and medical costs.

The DM prevalence reported in Nicaragua and Costa Rica is 11.5% [6, 8]. However, there are still many gaps in knowledge regarding risk factors and epidemiology of DM and the effectiveness of prevention guides which would allow to control this health problem and its complications in both countries.

In a multiregional study of adult populations in urban areas, there was evidence of high DM prevalence in Guatemala (8%) and Nicaragua (9%) [8]. In 2002, DM accounted for 24% (4273) of all hospital charges for chronic diseases (CDs) in Nicaragua. During the period between 1993 and 2002, mortality from diabetes increased rapidly, especially, in people aged above 50 years. The described Nicaraguan trend for DM is that the disease is affecting younger ages (15–34 years) and productive ages (35–49 years), which will result in lost life-years, as well as business days. The lack of optimal diabetes care favors the development of complications.

The estimated prevalence of DM in 1998 in Costa Rica was 4.8% in those aged 20 years and above. In 2006, the percentage of diabetic patients raised to 5.3% in the same age range population [6]. If the population is divided by age groups, the prevalence for people above 40 years is 9.4% and for older adults is 23.4% [6]. In Mexico, chronic disease (CDs) is a public health problem, as well as in other Latin American countries, which is the result of change in the epidemiological behavior and cardiovascular diseases (CVDs). They are conditions that prevail among adults and constitute the main causes of overall mortality [9, 10]. Heart disease, diabetes, dyslipidemia, and hypertension stand among these conditions because of their high prevalence and serious complications, such as neoplasms, cerebrovascular disease, and renal disease. DM, as part of cardiovascular risk factors, is one of the most important points of the health agenda of Mexico, because of the increased prevalence and complications in addition to high costs (direct and indirect) for Mexican society. The prevalence of DM in Mexico, according to ENSANUT 2012, is 9.2% in individuals aged 20 years or more [11]. This prevalence varied with the age of the individuals. The highest prevalence is found in subjects between 60 and 69 years (25.3%). DM prevalence in Yucatan reported in ENSANUT 2012 is 9.2%, ranking eighth nationally [11].

The ADVANCE study showed that in people with DM after eight years of evolution, when hemoglobin A1c (HbA1c) level was reduced from 7.3 to 6.5, it decreased the development of nephropathy in 20–30% of microvascular complications [12]. However, even with metabolic control, there are still environmental factors that enhance the progression of organ damage; in many cases, renal deterioration is inevitable, demonstrating the involvement of genetic factors. Participation of these factors is evident in the results of family studies, linkage, and association with genetic variants in populations unrelated, conducted in different regions of the world [13]. The genesis and progression of early stages of the latest clinical stages of nephropathy are influenced by own genetic variation, age, sex, metabolic factors, such as hyperglycemia, elevated levels of triglycerides and cholesterol, high body mass index, high blood pressure (HBP), and metabolic control [10, 14].

1.1. Diabetic nephropathy and genetic susceptibility

Diabetic nephropathy (DN) is a complex multifactorial disease; the development of this complication depends on the additive effect of the variation in the genes and the interaction with environmental factors, such that it may have mutations or genetic variants that predispose to the progression to the disease.

Genetic susceptibility plays an important role in the pathogenesis of DN, and several genetic approaches, including association studies of candidate genes and genomics, have identified susceptibility genes for DN [15]. In addition, it has been reported that the inflammatory mechanisms contribute to the development and progression of DN. However, these mechanisms underlying the regulation of cytokines in the kidneys of patients with DM remain unclear. Genetic variations in genes encoding inflammatory cytokines can confer susceptibility to DN by altering functions or expressions [16]. Polymorphisms in the CCR5 receptor and MMP9 have also been associated with increased risk of nephropathy following these mechanisms [15, 17]. Another gene associated with risk of DN is the angiotensin-converting enzyme gene (ACE). This gene modulates the generation of angiotensin II, which increases intraglomerular pressure, leading to glomerulopathy. The course of DN can be considerably improved by treatment with ACE inhibitors, in patients with type 1 diabetes [18].

The DN is considered a complex polygenic disorder in some studies, in which the association of polymorphisms in individual genes can be small and sometimes not informative, while specific combinations of specific genotypes may generate significant changes [15, 19, 20].

Polymorphism /SNP	Mutation	Chromosome	Genotype	Symbol	Phenotype Effect	Pathologic Association	References
MTHFR Gene MTHFR 677C>T ***Rs 1801133***	Ala >Val 677C>T	Chromosome 1 (1p36.3)	CC (wild type) CT (heterozygous) TT (homozygous)	CC CT TT	**Homocysteine level** normal normal mild increased	**Associated with** hyperhomocisteinemia.	**19 ; 37; 41**
ACE Gene I/D ACE ***Rs1799752***	alu repeat insertion	Chromosome 17 (17q23) Intron 16	II (insertion) ID (insertion/deletion) DD (deletion)	II ID DD	ACE enzyme normal mild increased increased	**Associated with** DN in three different european population*	**21; 39**
CCR5 *delta*32 *Rs333*	chemokine (C-C motif) receptor 5	Chromosome 3 (3p21:31)	II (insertion) ID (insertion/deletion) DD (deletion)	wt/wt wt/ D32 D32/D32	Normal level of CRP Low levels of CRP,	The chemokine receptor gene CCR5 plays an important role in many immune-related processes. D32 **rs333**, designating the CCR5-D32deletion of 32 nucleotides from within the gene, is perhaps the most famous allele of CCR5	**19;25**

* Unknown effect.

Table 1. Characteristics of the different polymorphisms analyzed associated with diabetic nephropathy.

This chapter presented the results about the prevalence of known risk factors and some genetic variants, such as ACE I/D (Rs1799752), MTHFRC677T (Rs1801133) and CCR5 D32 (Rs333), see **Table 1**, associated with DN in DM patients belonging to urban areas of Costa Rica, Nicaragua, and Mexico.

1.2. Genetic mutations associated with DN

1.2.1. ACE gene (Rs1799752)

ACE gene is located on chromosome 17q23.3, and one molecular variant contains an insert (I) or a deletion (D) of 287 bp in intron 16 [21]. The DD genotype has been associated with higher levels of ACE and an activity four times higher than the II genotype, in addition to higher levels of blood pressure, obesity, and increased cardiovascular risk [21, 22]. Other studies suggest that polymorphism ID is an aggressive factor for developing kidney damage in type 1 diabetes [22, 23].

The renin-angiotensin-aldosterone system (RAAS) is a cascade of interactions culminating in the production of angiotensin II (Ang II), which is the peptide responsible for the effects of this physiological axis. ACE is a protein that may have pleiotropic effects and play a role in various diseases and not just in hypertension [24]. ACE is a regulatory enzyme in RAAS. Due to the activation of ACE, conversion of angiotensin I to angiotensin II is given, which is a vasoconstrictor. ACE is also known to inactivate bradykinin, and kallikrein, vasodilator molecules. For this purpose, ACE is an enzyme that increases blood pressure [22, 23]. It is considered one of hemodynamic and vascular factors like other genes such as AGT1q42-q43, NOS37q36, NPR11q21-q22, among others [19].

1.2.2. CCR5 gene (Rs333)

Recently, there have been identified variants in CC chemokine receptor (CCR) and its importance in infectious and autoimmune disorders, which are significantly linked to diabetes and its complications. These variants interact with other genes associated with the inflammatory cascade, including CCR5 3p21.31, CCR2 3p21.31, IL6 7p21, TNF 6p21.3, and SELL 1q23-q25 [16, 17, 19].

The CCR5 variant, in particular, is a CC, which recruits immune receptor sites of infection, inflammation, and injury including renal disease cells. CCR5 is expressed on dendritic cells derived from peripheral blood, macrophages, lymphocytes, and vascular endothelial cells and its activity average ligands RANTES, eotaxin smooth muscle, and macrophage inflammatory proteins (MIP-1, MIP-1) [19]. Moreover, CCR5 and their ligands, for example, MIP-1 and RANTES [25, 26], have been detected in muscle cells smooth and macrophages of the atherosclerotic plaque.

The CCR5 gene is located on chromosome 3p21.31 [19]. Previous studies have shown that a 32-bp deletion leads to loss of CCR5 expression and function, resulting in a truncated protein, which is not expressed on the cell surface. CCR5 mediates monocyte recruitment and differentiation of macrophages in the glomerulus and intestine. It has been associated to have a role in the development of fibrosis and glomerulosclerosis in DN [26]. The CCR5 D32 variant has been associated with low levels of CRP, decreased intima media thickness, and risk of cardiovascular disease [26].

Furthermore, it has been reported an association of this mutation with risk of myocardial infarction [26]. These studies are consistent with the hypothesis that CCR5 receptor is involved in mediating systemic low-grade inflammation and can participate in diabetes, atherosclerosis, and cardiovascular disease (CVD).

1.2.3. The MTHFR C677T (Rs1801133) and hyperhomocysteinemia

Methylenetetrahydrofolate reductase (MTHFR) is an enzyme encoded by a gene located on chromosome 1p36.3 in position. This sequence has a size of 2.2 kilobases (kb) and consists of 11 exons [27]. In humans, the product of this gene is a protein of 77 kilodaltons (kDa) that catalyses the irreversible conversion of 5,10-methylenetetrahydrofolate to 5-methyltetrahydrofolate, the major circulating form of folate [28, 29]. This form of folate participates in the transfer of one carbon atom during the nucleotide synthesis, the synthesis of S-adenosylmethionine and methylation of DNA, proteins, neurotransmitters, and phospholipids [28]. Furthermore, it also acts as a donor of methyl groups on primary methylation of homocysteine to methionine, catalyzed by the enzyme methionine synthase (MS) [28].

The MTHFR enzyme activity helps maintain reserves of 5-methyltetrahydrofolate and methionine and negatively regulates circulating plasma homocysteine concentration [28]. Homocysteine levels can increase due to environmental factors such as smoking, low intake of folate, and vitamin B12 and related genetic polymorphisms in genes encoding enzymes or transport proteins [30].

Defects in the MTHFR enzyme have also been linked to venous thrombosis [29], Alzheimer's disease [31], some types of cancer [32], pregnancy complications [33], and neural tube defects (NTDs) [34]. The latter condition has been one of the most studied [28] and is one of the most common birth defects worldwide [35].

The C677T allele is in a 23.7–37% of the Caucasian population in Europe, 30.5–47.5% of the Hispanic population, 8.3–14.6% of African American population, in a homozygous state in 11% of the Australian population [36], and 26.8% in a Costa Rican population [37].

The main aim of this research was to determine the prevalence of some polymorphisms as ACE (I/D) Rs1799752; CCR5 D32 Rs333, and MTHFR (C677T) Rs1801133 and known risk factors associated with DN in DM patients belonging to urban areas of Costa Rica, Nicaragua, and Mexico.

2. Materials and methods

This research is descriptive and transversal, held from September to December 2012 in San Jose, Costa Rica; Leon, Nicaragua; and Yucatan, Mexico. The samples were from individuals who attended clinic centers from urban areas of Costa Rica, Nicaragua, and Mexico.

The Costa Rican samples were obtained from the DNA bank Research Center in Hematology and related disorders (CIHATA) of the University of Costa Rica. These samples were from DM patients who live in the areas covered by the basic care teams (EBAIS) within the program of comprehensive health care (PAIS)-CCSS-UCR region of Montes de Oca, Curridabat, and Tres Rios.

DNA samples were obtained from diabetic patients from Leon, Nicaragua, attending an attention program at different health territories, which are as follows: Maria Perla Health Center Norori, Sutiava, and Mantica. In the case of the Regional Research Center in Yucatan, Mexico, the samples were taken from patients attending consultation at the University Social Integration Unit of San José Tecoh. The samples were recollected anonymously with main clinical information and personal history of the individuals with the diagnosis. All participants gave informed consent according to a protocol approved by Bioethics on Human Subjects Research Committee and participating Universities.

2.1. Criteria samples of T2 DM patients

1. Adults between ages 20 and 80 years.

2. Any gender.

http://dx.doi.org/10.5772/64548

3. DM diagnosis, according to the criteria of the American Diabetes Association (ADA) or as directed by the attending physician on the ballot application of clinical laboratory diagnostic tests.

4. Clinical data, including cardiovascular and DN disease history.

5. Agreement to participate with signed written consent.

2.2. DNA analysis

DNA isolation was obtained following the standard NaCl precipitation method [38].

2.3. Mutation I/D ACE gene (Rs1799752)

Mutation study I/D ACE gene developed by polymerase chain (PCR) of intron 16 of the ACE gene, as primers the following sequence: 5′-3′-CTGGAGACCACTCCCATCCTTTCT 3′-5′-GATGTGGCCATCACATTCGTCAGAT [21], obtaining a 190 bp for DD genotype and a fragment of 490 bp in the presence of the corresponding insertion genotype II; heterozygous individuals have both bands (I/D). To avoid false-positive DD genotype, a second amplification [39] was performed, attempting to obtain a band of 300 bp for the heterozygous genotype (I/D) and the homozygous deletion allele (D/D) a band of 200 bp. The bands obtained were analyzed in agarose gels by electrophoresis.

2.4. CCR5 D32 mutation (Rs333)

CCR5 gene was performed by PCR with oligonucleotides 5′-CTTCATTACACCTG-CAGCTCTC CCR5 F-3′ and CCR5 R 5′-CTCACAGCCCAGTGCGACTTCTTCT-3′, which flank the deletion of 32 bp [40]. The reaction conditions were as follows: 10 mM Tris, 2.5 mM MgCl2, dNTPs 0.2 mm c/u, 0.25 μM oligonucleotide c/u, 1.5 GoTaq U (Promega). Amplification was performed with the following program: 94°C 2 min (1 cycle); 94°C 20 s, 55°C 20 s, 72 s 30 (35 cycles); 72°C 7 min (1 cycle). The products were detected by gel electrophoresis 8% polyacrylamide, stained with silver nitrate. The genotyping was performed according to the size of the amplification products (CCR5 wt/wt) a band of 184 bp was observed for the homozygous, deletion of 32 bp (D32/D32); the expected product was 152 bp and heterozygotes (wt/D32) 2 bands:184 and 152 bp.

2.5. MTHFR C677T (Rs1801133)

RFLP-PCR method [41] was used. The region of interest was amplified with the following oligonucleotides: 5′-AGGACGGTGCGGTGAGAGTG 1F-3′ and 2R-5′-TGAAGGA-GAAGGTGTCTGCGGGA-3′ (37). Amplification after digestion proceeded to the post-separation by agarose gel electrophoresis amplicon and 175-pb fragments which were obtained 23 pb and mutant homozygotes (T/T), a single fragment of 198 pb in wild homozygotes (CC) and the three fragments in heterozygous (C/T).

2.6. Statistical analysis

Statistical analysis was performed using SPSS version 16.1 program (SPSS Inc., USA). To determine the association between participating countries were compared, Pearson χ^2 value. The associations were tested for statistical significance; qualitative variables were assessed by OR, equivalent to relative risk, confidence interval, χ^2 value, and a value of $p < 0.05$ was considered. Yates correction for values in cells smaller than 5 was used. Later, analyses were performed to assess the possible association between the risk factors and the presence or absence of nephropathy or some of the complications listed in the questionnaire.

The association for quantitative variables was evaluated by Student's t-test for parametric data, previously applying the Levene's test of homogeneity of variances. Data were captured and analyzed in a database in Excel created for the case for each country and then were analyzed together and separately. Finally, allele frequencies of each polymorphism were determined according to the Hardy-Weinberg law, with χ^2-test. Statistically significant differences were set as $p < 0.05$.

3. Results

3.1. Demographic and clinical characteristics of the study cohort

A total of 521 DNA samples from DM patients were selected, 132 from San Jose, Costa Rica; 192 from Leon, Nicaragua; and 197 from Yucatan, Mexico. Demographic and clinical characteristics and the prevalence of risk factors are summarized in **Table 2**. The average age of the total group studied was 58.4 years, and it was not found a significant difference ($p > 0.05$), in terms of age distribution. Gender was a variant with statistically significant between the DM patients, there were more women (68.2%) than men (31.8%), $p = 0.005$, and the presence of DN was found with statistical significance, $p = 0.021$. The presence of HTA among all the studied patients was found as a risk factor with significant difference (OR of 25.1; $p < 0.000$). The same result was observed in the presence (+)/absence of dyslipidemia and history of CVD. The prevalence of DN is present in a 33.9% of the total 501 DM patient group studied (**Table 2**).

3.2. Prevalence of the genetic polymorphisms and DN risk factors association

The prevalence of polymorphisms and their distribution can be seen in **Table 3**. All polymorphisms were in Hardy-Weinberg equilibrium, to give an adequate composition and distribution of the polymorphisms analyzed in the populations remain in balance and natural selection.

The results of comparison of prevalence of genetic variants in the populations studied can be seen in **Table 3**, wherein the ACE I/D ($p < 0.001$) and CCR5 ($p < 0.001$) show differences between countries. Genotype I/I ACE is less prevalent in the Mexican population, compared to others ($p = 0.01$). A difference was also found in one homozygote Costa Rican patient in the CCR5 D32 polymorphism, which was not found in the other groups ($p = 0.001$). MTHFR C677T polymorphism, in the total group studied showed a higher frequency of the 677TT phenotype, but there was no significant difference ($p = 0.146$) between any of the groups.

The ACE polymorphism had a significance in the total group of DM patients with a history of CVD, $p = 0.02$, CCR5 with a history of dyslipidemia ($p = 0.008$) and presence of the HTA ($p = 0.022$).

Another analysis was performed between the presence of DN in patients with a history of CVD, and it was found a statistical association, $p < 0.001$ OR 3.1 (CI, 1.6–5.8).

The presence or absence of HTA with any of the polymorphisms analyzed was compared, obtaining statistical significance ($p = 0.042$) for Nicaraguan DM patients. In the presence or absence of dyslipidemia, there was a significant difference ($p = 0.031$) in the group of Nicaraguan patients and I/D polymorphism of the ACE gene.

The presence or absence of CVD in DM patients between the countries was compared, a significant difference ($p = 0.030$) was obtained in the group of Nicaraguan patients with CVD and MTHFR C677T gene, and also statistical difference was obtained ($p < 0.001$).

In the results of the interpopulation comparison, a significant difference ($p = 0.000$) between the onset of HTA in DM patients against Nicaraguans and similar behavior was found in the DM patients in Costa Rica ($p < 0.001$).

Variable/risk factor n (%)	Costa Rican (n = 132)	Nicaraguan (n = 192)	Mexican (n = 197)	p
Age, years	60.8 + 5.6	58.8 + 11.9	57.7 + 11.9	–
Gender	132	192	197	0.439
Male	38 (28.8)	61 (31.8)	69 (35.0)	
Female	94 (71.2)	131 (68.2)	128 (65.0)	
DN	132	192	197	0.009
DN+	54 (40.9)	71 (37.0)	50 (25.4)	
DN–	78 (59.1)	121 (63.0)	147 (74.6)	
Hypertension (HTA) (%)	132	192	104*	0.000
HTA+	104 (78.8)	106 (55.2)	37 (35.6)	
HTA–	28 (21.2)	86 (44.8)	67 (64.4)	
Dyslipidemia	132	192	101*	0.000
Yes	54 (40.9)	165 (85.9)	24 (23.8)	
No	78 (59.1)	27 (14.1)	77 (76.2)	
Cardiovascular disease	132	192	102*	0.000
Yes	45 (34.1)	187 (97.4)	06 (5.9)	
No	87 (65.9)	05 (2.6)	96 (94.1)	

DN, Diabetes nephropathy.
*Some data were not available in the Mexican cases. Age, mean + standard deviation. In the other rows, the values denote numbers of cases followed by percentage of the total group; p is significant <0.05

Table 2. Demographic and clinical characteristics of the study cohort.

The CR cases reported the use of glycemic control of DM, 10.9% of Nicaraguan cases reported that are not using any anti-glycemic drug, which is a significant difference ($p < 0.05$) between these Costa Rican and Nicaraguan populations. It was not possible obtain this information for the Mexican group.

The comparison was done according to genetic polymorphism and cases of each country. The following results were obtained: in the I/D ACE gene, there is a greater number of Nicaraguan cases with the heterozygous genotype ACE I/D, without this becomes significant, while a DM patient of Costa Rican cases showed a similar behavior. In relation to MTHFR C677T polymorphism, both Costa Rican and Nicaraguan DM patients showed a higher frequency of the C677T polymorphism, showing no significant difference ($p > 0.05$) between any of the groups. The CCR5 D32/D32 had very few cases with homozygous, and only one case was found in the Costa Rican group.

Polymorphisms	**Costa Rica**	**Nicaragua**	**México**	**p****
ACE	132	192	128*	
II (%)	41 (31.0)	39 (20.3)	12 (9.4)	0.000
ID (%)	55 (41.7)	97 (50.5)	80 (62.5)	
DD (%)	36 (27.3)	56 (29.2)	36 (28.1)	
Allelic frequency				
I	137 (0.52)	175 (0.46)	104 (0.41)	0.000
D	127 (0.48)	209 (0.54)	152 (0.59)	
MTHFR	132	192	197	
CC677 (%)	40 (30.3)	53 (27.6)	53 (26.9)	0.146
C677T (%)	67 (50.8)	83 (43.2)	82 (41.6)	
677TT (%)	25 (18.9)	56 (29.2)	62 (31.5)	
Allelic frequency				
C	147 (0.56)	189 (0.49)	188 (0.48)	0.122
T	117 (0.44)	195 (0.51)	206 (0.52)	
CCR5	132	192	197	
wt/wt (%)		183 (95.3)	161 (81)	–
	123 (93.2)			
wt/D32 (%)	8 (6.0)	9 (4.7)	36 (18.3)	0.000
D32/D32(%)	1 (0.8)	0	0	
Allelic frequency				
wt	254 (0.96)	375 (0.98)	358 (0.91)	–
D32	10 (0.04)	9 (0.002)		36 (0.09)

*Some Mexican DNA samples were without results for this polymorphism.
**p values were calculated by χ^2-test, p significant <0.05.
– Data not applicable.

Table 3. Prevalence of genotypes and allele frequency of the polymorphisms studied in type 2 DM patients from urban areas of San José, Costa Rica; León, Nicaragua; and Yucatán, Mexico.

4. Discussion

In this multicenter study from three Mesoamerican populations, we combined a metabolic disease as DM and a three genetic variants analysis to study their prevalence with the presence of DN. We found that DN in T2-DM patients was associated with the studied polymorphisms principally with ACE I/D and CCR5 d32 as well with HTA and dyslipidemia as risk factors. Our results related to I/D polymorphism are consistent with those reported in other studies [18], one meta-analysis [42], and with prospective follow-up studies [43]. We found that both, the *ACE* D allele and the CCR5 D 32 polymorphism, are prevalent in our type 2 DM patients, with statistical significance in the total studied group.

In an analysis of the total studied population, according to sex distribution, there was a prevalence of 67.6% (n = 339) females. This is a finding that could be explained given that in women, especially those who are near to menopausal age or those who live than this period, aging processes are complicated by hormonal, metabolic, and psychological changes that accompany them [44]. The fact that women are the majority population who assists to a primary health center in these countries; after menopause, pancreatic insulin secretion decreases and insulin resistance increases, and a further estrogen deficiency occurs. This deficiency also affects blood flow to the muscles, limiting the already reduced glucose uptake.

In the case of HTA variable, a significant difference ($p < 0.001$) with an OR of 25.1 was detected, demonstrating a strong association between the Costa Rican and Nicaraguan DM. It is clear that altering blood pressure contributes to the development and progression of chronic complications of this disease. In individuals with DM, HTA may be present in elemental diagnosis even before developing hyperglycemia and is often part of a syndrome that includes glucose intolerance, insulin resistance, obesity, dyslipidemia and coronary artery disease, constituting metabolic syndrome [45]. It is known that a strict control of blood pressure of 130/80 mmHg reduces cardiovascular morbidity and mortality, and renal complications than the control of other complications, hence the importance of maintaining strict control over the value of hypertension in DM patients [46].

On the other hand, 34.1% of Costa Ricans and 97.1% Nicaraguan had a history of some type of CVD, compared with 59% of Mexican patients, a difference that was statistically significant ($p = 0.001$), **Table 2**. These latter variables show similar behavior in other studies since it is known that the higher the value of blood pressure, the greater the probability of having a heart attack, heart failure, stroke, and/or kidney disease [47]. This applies especially for individuals aged between 40 and 70 years, since each increase of 20 mmHg in systolic blood pressure or 10 mmHg in diastolic in this population doubles in the risk of CVD over the range from 115/75 to 185/115 mmHg [48].

The 85.9% of DM Nicaraguan patients had dyslipidemia, it is also statistically significant ($p < 0.05$) compared with the full studied group, and this proportion is maintained by the value obtained for the OR of this study (OR = 9.54). This finding is consistent with other studies and is the association between DM and the presence of dyslipidemia [49]. The vasodilator action of insulin would frequently alter in the presence of insulin resistance; in these situations, by capillary recruitment, typical insulin target tissues (skeletal muscle) would be decreased. Insulin has different effects on the vascular tissues because it stimulates the activity of nitric oxide synthase enzyme endothelial and the endothelium-dependent vasodilatation. In theory, the alteration of the latter mechanism, insulin resistance as in the DM, contributes to endothelial vasomotor dysfunction and would lead to hypertension and atherogenesis [50]. All these variables, including the presence or absence of DM, tend to operate as a single entity, referred to as metabolic syndrome (MS), which is a complex entity, including risk factors predictors of CVD.

These associations found between hypertension, CVD, and dyslipidemia with DM confirm that the most important element in a strict treatment and followed program for DM patients is to avoid the complications as DN and CVD. If we discard the genetic components and rather focus solely on traditional risk factors, which can be prevented or improved, such as healthy lifestyle, together with existing drug therapy, they positively affect the quality of life of patients [51].

However, we found a higher prevalence of I/D ACE polymorphism in our DM patients and some association with DN, **Table 3**. It is important to know that DN is considered as a multicausal complication. Renal complications due to T2 DM owing to the multifactorial causes are a comprehensive expression of conditioning phenotype with the additive effect of multiple loci, and several environmental factors inherent to each population. More genetic regions are associated through sequencing techniques with the predisposition of developing diabetic complications. Around 69 genetic loci are described now, whereas binding studies have described more than 24 genes; therefore, more reports are required, given the genetic heterogeneity influences nephropathy, studies with more population are necessary to assume with greater relevance the interaction between multiple genetic loci and to get an association with a particular phenotype [19].

Comparing Costa Ricans against Nicaraguan and Mexican patients, a significant difference in some of the polymorphisms between these populations was found. One of those differences was CCR5 D32, with a significant difference ($p = 0.042$). This observation is consistent with that described in the literature where it is stated that there is an interaction in pathological states, including some classic risk factors (such as DM and overall metabolic syndrome) and some immunomodulatory factors (such as CCR5). However, the mechanism by which this process occurs had not been well described. An explanation is related to the obesity-associated insulin resistance, which is characterized by a chronic inflammation of tissues, including visceral adipose tissue, which recruits a large number of macrophages, T lymphocytes, and B lymphocytes; the interaction of these cells generates multiple cytokines secretions and autoantigens that predispose to the development of diabetic complications mainly of cardiometabolic type. The exact mechanism of how these interactions occur has not yet been elucidated nor the effects that are associated with this interaction [52].

For the variable of DN presence or absence of disease in Nicaraguan DM patients, two of the three polymorphisms showed statistical significance: MTHFR gene C677T genotype ($p = 0.030$) and genotype I/D ACE gene ($p < 0.001$). MTHFR C677T genotype literature does not describe associations between disease and this genotype, but rather a protective 677TT genotype of MTHFR gene [53] was documented effect. The differences obtained could be due to a small sample size or bias on the part of the information provided by the patient.

The genotype I/D ACE gene was found with significant difference in the distribution among Costa Rican and Nicaraguan populations and in association with the presence of DN. This finding is novel, because even that greater presence of individuals with the D/D genotype is described in the literature, the found difference is significant, therefore, and to confirm this finding, it is necessary to increase the sample size [24, 54].

A significant difference ($p = 0.031$) in the genotype I/D ACE gene was found among Nicaraguan patients with and without dyslipidemia. Similar to the comments on this genotype and an association with this risk factor was also found in the Nicaraguan population. This is an unreported (with statistical significance) finding; however, it had higher frequency of individuals with this polymorphism described in the studies [24].

Another important finding was the significant difference ($p < 0.001$) between the use or not of DM medicament by Nicaraguan patients, since 10.9% of the Nicaraguan population reported not using such medications to control serum glucose level. This finding is explained by a deficiency in the coverage of the Nicaraguan health system, which is a risk factor to take into account in the development of complications in the diabetic population.

In summary, the HTA and dyslipidemia are classic risk factors strongly linked to the DN disease to the T2 DM of the urban areas of San José, Costa Rica; Leon, Nicaragua; and Yucatan, Mexico. The molecular analysis of the genotype I/D ACE was the most important in T2 DM between the patients, principally in Nicaragua and Costa Rica. The polymorphism of the gene CCR5 was significant, with differences in its prevalence between the analyzed countries.

The highlights of the present study are that this is the first report of DN risk factors and three molecular variants in Mesoamerican T2 DM patients. Further studies are necessary to determine the exact impact of the genetics and environment on the risk and to define possible interaction with other candidates involved in the pathogenesis of DN in type 2 DM. These data prove the importance of continuation of this kind of research in order to consider the possibility of offering molecular analysis to type 2 DM population as a potential preventive diagnosis for DM patients with risk of DN.

Acknowledgements

This work was made possible by the support from Secretaria de Relaciones Exteriores de Mexico a través del Academic Exchange program ANUIES_CSUCA 2012, (Sa-2) and by Vicerrectoría de Investigación, University of Costa Rica (project No. 807-A5-311).

Author details

Lizbeth Salazar-Sanchez[1*], Juan Jose Madrigal-Sanchez[2], Pedro Gonzalez-Martinez[3], Edel Paredes[4], Ligia Vera-Gamboa[3], Norma Pavia Ruz[3] and Nina Valadez-Gonzalez[3]

*Address all correspondence to: Lizbeth.salazar@gmail.com

1 Medicine School, University of Costa Rica, San Jose, Costa Rica

2 CIHATA-Medicine School, University of Costa Rica, San Jose, Costa Rica

3 Hematology Laboratory, Regional Research Center, "Dr. Hideyo Noguchi," Autonomous University of Yucatán, Mérida, Mexico

4 Histoembriology Department, National Autonomous University of Nicaragua, Leon, Nicaragua

References

[1] OPS. ALAD 2006 diabetes mellitus type 2 diagnosis, control and treatment guides [Internet]. 2008 [Updated: Washington, OPS]. Available from: www.paho.org/

[2] King H, Aubert RE, Herman WH. Global burden of diabetes, 1995–2025: prevalence, numerical estimates an projections. Diabetes Care. 1998;21:1414–1431.

[3] PAHO. Diabetes shows an ascendent trend in the Americas [Internet]. 2014. Available from: www.paho.org

[4] WHO. Technical report of WHO study group. WHO: Geneva. 1985.

[5] Brenes G, Rosero L. www.ccp.ucr.ac.cr/creles/cientif.html. 2007.

[6] Roselló M, Araúz A, Padilla G, Morice A. Self-reported prevalence in Costa Rica, 1998. Acta Médica Costarricense 2004;4:190–195.

[7] Otiniano M, Ottenbacher K, Black S, Markides K. Lower extremity amputations in diabetic Mexican–American elders: incidence, prevalence and correlationes. J Diabetes. 2003;59–65.

[8] Ministry of Health of Nicaragua and Managua. Hypertension Care Protocol [Internet]. 2004. Available from: MSN. http://www.minsa.gob.ni/(2004).

[9] Guerrero RJ, Rodriguez MM.Complications related to the mortality: an analysis of multiple cause mortality. Med Interna Mex 1997;13:263–267.

[10] Cordova J, Lara A, Barquera S, Rosas M. Non-transmissible chronic diseases in Mexico: Epidemiologic sinopsis and integral prevention. Salud Pública México 2008;50:419–427.

[11] Gutiérrez JP, Rivera-Dommarco J, Shamah-Levy T, Villalpando-Hernández S, Franco A, Cuevas-Nasu L, Romero-Martínez M, Hernández-Ávila M. 2012 National Health and Nutrition National Results, Cuernavaca, Mexico: National Institute of Public Health (MX), 2012.

[12] ADVANCE1. The ADVANCE collaborative group. Engl J Med. 2008;358:2560–2572.

[13] Howard B, Rodríguez B, Bennett P, Harris M, Hamman R, Kuller L. Prevention conference VI: diabetes and cardiovascular disease: writing group I: epidemiology. Circulation. 2002;105:132–137.

[14] Laclé A, Valero J. Diabetic nephropathy prevalence and its risk factors in a marginal urban area of the central plateau of Costa Rica. Acta Médica Costarricense. 2009;51:26–33.

[15] Waters K, Hassanein M, LeMarchand L, Wilkens L. Consistent association of type 2 diabetes risk variants found in European in diverse racial and ethnic groups. PLoS Genet. 2010;6:8.

[16] Wilcox J, Nelken N, Coughlin S, Gordon D, Schall TH. Local expression of inflammatory cytokines in human atherosclerotic plaques. J Atheroscler Thromb. 1994 (Suppl):S10–S13.

[17] Prasad P, Tiwari AK, Kumar KM, Ammini AC, Gupta A, Gupta R, Thelma BK. Association of TGFbeta1, TNFalpha, CCR2 and CCR5 gene polymorphisms in type-2 diabetes and renal insufficiency among Asian Indians. BMC Med Genet. 2007;8(20):20.

[18] Kim S, Abboud HE, Pahl MV, Tayek J, Snyder S, Tamkin J, Alcorn H, Ipp E, Nast CC, Elston RC, Iyengar SK, Adler SG. Examination of association with candidate genes for diabetic nephropathy in a Mexican American population. Clin J Am Soc Nephrol. 2010;5:1072–1078.

[19] Roberto C, Rosales J, López N. Nephropathy due to type 2 diabetes : a multifactorial trait with threshold and cromosomal morbid map. Rev Med Inst Mex Seguro Soc. 2010;48(5):521–530.

[20] Murata M, Maruyama T, Suzuki Y, Saruta T. Paraoxonase 1 Gln/Arg polymorphism is associated with the risk of microangiopathy in type 2. Diabet Med. 2004;21(8):837–844.

[21] Rigat B, Hubert C, Alhenc F, Cambien F. I/D polymorphism in the angiotensin I-converting enzyme gene accounting for half the variance of serum enzyme levels. J Clin Invest. 1990;1343–1346.

[22] Coto E. Polymorphisms of the ACE gene and cardiovascular disease. Nefrologia. 2001;21(1):67–69.

[23] Marre M, Jeunemaitre X, Gallois Y. Contribution of genetic polymorphism in the renin-angiotensin system to the development of renal complications in insulin-dependent diabetes. J Clin Invest. 1997;7(99):1585–1595.

[24] Moya D, Madrigal J, Salazar L. I/D polymorphism of ACE gene and its association with some complications in patients with type 2 diabetes. Acta med Cost. 2012;54(2):102–108.

[25] Raport C, Gosling J, Schweickart V, Gray P. Molecular cloning and functional characterization of a novel human CC chemokine receptor (CCR5) for RANTES, MIP-1beta and MIP-1alpha. J Biol Chem. 1996;271:17161–17166.

[26] Ahluwalia T, Khullar M, Ahuja M, Kohli H. Common variants of inflammatory cytokine genes are associated with risk of nephropathy in type 2 diabetes among Asian Indians. PLoS One. 2009;4(4).

[27] Goyette P, Pai A, Milos R, Frosst P, Tran P, Chen Z, Chan M, Rozen R. Gene structure of human and mouse methylenetetrahydrofolate reductase (MTHFR). Mamm Genome. 1998;9:652–656.

[28] Botto LD, Yang Q. 5,10-Methylenetetrahydrofolate reductase gene variants and congenital anomalies: a HuGE review. Am J Epidemiol. 2000;151(9):862–877.

[29] Rajneesh T, Satyendra T, Prbhat K. Association of homocysteine and methylene tetrahydrofolate reductase (MTHFR C677T) gene polymorphism with coronary artery disease in the population of north India. Genet Mol Biol. 2010; 224–228.

[30] Zetterberg H. Methylenetetrahydrofolate reductase and transcobalamin genetic polymorphisms in human spontaneous abortion: biological and clinical implications. Reprod Biol Endocrinol. 2004;2:7.

[31] Clarke R, Smith AD, Jobst KA, Refsum H, Sutton L, Ueland PM. Folate, vitamin B12, and serum total homocysteine levels in confirmed Alzheimer disease. Arch Neurol. 1998;55(11):1449–1455.

[32] Wang ZG, Cui W, Yang LF, Zhu YQ, Wei WH. Association of dietary intake of folate and MTHFR genotype with breast cancer risk. Genet Mol Res. 2014;13 (3):5446–5545.

[33] Vollset SE, Refsum H, Irgens LM, Emblem BM, Tverdal A, Gjessing HK et al. Plasma total homocysteine, pregnancy complications, and adverse pregnancy outcomes: The Hordaland Homocysteine Study. Am J Clin Nutr. 2000;71, 962–996.

[34] van der Put NM, Gabreels F, Stevens EM, Smeitink JA, Trijbels FJ, Eskes TK, van den Heuvel LP, Blom HJ. A second common mutation in the methylenetetrahydrofolate reductase gene: an additional risk factor for neural-tube defects? Am J Hum Genet. 1998;62:1044–1105.

[35] Karalti MD, Inal M, Yildirim Y, Çoker I, et al. The relationship between maternal 5,10-methylenetetrahydrofolate reductase C677T polymorphism and the development of neural tube defects: a 5-year study in Aegean Obstetrics and Gynecology Training and Research Hospital. Turkiye Klinikleri J Gynecol Obst. 2007:337–341.

[36] Wilcken DE, Wang XL, Sim AS, McCredie RM. Distribution in healthy and coronary populations of the methylenetetrahydrofolate reductase (MTHFR) C677T mutation. Arterioscler Thromb Vasc Biol. 1996;16(7):878–882.

[37] Salazar-Sanchez L. Geographic and Ethnic differences in the prevalence of thrombophilia. In: InTech Open Access, editor. Thrombophilia, 1st ed. Rijeka, Croatia: InTech Publishers; 2011. p. 39–58.

[38] Miller S, Dykes D, Polesky H. A simple salting out procedure for extracting DNA from human nucleated cells. Nucleic Acid Res. 1998;16:1215.

[39] Odawara M, Matsunuma A, Yamashita K. Mistyping frequency of the angiotensin-converting enzyme gene polymorphism and an improved method for its avoidance. Hum Genet. 1997;100:163–166.

[40] Dean M, Carrington M, Winkler C, Huttley GA, Smith MW, Allikmets R, Goedert JJ. Genetic restriction of HIV-1 infection and progression to AIDS by a deletion allele of the CCR5 structural gene. Science. 1996;2739:1856–1862.

[41] Frosst P, Blom H, Milos R, Goyette P. A candidate genetic risk factor for vascular disease: a common mutation in methylenetetrahydrofolate reductase gene. Nat Genet. 1995;10:111–113.

[42] Ng DP, Tai BC, Koh D, Tan KW, Chia KS. Angiotensin-I converting enzyme insertion/deletion polymorphism and its association with diabetic nephropathy: a meta-analysis of studies reported between 1994 and 2004 and comprising 14,727 subjects. Diabetologia. 2005;48:1008–1016.

[43] Boright AP, Paterson AD, Mirea L, Bull SB, Mowjoodi A, Scheerer SW, Zinman B. Genetic variations of the ACE gene is associated with persistent microalbuminuria an severe nephropathy in type 1 diabetes: the DCC/EDIC genetics study. Diabetes. 2005;(54):1238–1244.

[44] SMNE. Diabetes and menopaue. Rev Endocrino Nutric. 2004;12(2):50–56.

[45] Araya-Orozco M. Hypertension and diabetes mellitus. Rev Costarric Cienc Med. 2004;25:3–4.

[46] Gorriz J, Marín R, Alvaro F, Martínez A. Arterial hypertension treatment in type 2 diabetes. NefroPLuS. 2008;1(1):16–27.

[47] Bertomeu V, Cordero A, Quiles J, Mazón P. Control of Risk Factors in and Treatment of Patients With Coronary Heart Disease: The TRECE Study. Rev Esp Cardiol. 2009:807–811.

[48] Alvarez A, Gonzalez J. Some risk factors oh hipertensive heart disease. Rev Cubana Med. 2009;48(4).

[49] Traversa M, Elbert A. Dyslipidemia, type 2 diabetes and kidney disease. Sep Línea Montpellier. 2009;17(2):36.

[50] Corbatón A, Cuervo R, Serrano M. Type 2 diabetes mellitus as a heart disease risk factor. Rev Esp Cardiol. 2007;7:9–22.

[51] Chowdury T, Dyer P, Kumar S, Barnett A. Genetic determinants of diabetic nephropathy. Clin Sci. 1999;96:221–230.

[52] Ammirati E, Bozzolo E, Contri R, Baragetti A. Cardiometabolic and immune factors associated with increased common carotid artery intima-media thickness and cardiovascular disease in patients with systemic lupus erythematosus. Nutr Metab Cardiovasc Dis. 2014;1(9).

[53] Garcia R, Ayala P, Villegas V, Salazar M. A study of MTHFR C677T polymorphism in newborns with isolated heart disease in a colombian population. Univ Med Bogota. 2011;3(53):269–277.

[54] Rubio JA, Rubio M, Alvarez J, Cancér E. ACE gene polymorphism and its asociation with the presence of albuminuria in a population with type 2 diabetes. AV Diabetol. 2001:156–160.

Chapter 8

Relevance of Personalized Health Care in Patients with Arterial Hypertension: Where are we now?

Carmen Binder, Hans Hendrik Schäfer,
Edelgard Kaiser, Martin Hund and Thomas Dieterle

Additional information is available at the end of the chapter

http://dx.doi.org/10.5772/63558

Abstract

Personalized health care (PHC) or precision medicine is a new medical concept that aids in treatment decisions for patients by tailoring them to their individual needs. It often employs genetic testing to select appropriate and optimal therapies (pharmacogenomics). Although this concept is widely applied in oncology, the field of hypertension is still in the early stages and "personalization" is currently limited to tailoring antihypertensive treatment according to age, comorbidities, and ethnicity. Despite the fact that incomplete/lack of treatment response occurs in 10–30% of hypertensive patients for angiotensin-converting enzyme (ACE) inhibitors and in 15–25% for β-blockers, major continental guidelines still recommend the use of antihypertensive agents in a "one-size-fits-all" approach, neglecting the 1977 postulation of the Joint National Committee that "all patients must receive individualized therapy programs." The arrival of molecular testing offers new possibilities to differentiate monogenetic from polygenetic disorders and to identify associations between hypertension and drug response to corresponding genes. Up to 50% of the variation in blood pressure (BP) is attributable to genetic factors. Polymorphisms have been identified and studied in genes for BP-modifying receptors, such as ADBR (β-adrenergic receptors), and pharmacological pathways (GNB3, RAAS system). Approximately, one-quarter of the currently analyzed gene polymorphisms demonstrate significant pharmacogenetic effects (ADD1 Gly460Trp and the insertion/deletion [I/D] polymorphism in intron 16 of the ACE gene). Several large screening studies are currently ongoing to assess the impact on efficacy of antihypertensive medication of variants in hypertension-susceptibility genes. The GenHAT substudy of the Antihypertensive and Lipid-Lowering Treatment to Prevent Heart Attack Trial (ALLHAT) assessed the predictive validity of the ACE I/D genotype for coronary heart disease. The Family Blood Pressure Program included 11,079 participants to map genetic variants associated with hypertension. In this review chapter, we display the current body of knowledge regarding PHC in the treatment of hypertension. In particular, we highlight genetic variants associated with hypertension and response/non-response to antihypertensive substance classes. Second, we describe technological aspects of PHC and display the most recent example of a PHC marker used in preeclampsia (PlGF/sFlt-1/PlGF). We then present the results of a guideline review, which included six international guidelines (the European Society of Cardiology/the European Society of Hypertension (ESC/ESH), the Joint National Committee (JNC)8, the Canadian Hypertension Education Program (CHEP), the National Institute for Health and Care Excellence (NICE) and the American Heart Association (AHA)/the American College of Cardiology (ACC)/the Centers for Disease Control and Prevention (CDC) and the American Society of Hypertension (ASH)/the International Society of Hypertension (ISH)) on recommendations regarding PHC in arterial hypertension and address contemporary governmental health agency perspectives on PHC. Finally, we present the view of physicians on the development of PHC.

Keywords: personalized health care, arterial hypertension, customer, technologies, genes

---

1. Introduction

The history of personalized medicine is as old as humankind. Attempts to identify which patients are prone to a particular disease and which patients will benefit from a particular treatment reach back to Hippocrates, who stated: "It is far more important to know what person the disease has than what disease the person has."

1.1. The term personalized health care

Personalized health care (PHC) describes attempts to tailor medical treatment to the characteristics of the individual patient. This creates a setting in which individuals can be allocated into subpopulations. PHC aims to allocate therapeutic and preventive interventions to that section of the population that is likely to respond [1]. Adequate treatment may lead to a significant reduction in disease burden by preventing a number of long-term problems, for example, caused by untreated hypertension including cerebrovascular disease, renal insufficiency, and coronary artery disease [2]. PHC can also reduce the response time to treatment and visit frequency. Drug intake itself can lead to adverse effects—a burden that is usually balanced against the beneficial effects of therapy [3]. Adverse events are a secondary source of costs and they increase the likelihood of therapy withdrawal and the risk of non-compliant behavior. PHC allows adverse events associated with ineffective treatment to be avoided and can reduce health-care costs significantly. **Table 1** exhibits the conceptual components of PHC. **Figure 1** displays the effects of PHC on the health-care environment.

1.2. Treating arterial hypertension

Hypertension is a major public health problem [4] and is the most common modifiable risk factor for vascular disease [5]. It affects around 992 million people worldwide [6] and has a high prevalence in Europe [7]. The response to antihypertensive therapy is very heterogeneous and this has driven much interest in the pharmacogenomics, which combines the fields of pharmacology and genomics to establish how a person's genetic makeup influences their response to drugs. In pharmacotherapy, on average only 50% of patients receiving a given drug will experience the expected therapeutic benefit [8]; the remaining 50% experience either insufficient effects or no effects at all [9]. In patients with hypertension, the rate of incomplete or absent responses ranges from 10 to 30% for angiotensin-converting enzyme inhibitors (ACEIs) and 15–25% for β-blockers reaching 30–70% for statins, and 40–70% for β2-agonists [10]. Overall, it is assumed that only approximately 30% of patients respond adequately to antihypertensive drugs [11].

Personalized Healthcare in arterial hypertension			
Detailed Assessment	**Comprehensive Assessment**	**Morphological Assessment**	**Functional Assessment**
Genomic Testing	Family History	Intima-Media Thickness	Endothelial Function
	Laboratory Testing		Heart Rate Variability
	Evidence on Gender/Age/Ethnicity		Stress Testing
	Risk Factors/Scores		

Table 1. Overview of components of PHC.

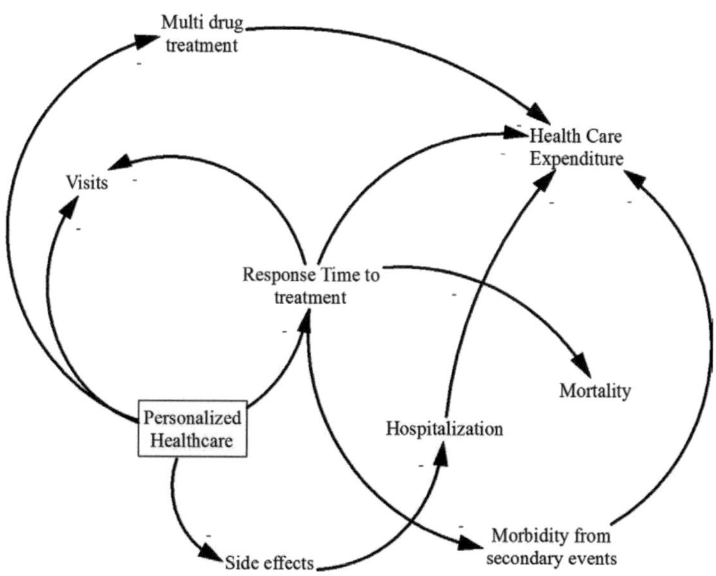

Figure 1. Effects of PHC on the health-care environment (causal loop).

1.3. Guideline recommendations and clinical practice

Individualized treatment approaches for patients with arterial hypertension have been recommended for several decades [12]. As early as 1977, the Joint National Committee (JNC)

Reports on the Detection, Evaluation, and Treatment of High Blood Pressure (BP) [13] stated predictively that "all patients must receive individualized therapy programs." In reality, this recommendation was replaced with a standardized advocacy of diuretics [14] and the only individualized component of contemporary blood pressure treatment remains clustering patients according to gender [15], race [16], end-organ damage, or comorbidities.

1.4. Genetic factors for blood pressure variability

The completion of the Human Genome Project [17] revolutionized medicine. Advances in the understanding of the human genome have enabled physicians to pursue optimal preventive health-care strategies instead of the rather reactive health-care approaches used in the past [18]. For the first time, it conclusively mapped all human genes, including those that may account for hypertension. Up to 50% of BP variation can be explained by either monogenetic or polygenetic factors [19]. However, it was disappointing that the influence of single gene polymorphisms was less than expected (<5%) while the impact of race and sex was considerably higher [20]. BP differences of <0.5 mmHg are normally associated with a single nucleotide polymorphism (SNP) [10].

1.5. Demand for better technologies

Parallel with these discoveries, breakthrough technologies came on the market, including the automated high-throughput sequencer [21], as well as new methodologies allowing less invasive diagnostics such as liquid biopsy [22]. These technologies were primarily driven by the need for better diagnostics in the oncology field and made the handling of genomic information more established and accepted.

1.6. Health economic aspects of PHC

Over the last couple of years, payers, health economists, and policy makers evolved as a new stakeholder group in the health-care landscape articulating an interest in a more cost-efficient treatment. Genomic investigation allows not only the early diagnosis of diseases but also the identification of disease sub-entities. Both components have an impact on the health-care expenditures. In recent years, other fields of medicine (e.g., neonatal diagnostics) have started using genetic information for patient management. Due to fairly low costs for antihypertensive therapy, PHC has been slow in entering this field of medicine. Thus, overall, the use of individualized treatment approaches in hypertension remains low (at around 7% in the USA [23]). A McKinsey ranking from 2010 [24] regarding the scientific and economic potential of companion diagnostics, which was based on expert interviews and other quantitative factors, yielded low values for antihypertensive assays (<1.7 on a scale from 0 to 2.7 for the economic potential and 1.1 on a scale from 0.4 to 2.8 for scientific potential), putting them in a "no-go" area for company investment. Not surprisingly, the analysis showed high values for oncology, anti-infectives, and autoimmune drugs. However, what is very often forgotten is the fact that a test, particularly one that is able to show high per-patient savings in a highly prevalent disease, can be a very attractive opportunity. Thus a test that can prevent or drastically delay an ischemic cardiac or a cerebral event can be considered as a favorable asset. In addition, PHC tests in hypertension are less likely to create microeconomic incentives for prescribing physicians. This is because the treatment of hypertension is a predominantly conservative discipline and not associated with costly procedures.

1.7. Pharmacogenetics

In more recent years, the International Haplotype Project contributed to better understanding of genetic polymorphisms by developing a map locating genes affecting health, disease, and responses to drugs (HapMap) [25]. However, in 2010 only around 10% of all Food and Drug Administration (FDA)-approved drugs include pharmacogenomic information in their labels [26], and a total of 39 FDA-approved drugs demanded genetic testing at that time [27]. By contrast, another study of 200 top-prescribed drugs showed that pharmacogenetic data were available for up to 71.3%, although only 24% of all cardiovascular drugs in the 200 top-prescribed drugs had pharmacogenetic data [28]. Of these, approximately 23 and 18% of pharmacogenetic data in the cardiovascular and hormone/hormone-modifier classes, respectively, were related to drug-metabolizing enzyme and drug transporter genes (i.e., pharmacokinetics) [28]. Trials investigating variants in hypertension-susceptibility genes and their interaction with antihypertensive therapy, for example, GenHat [29], have been initiated as well as biobanks and registries to assess information about pharmacogenomics of hypertension, including the Family Blood Pressure Program [30] and the Pharmacogenetics Knowledge Base (PharmGKB; https://www.pharmgkb.org/).

The following chapters review various aspects of PHC in arterial hypertension, namely genes in arterial hypertension, technologies used in PHC, guideline recommendations on PHC, and physician views on PHC. Finally, a case study of PHC displays the impact of a medical value assay on the management of preeclampsia.

2. Genes in arterial hypertension

BP is a complex physiological trait that is affected by complex interplays between genetic and environmental factors. Gene variants may affect BP variability by acting on gene and protein expression. Thus, the characterization of genes associated with BP may provide not only a deeper understanding of the cellular processes involved in BP regulation but also how transcripts mediate genetic and environmental effects.

Many trials have demonstrated a substantial heritability of BP. Adoption, twin, and family studies document a significant heritable component to BP levels and hypertension [31–33]. Estimates of the heritability of resting systolic and diastolic BPs, based on family studies, are thought to be generally in the range of 30–60% [34]. A heritable component to salt sensitivity of BP has been described in black Americans [35]. A large proportion of the phenotypic variation in BP appears to be inherited as a polygenic trait [36, 37]. A wide variety of approaches, such as linkage and candidate gene studies (CGSs) or studies of families with rare Mendelian high or low BP syndromes, were used for the search for genes associated with BP variability [38–42]. Nevertheless, the majority of genetic contribution to BP variation remained unexplained.

Systolic blood pressure			Diastolic blood pressure			Hypertension		
SNP	**Chr.**	**Nearest gene**	**SNP**	**Chr.**	**Nearest gene**	**SNP**	**Chr.**	**Nearest gene**
rs12046278	1	*CASZ1*	rs13423988	2	*GPR73/ARHGAP25*	rs17806132	2	*PMS1*
rs7571613	2	*PMS1*	rs13401889	2	*MSTN*	rs305489	3	*SYN2*
rs448378	3	*MDS1*	rs9815354	3	*ULK4*	rs7640747	3	*ITGA9*
rs2736376	8	*MTMR9*	rs7016759	8	*EFCAB1*	rs11775334	8	*MSRA*
rs1910252	8	*EFCAB1*	rs11014166	10	*CACNB2*	rs899364	8	*FAM167A/BLK*
rs11014166	10	*CACNB2*	rs11024074	11	*PLEKHA7*	rs11014166	10	*CACNB2*
rs1004467	10	*CYP17A1*	rs2681472	12	*ATP2B1*	rs2681472	12	*ATP2B1*
rs381815	11	*PLEKHA7*	rs3184504	12	*SH2B3*	rs278126	12	*CIT*
rs2681492	12	*ATP2B1*	rs2384550	12	*TBX3/TBX5*	rs11612893	12	*FZD10/PIWIL1*
rs3184504	12	*SH2B3*	rs6495122	15	*CSK/ULK3*	rs16982520	20	*ZNF831/EDN3*

SNP, single nucleotide polymorphism; Chr., chromosome.

Table 2. Meta-analysis of CHARGE and Global BPgen of top 10 loci for systolic and diastolic BP and hypertension (adapted from Levy et al. [43]).

It is conceivable that BP variation in the general population may be a reflection of the sum of multiple variants with small effects. Thus, very large studies might be needed to identify such effects. In fact, large-scale genome-wide association studies (GWAS) have identified numerous gene loci that are associated with BP [43–45]. As an example, the top 10 loci for systolic and diastolic BP as well as for arterial hypertension derived from the Cohorts for Heart and Aging Research in Genome Epidemiology (CHARGE) Consortium [46] and the Global BPgen Consortium [43] are summarized in **Table 2**.

The study of the genetic background of an individual may be helpful to analyze the intrinsic and extrinsic susceptibility for a disease as well as the effects of the disease on the individual. The potential of such a personalized, particularly genome-based approach to arterial hypertension is summarized in **Figure 2**. Obviously, the treatment of chronic conditions would not start before the earliest possible time of point detection. In many cases, it will only start with substantial delays after this time point and many chronic conditions, including hypertension, will only be detected when acute or chronic end-organ damage becomes clinically overt resulting in deleterious consequences for the patient [47]. In these conditions, genome-based information across the continuum of health and disease may complement and improve the current approach by early identification of individuals at risk for a disease and, at the same time, enabling early preventive and/or therapeutic interventions [48, 49].

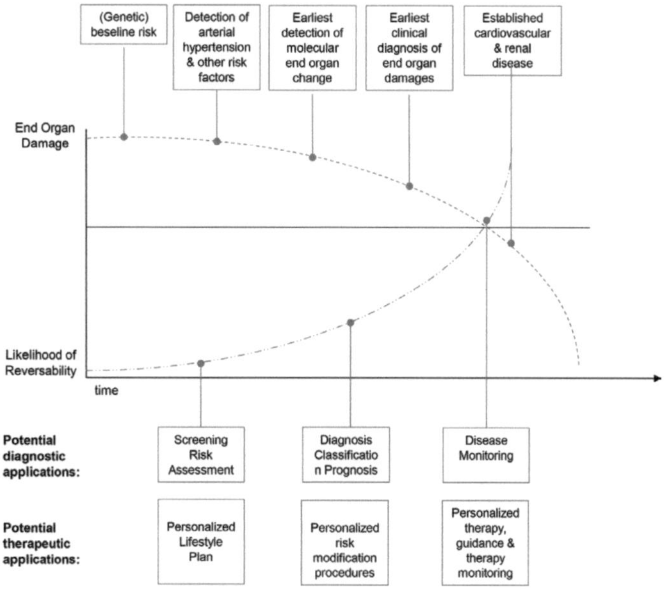

Figure 2. Opportunities for PHC in hypertension.

2.1. Potential application of genomics in risk stratification in arterial hypertension

Associations between genes and hypertension identified by GWAS or CGS are limited by small effect sizes limiting the ability of individual genes to predict the development of hypertension. This limitation can be overcome by constructing genetic risk scores that combine the effects of multiple genetic variants into a single variable. A potential application of genetic risk scores can be the early identification of patients at risk for developing hypertension. Published examples include a genetic risk score derived from data from the British Genetics in Hypertension (BRIGHT) study and a genetic risk prediction model derived from the Wellcome Trust Case Control Consortium (WTCCC) study [50–52]. Unfortunately, genetic risk scores for hypertension only have a very limited predictive power [51] and therefore add little additional information compared to non-genetic risk prediction models.

2.2. Potential application of genomics in therapy guidance

More promising applications of genetic testing are expected from the field of pharmacogenomics (i.e., the study of genetic predisposition to drug response). It is estimated that 1.56 billion adults worldwide will be diagnosed with arterial hypertension by 2025 [6]. Being a chronic condition, hypertension usually requires lifelong therapy. However, despite a wide variety of available antihypertensive drugs, BP is controlled in only approximately 50% of patients. Moreover, therapeutic strategies in the general population have not been as effective as expected from clinical trial results [53]. These data indicate that the optimal approach to antihypertensive therapy has not yet been established and that further improvements in patient care and treatment efficacy need to be achieved.

Drug class	Gene	Population	Drug	Data source	Reference
Diuretics	*YEATS4*	White-/African-Americans/Others	Hydrochloro-thizide	GWAS, CGS	[56, 57]
	PRKCA	Swedish/Norwegian, Finnish		GWAS	[58]
	NEDDL4	Swedish/Norwegian, White-/ African-Americans/Others, White-/African-Americans/ Hispanics		CGS	[59, 60]
	FGF5 *SH2B3* *EBF1*	White-/African- Americans/Others		CGS	[61]
	CLIC5 *RUNX2*	Finnish		GWAS	[62]
	TET2 *CSMD1*	Italian		GWAS	[63]
ACE Inhibitors / Angiotensin II Receptor Blockers	*AGT*	Chinese, Indian	Enalapril/ Inidapril, Benazepril	CGS	[64–66]
	AGTR1 *NR3C2*	Chinese	Enalapril	CGS	[67]
	ABCC9 *YIPF1*	Japanese	Not specified	GWAS	[68]
	FUT4	White-/African- Americans	Candesartan	GWAS	[69]
	GPR83 *SCNN1G* *CYP11B2*	Not specified		CGS	[70]
	STK39	Finnish	Losartan	GWAS	[71]
	CAMK1D	Italian		GWAS	[72]
	GRK4	Japanese	Losartan, Candesartan, Telmisartan	GCS	[73–75]
Beta-Blockers	ADRB1	White-/African- Americans Hispanics	Metoprolol	CGS	[76]
	FGF5 CHIC2 MOV11 HFE	White-/African-Americans/Others	Atenolol	CGS	[61]
	GNB3	Italian		CGS	[77]
	GRK4	White-/African- Americans/Hispanics		CGS	[78]
	LPL PPARA	Europe, Africa, Asia		CGS	[79]

Drug class	Gene	Population	Drug	Data source	Reference
	TNFRSF11B APOB ADRA1A CACNB2 LIPC CASR				
Calcium Channel Blockers	PICALM TANC2 NUMA1 APCDD1	Japanese	Not specified	GWAS	[68]
	KCNMB1	White-/African-Americans/Hispanics	Verapamil	CGS	[80]
	CACNA1C	White-/African-Americans/Hispanics		CGS	[81]
	PLCD3	Swedish/Norwegian	Diltiazem	CGS	[82]

GWAS, genome-wide association study; CGS, candidate-gene study.

Table 3. Pharmacogenetics/genomics studies in arterial hypertension by drug class.

In this respect, pharmacogenomic approaches have the potential to lead to the development of diagnostic tools for predicting the most effective therapeutic approach to hypertension. In fact, an increasing number of studies have revealed and continue to reveal genetic variants that are associated with response or non-response to antihypertensive drug classes such as diuretics, β-blockers, calcium channel blockers (CCBs), ACE inhibitors, and angiotensin II receptor blockers (**Table 3**). While parameters obtained from anthropometric, biochemical, or technical examinations are helpful for the adequate selection of drug classes that will provide optimal end-organ protection, they are of limited value for predicting the individual response to antihypertensive therapy [54, 55]. Unfortunately, despite promising data, information on interactions between gene variants and antihypertensive drug efficacy is not yet part of the routine evaluation of hypertensive patients. This may be due to confounding factors (e.g., environmental or epigenetic factors). Their effect is far less well understood and more research is needed to further clarify the interplay between genes, environment, and response to antihypertensive therapy.

3. Technologies for PHC in essential hypertension

BP has a significant genetic component, but only a minority of cases is attributed to genetic variants identified to date [83]. There is a general belief, however, that by further understanding these interactions, there is high potential in PHC for the prevention and treatment of essential hypertension. While most studies focus on the types of analytes that could be relevant, such as nucleic acids and proteins, here we investigate the technologies currently in use and those with the biggest potential for PHC in hypertension.

3.1. Real-time quantitative PCR and digital PCR

Polymerase chain reaction (PCR) has become an indispensable tool in biomedical research. Real-time quantitative PCR (qPCR) allows measurement of the amplification of a targeted DNA molecule in real time based on fluorescence [84]. The resulting PCR curve is used to define the exponential phase of the reaction, which is a prerequisite for the accurate calculation of the initial copy number at the beginning of the reaction [84, 85]. One study developed a screening test based on six multiple SNP loci associated with essential hypertension and was able to demonstrate significant correlation between one SNP and patients with hypertension [86].

Although qPCR is still the technology of choice, the latest PCR technology—the so-called digital PCR (dPCR)—now offers measurement of nucleic acids with generally superior precision, sensitivity, and reproducibility over qPCR [87, 88]. In dPCR, the sample is separated into a large number of partitions, allowing for simultaneous template amplification separately in each partition. The latest development of dPCR technology employs thousands to millions of reaction partitions, thus providing a scalable multiplexing environment [89]. The advantages in terms of sensitivity and reliability demonstrate the potential of dPCR for molecular diagnostics, for example, in the cell-free DNA fraction of blood plasma, but the technology has not yet been introduced into mainstream clinical practice, and hence no reference was found for the use of dPCR with regard to genetic testing for hypertension.

3.2. Next-generation sequencing (NGS)

In the past decade, there has been extraordinary progress in our ability to sequence the human genome and the price of sequencing an average human genome has dropped from approximately US$10 million to below US$1000 [90, 91]. Most sequencing technologies use similar protocols with common methods for template preparation (building and amplifying a library of nucleic acids), nucleic acid sequencing using library fragments as template from which a new complementary DNA fragment is synthesized, and imaging and data analysis [92]. The actual sequencing occurs through a cycle of washing and flooding the fragments with known nucleotides in a sequential order, and digital recording of incorporated nucleotides [92]. Raw sequencing data then undergo several layers of data analysis to rebuild the sequence from a multitude of DNA fragments, after which the compiled sequence can be analyzed [93]. Targeted sequencing, such as whole-exome sequencing, allows us to investigate the coding part of the genome, which represents only about 1.5% of the genetic code. The exome can be sequenced at a much lower cost compared with the whole genome, and with deeper coverage (>100× vs. 30–40× coverage), which increases accuracy [94]. Technological advances in high-throughput genomic sequencing enabling genome-wide association studies and whole-exome sequencing are expected to bring greater insights into the genetic causes of essential hypertension and will eventually bring those technologies into clinical practice [79]. Numerous companies are working on the development of high-throughput genomic technologies in order to make genomics information universally available.

Examples include Genia, with its nanopore technology for single molecule sequencing, and Illumina Inc., which has developed large-scale whole-genome sequencing on the HiSeq X Series and Thermo Scientific (http://www.pacb.com/products-and-services/; https://www.thermofisher.com/ch/en/home.html) [95, 96].

To fully reveal the potential of NGS, it is important to consider multiple sources of genetic information, such as inheritance and association studies, and bioinformatics. For example, the application of next-generation linkage and association methods to hypertension demonstrated that OSBPL10—a disease-susceptibility gene for dyslipidemia—might also influence systolic BP [97]. A novel statistical approach to detect genetic associations between a trait and SNP regions across the entire genome (whole-genome sliding-window-based optimal weighted approach) revealed three highly susceptible windows across chromosome 3 for diastolic BP and identified 10 of 48,176 windows as the most promising for influencing both diastolic and systolic BP [98]. A recent analysis of functional differences in hypertension pharmacogenes was conducted by investigating human genomic variation using data from the 1000 genomes project, coupled with a functional prediction analysis [79]. Results indicated significant interpopulation differences depending on geographical origin, giving insights into interindividual differences in antihypertensive drug response and suggesting that rare variants mainly determine the functionality of hypertension pharmacogenes [79]. However, there have been few of these studies and more research based on NGS technologies is necessary to further understand hypertension pharmacogenomics and to fully leverage them for PHC [79].

3.3. Bioinformatics

The above examples underline the fundamental role played in PHC of the ability to process and analyze huge volumes of data, such as electronic medical records, in vivo imaging, genomics, and other "-omic" technologies [94, 99]. Millions of genetic polymorphisms are identified with NGS technology; but in order to find an association between a polymorphism and a phenotype, a large number of statistical tests have to be performed and then require correction for multiple testing [100]. A methodology was recently proposed for unified analysis of NGS data. A pipelined series of statistical and bioinformatics methods was used to analyze associations between genetic polymorphisms and a disease phenotype, using hypertension as the example, and to identify statistically significant pathways of genes that may play a role in the disease [100].

3.4. Epigenomics

Rather than just being affected by variations in the coding genome, epigenetic mechanisms, including microRNAs, histone modification, and methylation, are increasingly seen to play a role in the development of hypertension [101]. Non-coding areas of the human genome, which make up almost 99% of it, were long regarded as "junk DNA" [102]. In contrast, the Encyclopedia of DNA Elements (ENCODE) project has shown that non-coding DNA is a critical element of gene function regulation across cell, tissue, and organ types [103, 104]. The ENCODE project systematically mapped regions of transcription, transcription factor association, chromatin structure, and histone modification, which enabled them to assign biochemical functions for 80% of the genome [103]. Regulatory elements, such as transcription-factor-binding sites, histone modification, chromatin structure, and DNA methylation, are highly cell-type specific. Those non-coding regions are extensively transcribed into non-coding RNAs, such as microRNAs and long-non-coding RNAs (lncRNA), with various functions including the influence of the pathophysiology of hypertension [102]. For example, microRNAs seem to be associated with hypertension via sympathetic nerve activity, ion transporters in the kidney, endothelial function, vascular smooth muscle phenotype transformation, and communication between cells [102]. In another study, expression levels of microRNAs implicated in vascular smooth muscle cell phenotypic modulation were assessed in patients with hypertension and healthy controls. Changes in vascular smooth muscle cells play a critical role in the pathophysiology of arterial remodeling in essential hypertension. Levels of hsa-miR-143, hsa-miR-145, and hsa-miR-133a were downregulated, and hsa-miR-21 and hsa-miR-1 upregulated in peripheral blood mononuclear cells of patients with hypertension compared with normotensive subjects [105]. There also seems to be potential for clinical use of non-coding RNAs to identify or treat patients with cardiovascular diseases [106, 107]. As non-coding RNAs are a relatively new field of research for hypertension, the number of supporting studies is small, and further research is needed [107].

3.5. Other "omic" studies and technologies

Despite the leading role of genomics, other new "omics" technologies have been developed that allow us to bridge between genotype and phenotype [92].

3.5.1. Transcriptomics and differential gene expression

Transcriptomic approaches allow us to study the complete set of RNA transcripts, for example, through microarray or RNA sequencing. Microarray chips can hold tens of thousands of genes and can be used to compare gene expression levels in certain disease states [108, 109]. However, our literature review did not reveal any transcriptome studies addressing PHC in essential hypertension.

3.5.2. Proteomics

Proteomics gives a snapshot of the proteins present at a given time in a cell or an organism and might help to reveal novel diagnostic and therapeutic approaches in hypertension. A study aiming to identify urinary proteins involved in the pathogenesis of hypertension and salt sensitivity revealed different uromodulin protein levels in individuals with hypertension versus healthy individuals [110]. Patients with higher levels of uromodulin were homozygotes for specific UMOD gene variants and displayed a decreased level of salt excretion [110]. Another study assessing the correlation between hypertension with γ-glutamyltransferase (GGT) and alanine aminotransferase (ALT) levels in a Chinese population revealed that elevated GGT was associated with hypertension but not ALT [111].

http://dx.doi.org/10.5772/63558

3.5.3. Metabolomics

Metabolomics studies the metabolites resulting from biochemical degradation processes and allows conclusions to be drawn on the prevalence of such processes. Several studies highlighted distinctions in the metabolic footprint of patients with hypertension and hence the potential in its analysis (e.g., through gas chromatography-mass spectrometry and liquid chromatography-mass spectrometry) [112–114]. One study pointed out that the metabolic perturbation associated with alcohol abuse may contribute to the development of hypertension, probably by a shift in the ratio of the oxidized:reduced forms of nicotinamide adenine dinucleotide (NADH:NAD^+) [112]. Other results suggest that disorders in amino acid metabolism might play an important role in the pathogenesis of juvenile hypertension and circulating levels of uridine adenosine tetraphosphate are strongly associated with the disease [113, 115]. In another study, sex-steroid pattern was significantly associated with the risk of incident hypertension [116]. However, more clarity about the different metabolic influences is needed to translate these findings into clinical practice.

3.6. Importance of mobile technologies

With the omnipresence of new mobile technologies and connected devices, patient self-monitoring is becoming an increasingly important and promising topic across various diseases. Despite a large number of mobile apps and devices designed to track general health and well-being and also BP specifically [117], formal clinical research on such self-monitoring devices still seems to be limited. Some initial studies focused on patient education in patient-centered hypertension care [118, 119]. The FDA has cleared some mobile apps for BP and cardiac monitoring (e.g., the Withings BP Monitor) [120]. Initial studies dealing with patients' self-monitoring conclude that in order to motivate patients to self-manage their hypertension, engage with their devices, and communicate through them with health-care providers, it is crucial that the technology is both flexible and secure [119].

In the following chapter, we compare the content of important international guidelines regarding PHC in hypertension.

4. Guidelines on PHC in arterial hypertension

4.1. Status quo and guidance in hypertension on personalized medicine: hypertension guideline perspectives

In this section, we review the content of six international hypertension guidelines regarding evidence and recommendations on how to execute PHC in the management of high blood pressure. While the majority of guidelines still emphasize the importance of comprehensive PHC, only little evidence is displayed on detailed PHC. The guidelines reviewed here are summarized in **Table 4**.

Guideline	Specific condition	Treatment				Notes
		Initial	2nd line	3rd line	4th line	
ESC/ESH	**Asymptomatic organ damage**					
	LVH	ACE inhibitor, calcium antagonist, ARB				
	Asymptomatic atherosclerosis	Calcium antagonist, ACE inhibitor				
	Microalbuminuria	ACE inhibitor, ARB				
	Renal dysfunction	ACE inhibitor, ARB				
	Clinical CV event					
	Previous stroke	Any agent effectively lowering BP				
	Previous MI	BB, ACE inhibitor, ARB				
	Angina pectoris	BB, calcium antagonist				
	HF	Diuretic, BB, ACE inhibitor, ARB, mineralocorticoid receptor antagonists				
	Aortic aneurysm	BB				
	Atrial fibrillation, prevention	Consider ARB, ACE inhibitor, BB, or mineralocorticoid receptor antagonist				
	Atrial fibrillation, ventricular rate	BB, non-dihydropyridine calcium antagonist				
	ESRD/proteinuria	ACE inhibitor, ARB				
	Peripheral artery disease	ACE inhibitor, calcium antagonist				
	Other					
	Isolated systolic hypertension (elderly)	Diuretic, calcium antagonist				
	Metabolic syndrome	ACE inhibitor, ARB, calcium antagonist				
	Diabetes mellitus	ACE inhibitor, ARB				
	Pregnancy	Methyldopa, BB, calcium antagonist				
	Blacks	Diuretic, calcium antagonist				
JNC8						
	Nonblacks, including T2D	Initiate thiazide-type diuretic or ACEI or ARB or CCB, alone or in combination				
	CKD ± diabetes, all races	Initiate ACE inhibitor or ARB, alone or in combination with other drug class				
	Blacks, including T2D	Initiate thiazide-type diuretic or CCB, alone or in combination				
CHEP 2015	Diastolic hypertension ± systolic hypertension (target BP <140/90 mmHg)	Thiazide/thiazide-like diuretics, BBs, ACE inhibitors, ARBs, or long-acting CCBs (consider ASA and statins in selected patients). Consider initiating therapy with a combination of first-line drugs if the BP is 20 Hg	Combinations of first-line drugs			Not recommended for monotherapy: α-blockers, BBs in those 60 years of age, ACE inhibitors in black people. Hypokalemia should be avoided in those prescribed diuretics. ACE inhibitors, ARBs, and direct renin inhibitors are

Guideline	Specific condition	Treatment				
		Initial	2nd line	3rd line	4th line	Notes
		systolic or 10 mmHg diastolic above target				potential teratogens, and caution is required if prescribing to women with child-bearing potential. Combination of an ACE inhibitor with an ARB is not recommended
	LVH (target BP <140/90 mmHg)	ACE inhibitor, ARB, long-acting CCB, or thiazide/thiazide-like diuretics	Combination of additional agents			Hydralazine and minoxidil should not be used
	Nondiabetic CKD (target BP <140/90 mmHg)					
	Renovascular disease	Does not affect initial treatment recommendations. Renal artery stenosis should be primarily managed medically	Combinations of additional agents			Caution with ACE inhibitors or ARB if bilateral renal artery stenosis or unilateral disease with solitary kidney. Renal artery angioplasty and stenting could be considered for patients with renal artery stenosis and complicated, uncontrolled hypertension
	Cardiovascular disease (target BP <140/90 mmHg)					
	Past stroke or TIA	ACE inhibitor and a thiazide/thiazide-like diuretic combination	Combination of additional agents			Treatment of hypertension should not be routinely undertaken in acute stroke unless extreme BP increase. Combination of an ACE inhibitor with an ARB is not recommended
	Recent MI	BBs and ACE inhibitors (ARBs if ACE inhibitor intolerant)	Long-acting CCBs if BB contraindicated or not effective			Nondihydropyridine CCBs should not be used with concomitant HF
	CAD	ACE inhibitors or ARBs; BBs for patients with stable angina	Long-acting CCBs. When combination therapy is being			Avoid short-acting nifedipine. Combination of an ACE inhibitor with an ARB is specifically not

Guideline	Specific condition	Treatment				
		Initial	2nd line	3rd line	4th line	Notes
			used for high-risk patients, an ACE inhibitor/dihydropyridine CCB is preferred			recommended. Exercise caution when lowering SBP to target if DBP is ≤ 60 mmHg
		For patients with stable angina, BBs are preferred as initial therapy (Grade B). CCBs may also be used (Grade B)				
	HF	ACE inhibitors (ARBs if ACE inhibitor intolerant) and BBs. Aldosterone antagonists (mineralocorticoid receptor antagonists) may be added for patients with a recent cardiovascular hospitalization, acute MI, increased BNP or NT-proBNP level, or NYHA class II -IV symptoms	ACE inhibitor and ARB combined. Hydralazine/isosorbide dinitrate combination if ACE inhibitor and ARB contraindicated or not tolerated. Thiazide/thiazide-like or loop diuretics are recommended as additive therapy. Dihydropyridine CCB can also be used			Titrate doses of ACE inhibitors and ARBs to those used in clinical trials. Carefully monitor potassium and renal function if combining any of ACE inhibitor, ARB, and/ or aldosterone antagonist
	Nondiabetic CKD with proteinuria ** (target BP <140/90 mmHg)	ACE inhibitors (ARBs if ACE inhibitor-intolerant) if there is proteinuria, diuretics as additive therapy	Combinations of additional agents			Carefully monitor renal function and potassium for those receiving an ACE inhibitor or ARB. Combinations of an ACE inhibitor and ARB are not recommended in patients without proteinuria
	Peripheral arterial disease	Does not affect initial treatment recommendations	Combinations of additional agents			Avoid BBs with severe disease
	Isolated systolic hypertension without other compelling indications (target BP for age	Thiazide/thiazide-like diuretics, ARBs, or	Combinations of first-line drugs			Same as diastolic hypertension ± systolic

http://dx.doi.org/10.5772/63558

Guideline	Specific condition	Treatment				
		Initial	2nd line	3rd line	4th line	Notes
	<80 years is <140/90 mmHg; for age ≥ 80 years: target SBP is <150 mmHg)	long-acting dihydropyridine CCBs				hypertension
	Dyslipidemia	Does not affect initial treatment recommendations	Combinations of additional agents			
	Diabetes mellitus (target BP <130/80 mmHg) Diabetes mellitus with microalbuminuria,* renal disease, cardiovascular disease, or additional cardiovascular risk factors	ACE inhibitors or ARBs	Addition of a dihydropyridine CCB is preferred over a thiazide/thiazide-like diuretic			A loop diuretic could be considered in hypertensive CKD patients with extracellular fluid volume overload
	Diabetes mellitus not included in the above category	ACE inhibitors, ARBs, dihydropyridine CCBs or thiazide/ thiazide-like diuretics	Combination of first-line drugs. If combination with ACE inhibitor is being considered, a dihydropyridine CCB is preferable to a thiazide/thiazide-like diuretic			Normal urine microalbumin to creatinine ratio <2.0 mg/mmol
	Blacks	ACE inhibitors are not recommended as first-line therapy for uncomplicated hypertension in black patients				
	Overall vascular protection	Statin therapy for patients with 3 or more cardiovascular risk factors or atherosclerotic disease. Low-dose ASA in patients 50 years of age. Advise on smoking cessation and use pharmacotherapy for smoking cessation if indicated				Caution should be exercised with the ASA recommendation if BP is not controlled
NICE 2011	Aged <55 years, non-black: target BP below: 140/90 mmHg in people aged <80	Step 1: ACE inhibitor or ARB	Step 2: CCB in combination with	Step 3: Step 2 optimal or best	Step 4: Low-dose	BBs not preferred initial therapy, maybe in

Guideline	Specific condition	Treatment				
		Initial	2nd line	3rd line	4th line	Notes
	years (http://www.nice.org.uk/guidance/cg127)		ACE inhibitor or ARB	tolerated doses or combination of ACE inhibitor or ARB, CCB, and thiazide-like diuretic	spironolactone (25 mg/d) if blood potassium level ≤4.5 mmol/L; higher-dose thiazide-like diuretic if blood potassium level >4.5 mmol/L. If further diuretic therapy not tolerated, contraindicated, or ineffective: α-blocker or BB	younger people '… with intolerance or contraindication to ACE inhibitor or ARB '… women of child-bearing potential or '… increased sympathetic drive Initial therapy with BB + second drug CCB not thiazide-like diuretic reduce risk of developing diabetes NICE new evidence uncertainties: 'Different antihypertensive strategies in patients with diabetes, nephropathy and a history of MI for the treatment of hypertension and prevention of HF'
	Diabetes and kidney disease: BP target <130/80 mmHg (nice.org.uk/guidance/ng28, nice.org.uk/guidance/cg182)	RAS antagonist to: '- patients with CKD and diabetes and ACR ≥3 mg/mmol '- patients with CKD and hypertension and ACR ≥30 mg/mmol '- all patients with ACR ≥70 mg/mmol (irrespective of hypertension or CVD) In patients with CKD, hypertension and ACR <30 mg/mmol but no diabetes treat according to hypertension guidelines				Do not offer a combination of RAS antagonists to people with CKD [new 2014]
	Diabetes and cerebrovascular damage: BP target <130/80mmHg					

http://dx.doi.org/10.5772/63558

Guideline	Specific condition	Treatment				
		Initial	2nd line	3rd line	4th line	Notes
	(nice.org.uk/guidance/ng28)					
	HF (nice.org.uk/guidance/cg108; http://www.nice.org.uk/guidance/cg127)	Amlodipine Step1: to people aged > 55 years and to black people of African or Caribbean family origin of any age. If there is edema or intolerance, or evidence of HF or a high risk of HF, offer a thiazide-like diuretic	If a CCB is not suitable for step 2 treatment, for example because of oedema or intolerance, or if there is evidence of heart failure or a high risk of heart failure, offer a thiazide-like diuretic.			Verapamil, diltiazem or short-acting dihydropyridine agents should be avoided
	BP <140/80 mmHg (nice.org.uk/guidance/ng28)	ACE or if intolerant ARB African or Caribbean family origin ACE inhibitor + plus either diuretic or CCB.	CCB or diuretic (thiazide or thiazide-related diuretic)	Add the other drug (ie CCB or diuretic)	α-blocker, a BB or a potassium-sparing diuretic (caution if already taking ACE inhibitor or ARB)	not combine ACE inhibitor with ARB
	Women of child-bearing potential	BBs or see hypertension guidelines in specific situations (eg preeclampsia, diabetes (CCB) etc.) (nice.org.uk/guidance/cg107)				
	Black people of African or Caribbean family origin, age >55 years	CCB If CCB not suitable, eg edema or intolerance, HF, or high risk of HF: thiazide-like diuretic	Black people of African or Caribbean family origin, consider an ARB in preference to an ACE inhibitor, in combination with CCB			
	Age >80 years: BP target 150/90 mmHg	same antihypertensive drug treatment as age >55 years, taking into account any				

Guideline	Specific condition	Treatment				
		Initial	2nd line	3rd line	4th line	Notes
		comorbidities				
	Diabetes and eye: BP target <130/80 mmHg (nice.org.uk/guidance/ng28)					
AHA/ACC/CDC	Systolic 140–159 or diastolic 90–99 mmHg	Thiazide	Thiazide for most patients or ACE inhibitor, ARB, CCB or combination	Optimize dosage or add medications		
	Systolic >160 or diastolic >100 mmHg	Thiazide and ACE inhibitor, ARB, or CCB or consider ACE inhibitor and CCB				
	Kidney disease	ACE inhibitor, ARB				
	Stroke and TIA	Thiazide, ACE inhibitor				
	CAD/post MI	BB, ACE inhibitor				
	Systolic HF Diastolic HF	ACE inhibitor or ARB, BB, aldosterone antagonist, thiazide ACE inhibitor or ARB, BB thiazide				
	Diabetes	ACE inhibitor or ARB, thiazide, BB				
ASH/ISH	Nonblack, stage 1, age <60 years	ACE inhibitor or ARB	CCB or thiazide	CCB + Thiazide + ACE inhibitor or (ARB),	spironolactone, centrally acting agents, BBs	
	Stage 2	Start with 2 drugs: CCB or thiazide + ACE inhibitor or ARB		CCB + thiazide + ACE inhibitor or (ARB),	spironolactone, centrally acting agents, BBs	
	CAD	BB + ACE inhibitor or ARB	CCB or thiazide	CCB or thiazide		
	Stroke	ACE inhibitor or ARB	Thiazide or CCB	CCB or thiazide		
	HF	ACE inhibitor or ARB + BB + diuretic + spironolactone regardless of BP	Dihydropyridine CCB			
	CKD	ACE inhibitor or ARB, in blacks ACE inhibitor	CCB or thiazide	Thiazide or CCB		
	Diabetes	ARB or ACE inhibitor, in blacks CCB or thiazide	CCB or thiazide, in blacks ACE inhibitor or ARB	Thiazide or CCB		
	Blacks, stage 1, all ages	CCB or thiazide	ACE inhibitor or	CCB + thiazide	spironolactone,	
			ARB or combine CCB + thiazide	+ ACE inhibitor or (ARB),	centrally acting agents, BBs	
	Non-black, age ≥60 years	CCB or thiazide	ACE inhibitor or ARB	CCB + thiazide + ACE inhibitor or (ARB),	spironolactone, centrally acting agents, BBs	

*Microalbuminuria defined as persistent ACR > 2.0 mg/mmol;** Proteinuria defined as urinary protein > 500 mg per 24 hours or ACR > 30 mg/mmol in 2 of 3 specimens.
ACC = American College of Cardiology; ACE = angiotensin-converting enzyme; ACR = albumin:creatinine ratio; AHA = American Heart Association; ARB = angiotensin receptor blocker; ASA = acetylsalicylic acid; ASH = American Society of Hypertension; BB = β-blocker; BP = blood pressure; CAD = coronary artery disease; CCB = calcium channel blocker; CDC = Centers for Disease Control and Prevention; CHEP = Canadian Hypertension Education Program; CKD = chronic kidney disease; CV = cardiovascular; CVD = cardiovascular disease; ESRD = end-stage renal disease; ESC = European Society of Cardiology; ESH = European Society of Hypertension; HF = heart failure; ISH = International Society of Hypertension; JNC = Joint National Committee; LVH = left ventricular hypertrophy; MI = myocardial infarction; NICE = National Institute for Health and Care Excellence; NT-proBNP = *N*-terminal pro-brain natriuretic peptide; NYHA = New York Heart Association; RAS = renin–angiotensin system; T2D = type 2 diabetes; TIA = transient ischemic attack.

Table 4. Summary of hypertension treatment guidelines.

4.1.1. European Society of Cardiology/European Society of Hypertension

The European Society of Cardiology/European Society of Hypertension (ESC/ESH) guidelines [121] categorize patients with hypertension according to their BP, medical history, physical

http://dx.doi.org/10.5772/63558

examination, and laboratory parameters. The ESC/ESH guideline recommends that physicians detect causes of secondary hypertension, record cardiovascular risk factors, and identify other cardiovascular diseases. It further advises the evaluation of familial (genetic) predisposition to hypertension and cardiovascular disease and alludes to 29 SNPs that are associated with systolic and/or diastolic BP and could be useful contributors to risk scores for organ damage. Methodologies to detect asymptomatic organ damage in the individual patient are described. The focus for the heart is on left ventricular hypertrophy; for the vessels, it is on arterial stiffness and carotid plaque load; for kidney function, on glomerular filtration rate and the existence of established renal parenchymatous disease on proteinuria. For the brain, the guidelines refer to silent infarctions, white matter hyperintensities, and microbleeds.

In general, the ESC/ESH guideline concludes that the main benefits of antihypertensive treatment are due to lowering of BP per se and are largely independent of the drugs employed. Thus, all drug classes are suitable for the initiation and maintenance of antihypertensive treatment, either as monotherapy or in combination. The guideline discusses the hypotheses behind BP recommendations (i.e., the "lower the better" vs. J-shaped curve theories) and suggests that targeted BP will have to be revisited with additional data concerning associated organ damage and evaluating different end points (left ventricular hypertrophy, new-onset microalbuminuria, renal failure, cardiovascular events, etc.). Despite this uncertainty, the ESC/ESH guideline recommends continued monitoring for asymptomatic organ damage. It suggests therapy stratification of antihypertensive drugs for specific conditions and organ damage types (e.g., with some organ damage certain hypertension medications are discouraged because of contraindications, while others are recommended, as they show a greater effectiveness). Monitoring of end-organ damage with (bio)markers (e.g., serum creatinine level, electrocardiograph, echocardiograph, ankle-brachial index, etc.) to detect regression with treatment, progression of hypertension-dependent abnormalities, as well as the appearance of conditions requiring additional therapeutic interventions (such as arrhythmias, myocardial ischemia, stenotic plaques, and heart failure) is valued in the ESC/ESH guidelines. Further detail is given on the combinatory possibilities of the drug classes.

4.1.2. US Eighth Joint National Committee

The US Eighth Joint National Committee (JNC8) guideline [122] presents an evidence-based approach for the management of hypertension in adults to recommend treatment thresholds, goals, and medications. JNC8 stratifies its blood-pressure-lowering therapy recommendations based on age, ethnicity (black vs. non-black), diabetes, and chronic kidney disease (CKD).

JNC8 gives eight recommendations based on systematic review of the literature. A ninth recommendation was developed by the panel members based on expert opinion to aid physicians in implementing JNC8. It includes an algorithm summarizing recommendations 1–8 and advice on combining antihypertensive drugs. JNC8 acknowledges that recommendation 9 has not been validated with respect to achieving improved patient outcomes and there will likely be no supporting evidence from well-designed randomized controlled trials.

The JNC8 dosing regimen proposes three strategies:

- Start one drug, titrate to maximum dose, and then add a second drug.
- Start one drug and then add a second drug before achieving maximum dose of the initial drug.
- Begin with two drugs at the same time, either as two separate pills or as a single pill combination.

If BP goals are not achieved, then JNC8 urges that second and third drugs are added from the list. Continuous monitoring of BP is advised to adjust the treatment regimen until target BP is reached. The combination of an ACEi and angiotensin receptor blocker should not be used. If an antihypertensive drug is not effective in a specific situation or has an adverse effect, it can be replaced.

4.1.3. Canadian Hypertension Education Program guideline

The Canadian Hypertension Education Program (CHEP) treatment guidelines [123] provide recommendations for the indication of drug therapy, therapy goals, and detailed patient categorization according to their organ damage or comorbidities. For individuals with diastolic and/or systolic hypertension, no rigid specification is provided for initial therapy. The physician can chose from β-blocker, thiazide/thiazide-like diuretic, long-acting calcium channel blocker (CCB), or ACEi/ARB taking into consideration patient age (β-blocker only in patients aged <60 years) and ethnicity (ACEi in non-black patients).

In isolated hypertension, β-blockers are no longer part of first-line therapy if patients are aged ≥60 years.

In general, the CHEP guideline recommends global vascular protection therapy for adults with hypertension without compelling indications for specific agents, including statin therapy in hypertensive patients with ≥3 cardiovascular risk factors and acetylsalicylic acid therapy in hypertensive patients aged ≥50 years.

Additional hypertension treatment categories are ischemic heart disease (coronary artery disease or a recent myocardial infarction), heart failure, stroke (acute and non-acute management), left ventricular hypertrophy, non-diabetic CKD, renovascular disease, and diabetes mellitus. The specific and detailed BP targets and pharmacological recommendations specifying initial therapy, second-line therapy, and notes and/or cautions for hypertension are summarized.

4.1.4. UK National Institute for Health and Care Excellence hypertension guideline

The UK National Institute for Health and Care Excellence (NICE) hypertension guideline (http://www.nice.org.uk/guidance/cg127) uses patient age as the starting point for their recommendations, with treatment escalation in a stepwise fashion if BP is not adequately controlled. If the patient is aged <55 years, step 1 antihypertensive treatment is an ACEi or a low-cost ARB. In patients aged ≥55 and black people of African or Caribbean family origin of any age, NICE recommends a CCB. A thiazide-like diuretic (chlorthalidone, indapamide) can be selected instead of a CCB if the patients present with edema, intolerance, heart failure, or a high risk of heart failure.

In step 2, NICE recommends the addition of a CCB to the ACEi or ARB. Alternatively, a thiazide-like diuretic can be used. In step 3, the combination of ACEi (ARB), CCB, and thiazide-like diuretic should be used. Resistant hypertension is treated at step 4 by adding diuretics (low-dose spironolactone, higher-dose thiazide-like diuretic) or a β-blocker or an α-blocker to the treatment regimen.

NICE recommends that patients aged ≥80 years should receive the same antihypertensive regimen as people aged >55, taking into account any comorbidities. Patients with isolated systolic hypertension (systolic BP ≥160 mmHg) should be treated with the same regimen as those with both raised systolic and diastolic BP. β-Blockers are not preferred for initial therapy in hypertension, but could be considered in younger patients with evidence of increased sympathetic drive, intolerance, or contraindication to ACEi and ARB, or for women of child-bearing potential. If β-blockers are required, then a CCB rather than a thiazide-like diuretic should be added to reduce the risk of developing diabetes.

BP targets and therapy recommendations for hypertensive patients with diabetes and/or CKD are not given in the NICE hypertension guideline but appear separately in the NICE guidelines for type 2 diabetes (NG28; http://www.nice.org.uk/guidance/ng28) and CKD (CG182; chronic-kidney-disease-in-adults-assessment-and-management-35109809343205). Since publication of the hypertension guidelines in 2011, there has been an evidence update (https://www.nice.org.uk/guidance/cg127/evidence/evidence-update-248584429).

In brief, current NICE treatment recommendations for patients with diabetes (http://www.nice.org.uk/guidance/ng28) comprise first-line treatment with an ACEi or an ARB. If the patient is of African or Caribbean family origin, an ACEi/ARB should be combined with a diuretic or a CCB. Second and third steps could be a CCB and/or a diuretic. BP targets are 140/80 mmHg (or 130/80 mmHg if there is kidney, eye, or cerebrovascular damage). Patients with CKD (albumin:creatinine ratio (ACR) ≥30 mg/mmol) and hypertension should be started on an ACEi/ARB. Patients with CKD and an ACR <30 mg/mmol and no diabetes should follow NICE hypertension guideline recommendations (http://www.nice.org.uk/guidance/cg182). Patients with diabetes and an ACR ≥3 mg/mmol or an ACR ≥70 mg/mmol (irrespective of hypertension or cardiovascular disease) should also be treated with an ACEi/ARB. In patients with CKD, target systolic BP should be <140 mmHg and diastolic <90 mmHg (unless they also have diabetes, see above).

4.1.5. American Heart Association/American College of Cardiology/Centers for Disease Control and Prevention treatment algorithm

The AHA, American College of Cardiology, and CDC hypertension management algorithm recommends stratifying treatment according to hypertension stages [124]. Patients with stage 1 hypertension should start with lifestyle modification and treatment with a thiazide diuretic should be considered. Patients with stage 2 hypertension should immediately start a thiazide with either an ACEi or ARB or a CCB. Alternatively, an ACEi and CCB combination could also be used. If BP cannot be controlled, they recommend a thiazide for most patients or an ACEi, ARB, or a CCB, or a combination. The next treatment step involves using the highest tolerated dose or adding another antihypertensive.

The AHA/ACC/CDC algorithm recommends different medications depending on the medical conditions associated with hypertension as follows:

- Coronary artery disease/post-myocardial infarction: β-blockers, ACEi.
- Systolic heart failure: ACEi or ARB, β-blockers, aldosterone receptor blocker, thiazide.
- Diastolic heart failure: ACEi or ARB, β-blockers, thiazide.
- Diabetes: ACEi or ARB, thiazide, β-blockers, CCB.
- Kidney disease: ACEi or ARB.
- Stroke or transient ischemic attack: thiazide, ACEi.

4.1.6. American Society of Hypertension/International Society of Hypertension clinical practice guidelines

In the American Society of Hypertension and International Society of Hypertension clinical practice guidelines, the BP targets are defined according to age and comorbidities [125]. The target is 140/90 mmHg in the general hypertensive population. In older patients (aged >80 years), the goal is <150/90 mmHg unless these patients have CKD or diabetes, in which case <140/90 mmHg can be considered. With most patients requiring more than one drug, the increase of the dose and/or adding a new drug to achieve BP control is required. If the untreated BP is ≥20/10 mmHg above the target BP, treatment should be started with two drugs simultaneously. The choice of drug is dependent on age, ethnicity/race, and other clinical characteristics and comorbid conditions (e.g., diabetes, coronary artery disease, etc.) of the patient.

4.2. Government health agencies' perspectives on personalized medicine

The European Health Research Directorate of the European Commission defined PHC as a medical model using molecular profiling for tailoring the right therapeutic strategy for the right person at the right time, and/or to determine the predisposition to disease and/or to deliver timely and targeted prevention with fewer side effects. In support of the 2020 vision for PHC in Europe, the Health Research Directorate of the European Commission started with a series of four preparatory workshops (http://ec.europa.eu/research/health/pdf/towards-personalised-medicine-leaflet_en.pdf; http://ec.europa.eu/research/health/index.cfm?pg=policy&policyname=personalised, PerMed: http://www.permed2020.eu/) on personalized medicine covering

- The role of "-omics" technologies for personalized medicine (http://ec.europa.eu/research/health/pdf/summary-report-omics-for-personalised-medicine-workshop_en.pdf).
- Stratification biomarkers (http://ec.europa.eu/research/health/pdf/biomarkers-for-patient-stratification_en.pdf).

- Clinical trials and regulatory aspects.
- Opportunities and challenges for European health care (http://ec.europa.eu/research/health/pdf/13th-european-health-forum-workshop-report_en.pdf).

This was followed by a conference entitled "European Perspectives in Personalized Medicine" in 2011, acknowledging the huge potential for PHC and the multitude of challenges (http://ec.europa.eu/research/health/pdf/personalised-medicine-conference-report_en.pdf). In 2013, the Commission developed a staff working document on "-omics" technologies in PHC (http://ec.europa.eu/research/health/pdf/2013-10_personalised_medicine_en.pdf). In 2014, an additional workshop for Regulatory Aspects and Early Dialogue EHFG Forum 4 "Personalised Medicine 2020" – October 2, 2014, Bad Hofgastein, Austria (http://www.permed2020.eu/_media/2_EMA_02-10-14_Ehmann.pdf), was held.

As part of the Horizon 2020 program, a call for a proposal has been issued for "Coordinating personalized medicine research" (http://ec.europa.eu/research/participants/portal/desktop/en/opportunities/h2020/topics/2449-sc1-hco-05-2016.html). Thus, the European Commission attributes great importance to the topic of PHC in general.

Expectations regarding potential benefits for patients, clinicians, and health-care systems are as follows:

- Ability to make better-informed medical decisions,
- Higher probability of desired outcomes owing to better-targeted therapies,
- Reduced probability of adverse reactions to medicines,
- Focus on the prevention and prediction of disease rather than on reaction to it,
- Earlier disease intervention than has been possible in the past, and
- Improved health-care cost containment.

4.3. Assessment of guideline content

Although some therapy guidance is provided by the guidelines, the method of selection for antihypertensive therapy is largely empirical [126] and an individual cardiovascular and renal event risk assessment is yet not possible. In the various guidelines, different approaches have been taken to stratify patients and integrate BP with either age and ethnicity or other risk factors. Some guidelines (e.g., NICE) focused primarily on the age and ethnicity most likely associated with differences in plasma renin activity, while others provide specific recommendations to integrate different asymptomatic organ damage, metabolic conditions, and cardiovascular and renal comorbidities to establish an individual patient regimen (e.g., CHEP 2015). This approach is based on the finding that BP reduction is not considered to be the only mechanism acting to reduce cardiovascular risk, as BP-independent, probably class-specific effects seem to contribute to the effects of risk reduction with BP-lowering drugs. In a recent meta-analysis, the evidence of risk reduction for congestive heart disease and heart failure, and particularly mortality, was found with some drug classes only [127].

There are efforts to understand the molecular underpinnings of BP regulation. The hope is that this will improve the prediction of cardiovascular susceptibility and thus could in the future offer insight into personalized hypertension treatment. As hypertension is a difficult phenotype to access, owing to its variability and susceptibility to other environmental factors and physiological pathways, another approach could be to search for predictors of antihypertensive drug responses. If robust predictors of BP response are available, therapy stratification will be feasible, which could facilitate treatment success.

The available data on genetic markers have been promising in terms of defining genetic determinants of response to antihypertensive drugs. However, no studies to date have been sufficiently powered with an effect size large enough to allow genetic markers of antihypertensive drug responses to be included in the guidelines to inform individualized antihypertensive treatment decisions. Despite a lack of pharmacogenomics for personalized antihypertension treatment-guided approaches, Clinical Pharmacogenetics Implementation Consortium guidelines [128] are available for other cardiovascular drugs (i.e., clopidogrel [129], warfarin [130], and simvastatin [131]).

To overcome the challenges (small sample sizes in available studies with well-characterized BP responses and genetic data, replication of genomic signals in independent cohorts, identification of the biological basis for the genetic association, etc.), the International Consortium for Antihypertensive Pharmacogenomics Studies was formed in 2012. In addition, the US President Barack Obama has announced a research initiative that aims to accelerate progress toward a new era of precision medicine ([132], www.whitehouse.gov/precisionmedicine) and the National Institutes of Health and other partners are implementing this vision (http://www.nih.gov/precision-medicine-initiative-cohort-program).

5. PHC from a physician's perspective

Despite advances in research and technologies, the PHC concept is still new for a number of physicians and it remains unclear how quickly the adoption of PHC into routine practice will occur.

5.1. Warfarin and statins: a field study on genetic testing

There is wide variation in inter-individual responses to anticoagulants, such as clopidogrel, as well as to statin therapy with underlying genetic differences assumed to be responsible [133, 134]. In fact, of patients with an acute myocardial infarction treated with clopidogrel, those carrying CYP2C19 loss-of-function alleles had a higher rate of subsequent cardiovascular events than non-carriers of that allele [135]. The FDA even published a black-box warning regarding clopidogrel administration, as 2–14% of the population are poor CYP2C19 metabolizers and hence require alternative clopidogrel dosing in order to effectively prevent clotting, heart attacks, and strokes [136].

Also for the target molecule of statins, 3-hydroxy-3-methylglutaryl-coenzyme A reductase, it is known that, compared with individual homozygous for the major allele of one of the SNPs, individuals with a single copy of the minor allele had up to 22% less reduction in total cholesterol levels [133].

Genetic screening to guide selection of anticoagulation and lipid-lowering therapy has been limited to date, because solid clinical data to support its use are not yet available [133, 137, 138]. However, it is believed that the formal integration of genetic testing to optimize warfarin dosage would reduce over- or under-coagulation of patients. In the US alone, optimal coagulation has been estimated to translate into an annual reduction of 85,000 serious bleeding events and 17,000 strokes, leading to a reduction in health-care spending of about $1.1 billion [139]. In order to investigate the current use and evolution of genetic testing in clinical practice, interviews with cardiologists in the USA and Germany have recently been conducted.

In a substudy of a recently published analysis [140], we interviewed 39 cardiologists in private practices, community hospitals, and academic centers in the USA and Germany about their use of genetic testing for diagnosis and treatment, and treatment guidance. Physicians were initially asked about how frequently they order genetic (genotyping) tests for cardiovascular risk factors in patients with heart failure: (i) before prescribing warfarin or clopidogrel and (ii) before prescribing statin drugs or hydralazine. They were also asked (iii) how frequently they order genetic tests to diagnose or assess the risk of long QT syndrome and various cardiomyopathies or to monitor transplant rejection in heart-transplant patients. In conclusion, the cardiologists were asked (iv) how they expect the use of personalized medicine tests to change in the area of heart failure and hypertension. These interviews were conducted by three neutral, interview-experienced researchers employed by Enterprise Analysis Corporation (EAC; Stamford, CT, USA), all of whom had strong diagnostic knowledge (one MD, one PhD, and one BS, MBA).

The results of our interviews are summarized in **Table 5** and **Figure 3**. Only one US cardiologist routinely ordered genotyping tests to determine patient response to clopidogrel or warfarin. The majority of interviewees indicated that they never or rarely ordered these tests in cases of non-response to treatment, with numbers being close to equal in the USA and Germany. Functional thrombocyte tests were ordered as they were reimbursed. In the case of statins, only one cardiologist in the USA and two in Germany ordered genetic tests frequently for all patients to assess responsiveness to statin drugs or for inheritance of familial hypercholesterolemia. About 10% of interviewees ordered these tests occasionally but more than 80% never or rarely ordered these types of tests. Limited clinical benefit, cost, and reimbursement were mentioned as the main reasons for not using these tests. Although patients with cardiomyopathies, such as long QT syndrome, and transplant patients, were rare compared with anticoagulation patients, physicians seem to be aware of the genetic tests that have been developed for those conditions. Fifteen percent of the physicians mentioned that they ordered these genetic tests occasionally when they see such a case, but 44% said that they never ordered these tests. Physicians in private practice often indicated that they referred their patients to an academic center for specialized evaluation.

	never	rarely	occasionally	frequently	all patients	total
Warfarin / Plavix						
Germany	12 (60%)	7 (35%)	1 (5%)	0 (0%)	0 (0%)	20 (100%)
USA	10 (53%)	7 (37%)	1 (5%)	0 (0%)	1 (5%)	19 (100%)
Total	**22 (56%)**	**14 (36%)**	**2 (5%)**	0 (0%)	**1 (3%)**	**39 (100%)**
Statins						
Germany	10 (50%)	6 (30%)	2 (10%)	1 (5%)	1 (5%)	20 (100%)
USA	10 (53%)	6 (32%)	2 (10%)	0 (0%)	1 (5%)	19 (100%)
Total	**20 (51%)**	**12 (31%)**	**4 (10%)**	**1 (3%)**	**2 (5%)**	**39 (100%)**
Cardiomyopathies / long QT						
Germany	9 (45%)	4 (20%)	3 (15%)	2 (10%)	2 (10%)	20 (100%)
USA	8 (42%)	6 (32%)	3 (16%)	2 (10%)	0 (0%)	19 (100%)
Total	**17 (44%)**	**10 (26%)**	**6 (15%)**	**4 (10%)**	**2 (5%)**	**39 (100%)**

Table 5. Physician responses concerning the use of genetic testing for warfarin/clopidogrel prescription, statin prescription, and in cardiomyopathies such as long QT syndrome.

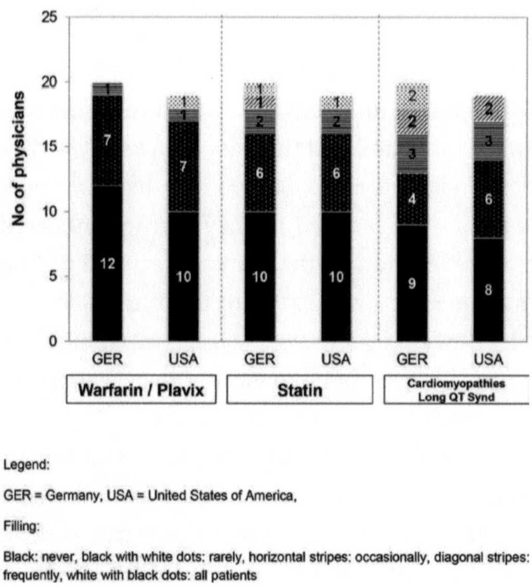

Figure 3. Physicians' responses concerning the use of genetic tests in cardiology.

Despite the fact that currently most cardiologists barely use PHC tests, most believe that the use of such tests will increase over the next decade. In the USA, 89% anticipate growth in the use of these tests, with 37% expecting a slight, 47% a moderate, and 5% a substantial growth. In Germany, 85% of physicians predict an increased usage of personalized medicine in cardiology, with 20% expecting a substantial, 60% a moderate, and 5% a slight growth. Only 15% of the German cardiologists and 11% of the US cardiologists do not anticipate any change in the use of these tests (see **Table 6**).

Country	**Expected change, No. of responses (%)**			
	Substantial	**Moderate**	**Slight**	**No change**
Germany (n=20)	4 (20%)	12 (60%)	1 (5%)	3 (15%)
USA (n=19)	1 (5%)	9 (47%)	7 (37%)	2 (11%)
Total (n=39)	**5** **(13%)**	**21** **(54%)**	**8** **(21%)**	**5** **(13%)**

Table 6. Expected change in the use of personalized medicine in cardiology.

Despite the fact that the concept of personalized medicine has been discussed in cardiology for over a decade, our study has confirmed that there is still no regular use of genetic tests for pharmacogenomic-guided treatment in cardiovascular disease [139]. Although cardiologists are known to order general in vitro diagnostic (IVD) tests in 60% of their consultations with the results of these tests influencing diagnosis or treatment decisions in 70% of cases [140], the use of genetic testing is still rare in routine cardiology. Our study has shown that only one to three cardiologists out of 39 ordered genetic tests on a regular basis before prescribing anticoagulation or statins. For long QT syndrome and other rare cardiomyopathies, physicians indicated more frequent use of genetic testing, with 15% of cardiologists using them occasionally.

One reason for the limited use of genetic testing for pharmacogenomics in cardiology seems to be a lack of sufficient clinical evidence. Physicians often indicate that there is no adequate benefit to be gained from these tests, which has been mentioned in earlier studies [139]. Even though newer studies have demonstrated the value of genetic testing (e.g., identifying CYP2C19*2 carriers for antiplatelet treatment with prasugrel rather than with clopidogrel to reduce high on-treatment platelet reactivity after percutaneous coronary intervention [141]), larger clinical utility studies might be needed. Another reason stated by the physicians is the cost of these tests or the lack of reimbursement. Both reasons highlight little awareness of the value of genetic testing in terms of economic benefits, which would equal clinical utility and cost-effectiveness [142]. This indicates that more studies are needed to generate clinical evidence and proof of economic value for genetic testing in patients with cardiovascular diseases.

To showcase a successful example of how PHC is used in a sub-entity of HT, the next chapter focuses on the development of the sFlt-1/PlGF ratio, used to guide treatment decisions in patients with preeclampsia. Despite being a secondary form of hypertension, its prevalence is associated with the existence of chronic hypertension in women. While in the general population the risk of preeclampsia is 3–5%, around 17–25% of women with chronic hypertension develop superimposed preeclampsia [143].

6. PHC in preeclampsia

6.1. Hypertension in pregnancy

Hypertension is the most common complication of pregnancy [144]. Although many pregnant women with high BP have healthy babies, hypertension during pregnancy can be dangerous for both mother and fetus. Hypertensive disorders of pregnancy can be classified as follows: (a) chronic hypertension (high BP that either precedes pregnancy, is diagnosed within the first 20 weeks of pregnancy, or does not resolve by the 12-week postpartum checkup), (b) gestational hypertension (transient hypertension of pregnancy or chronic hypertension identified in the latter half of pregnancy), (c) preeclampsia-eclampsia, or (d) preeclampsia superimposed on chronic hypertension [144]. Effects of high BP range from mild to very severe, with serious cases causing maternal and fetal harm. Preeclampsia and eclampsia, in particular, can be life-threatening for mother and baby.

6.2. What is preeclampsia?

Preeclampsia is a heterogeneous, multi-organ disorder, which affects 3–5% of pregnancies worldwide and is a leading cause of maternal death [145–148]. It is associated with placental dysfunction and can result in adverse outcomes for mother and child. Maternal adverse outcomes include eclampsia (seizures), HELLP syndrome (hemolysis, elevated liver enzymes, low platelets), early delivery, placental abruption, renal failure, and death [149–151]. Adverse outcomes for the child include intrauterine growth restriction (IUGR), intraventricular hemorrhage, necrotizing enterocolitis, and perinatal death.

The clinical features of preeclampsia are often variable and non-specific. Hypertension is often present, and is associated with convulsions and other severe cerebral manifestations, but it is not easily differentiated from gestational hypertension or undiagnosed pre-existing chronic hypertension. Other signs include headache, proteinuria, visual disturbances, abdominal pain, edema, sudden weight gain, and vomiting. It is difficult to predict which women who present with these signs and symptoms during pregnancy will develop preeclampsia. There has been an unmet medical need to improve current predictive tools in order to better tailor the provision of specialized management and care to those women who require it.

6.3. Management of preeclampsia

Currently, there is no cure for preeclampsia, other than delivery of the baby. Available pharmacological interventions are limited and are generally aimed at treating the complications of the syndrome. Such treatments include anticonvulsive medication (magnesium sulfate [152]) and antihypertensive medications (e.g., labetalol), and the use of corticosteroids to promote fetal lung maturation ahead of preterm delivery. Clinical experience suggests that early detection, monitoring, and supportive care are important to improve maternal and fetal outcomes in this progressive syndrome, by allowing expeditious decision making and referral to specialist perinatal care centers [153–155]. This requires a reliable model of preeclampsia prediction in order to appropriately tailor management plans.

6.4. Clinical benefits of preeclampsia prediction: tailoring health care

The use of a clinical measurement (a biomarker) for the prediction of preeclampsia in women with signs of preeclampsia could facilitate PHC, and ensure that the right patients are identified for monitoring, for referral to specialist perinatal centers (if required), and to receive appropriate interventions. Furthermore, the ability to accurately rule out a diagnosis of preeclampsia could help prevent unnecessary hospitalization and the emotional stress for patients and their families that this entails. Targeted monitoring and management could also provide economic benefits for health-care providers, by reducing the level of monitoring required for those women unlikely to develop the syndrome. Advances in the understanding of preeclampsia pathogenesis have enabled the identification of potential biomarkers.

6.5. Pathology of preeclampsia

Historically, preeclampsia was defined by the new onset of hypertension and proteinuria during pregnancy. However, the definition of preeclampsia has recently been revised to include women with new-onset hypertension without new-onset proteinuria, provided that there are other new-onset manifestations (e.g., IUGR or maternal renal, hepatic, or neurologic dysfunction) [156]. In fact, preeclampsia is part of a wider spectrum of conditions, which involve placental dysfunction, decreased perfusion of the placenta, and inflammation (**Figure 4**).

In preeclampsia, incomplete remodeling of maternal spiral arteries can lead to intermittent placental hypoperfusion and oxidative stress, which in turn leads to an exaggerated maternal inflammatory response [157]. Immune factors (e.g., AT1-AA), oxidative stress, natural killer cell abnormalities, and other factors may cause placental dysfunction, leading to the release of anti-angiogenic factors, such as soluble fms-like tyrosine kinase-1 (sFlt-1) and soluble endoglin (sENG). Conversely, circulating maternal serum concentrations of pro-angiogenic placental growth factor (PlGF) are decreased (relative to normotensive pregnancies) [157]. This angiogenic imbalance is thought to cause vasoconstriction and generalized endothelial dysfunction, which may lead to preeclampsia and fetal growth restriction [158–160]. PlGF has been investigated as a potential diagnostic and predictive biomarker for preeclampsia [161–163]. The ratio of circulating maternal serum levels of sFlt-1 and PlGF has also been proposed as an indicator of preeclampsia; a high sFlt-1/PlGF ratio is associated with an increased risk of preeclampsia [164–170], and the ratio is elevated in pregnant women 4–5 weeks before the clinical onset of preeclampsia [166]. There has been evidence to suggest that the sFlt-1/PlGF ratio (which reflects the in situ balance of an anti-angiogenic factor and a pro-angiogenic factor) may be a better indicator of preeclampsia than either sFlt-1 or PlGF alone [171].

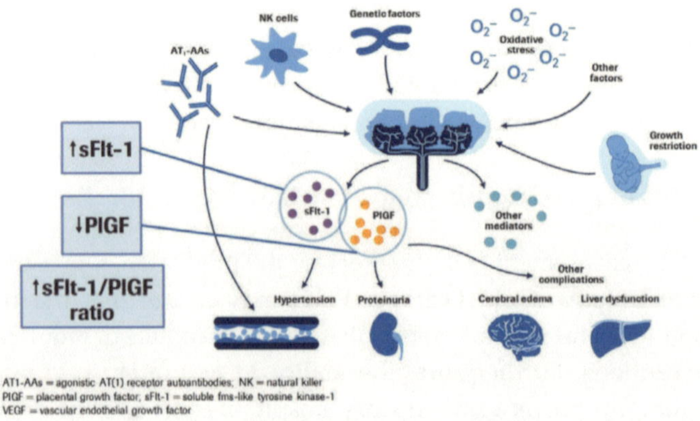

Figure 4. Pathophysiological features of preeclampsia (adapted from Wang A, Rana S, Karumanchi SA. Preeclampsia: the role of angiogenic factors in its pathogenesis. Physiology [Bethesda]. 2009;24:147–158).

6.6. Measurement of sFlt-1, PlGF, and the sFlt-1/PlGF ratio

There are a variety of commercially available tests for PlGF, which include the Elecsys® PlGF immunoassay (cobas e platform; Roche Diagnostics, Mannheim, Germany, **Table 7** [172]), Triage® PlGF test (Alere International, Waltham, MA) [173], DELFIA® Xpress PlGF 1-2-3 test (Perkin Elmer, Waltham, MA) [162, 163], and the BRAHMS PlGF Kryptor™ (Thermo Fisher Scientific, Waltham, MA) [174]. There are two sFlt-1 assays available: the Elecsys®sFlt-1 (cobas e platform; Roche Diagnostics) and the BRAHMS sFlt-1 Kryptor™ (Thermo Fisher Scientific) [175]). These are automated assays that use maternal serum.

	Elecsys® sFlt-1	Elecsys® PlGF
Assay time	18 min	18 min
Sample material	Serum	Serum
Sample volume	20 μL	50 μL
Detection limit	Approx. 6 pg/ml	< 2 pg/ml
Measuring range	10–85 000 pg/ml	3–10 000 pg/ml
Imprecision	< 5%	< 5%

Table 7. Product characteristics of the Elecsys® sFlt-1 and PlGF assays [172, 175].

http://dx.doi.org/10.5772/63558

The sFlt-1/PlGF ratio can be calculated using the Roche Elecsys® test or the BRAHMS Kryptor™ assays. It is important to note that the testing methods from different companies are not interchangeable, and the cutoff levels established with a one-assay ratio are not applicable to the other assays.

6.7. PlGF and the sFlt-1/PlGF for preeclampsia diagnosis

An Alere Triage® PlGF level of <36 pg/mL supports a diagnosis of preeclampsia [173]. In a method comparison study the Elecsys® immunoassay sFlt-1/PlGF ratio showed improved diagnostic utility over the Triage® PlGF assay with improved specificity as a diagnostic aid of preeclampsia [176].

For the Elecsys® sFlt-1/PlGF ratio, the reference median values during an uneventful pregnancy have been published (**Figure 5**). The analysis of elevated Elecsys® sFlt-1/PlGF ratios in women with preeclampsia has been used to establish recommended cutoff levels for preeclampsia diagnosis by gestational age [177]. For the early gestational phase (week 20 + 0 days to week 33 + 6 days), women with an sFlt-1/PlGF ratio of ≤33 had the lowest likelihood of a positive preeclampsia diagnosis (sensitivity/specificity of the test: 95/94%), and women with a ratio of ≥85 had the highest likelihood of a positive preeclampsia diagnosis (sensitivity/specificity: 88/99.5%). For the late gestational phase (week 34 to delivery), a cutoff of ≤33 to rule out diagnosis and a cutoff of ≥110 to rule in diagnosis has been recommended (sensitivity/specificity of 89.6/73.1% and 58.2/95.5%, respectively) [172, 175]. The Elecsys® sFlt-1/PlGF ratio is CE-IVD (Conformité Européenne–In Vitro Diagnostics) approved for use as an aid in the diagnosis of preeclampsia in conjunction with other diagnostic and clinical information.

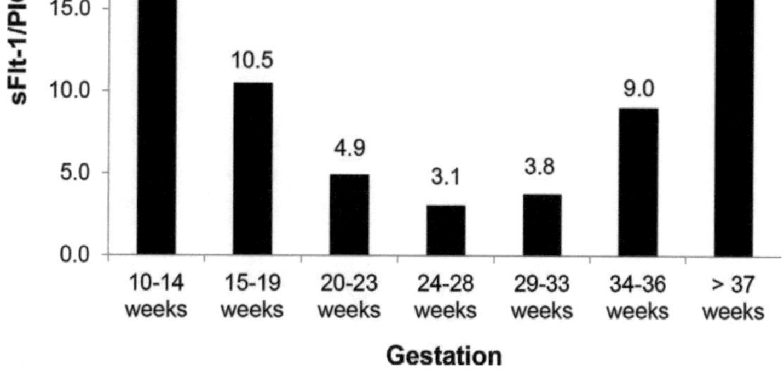

Figure 5. Median values of the Elecsys® sFlt-1/PlGF ratio in uneventful pregnancies [177].

The BRAHMS Kryptor™ sFlt-1/PlGF ratio was assessed for preeclampsia diagnostic utility in a recent small study ($n = 39$ women who developed preeclampsia including $n = 30$ women with late-onset preeclampsia; 76 controls). To diagnose preeclampsia (rule in preeclampsia), a BRAHMS Kryptor™ sFlt-1/PlGF ratio of >110 had a 67.7% specificity (late-onset preeclampsia), compared with the Roche Elecsys® sFlt-1/PlGF ratio showing 85.5% specificity [178].

6.8. The sFlt-1/PlGF ratio and preeclampsia prediction

To date, the BRAHMS sFlt-1/PlGF ratio has been assessed only for the diagnosis of preeclampsia [174, 178]. By contrast, the Elecsys® sFlt-1/PlGF ratio has been validated for both the diagnosis and the prediction of preeclampsia [172, 175]; it is the *predictive* role of the biomarker that is anticipated to guide PHC for preeclampsia, and so the results of studies examining the Elecsys® sFlt-1/PlGF ratio for preeclampsia prediction are discussed subsequently.

The Prediction of Short-Term Outcome in Pregnant Women with Suspected Preeclampsia Study (PROGNOSIS) was a large, non-interventional, multicenter study, designed to derive and validate a cutoff-based prediction model for the short-term prediction of the absence or the presence of preeclampsia using the sFlt-1/PlGF ratio [171]. In this study, 1050 women with singleton pregnancies between 24 + 0 and 36 + 6 weeks of gestation, and one or more symptoms of preeclampsia (but no confirmed diagnosis), were enrolled and split into two cohorts. Data from the first cohort of 500 women (development cohort) were used to develop a model and identify the optimum sFlt-1/PlGF cutoff level of 38, which was independent of gestational age (**Table 8**). The second cohort (validation cohort, $n = 550$) was used to validate this proposed optimum level.

	Development Cohort	Validation Cohort
Preeclampsia within 1 week, % (95% CI)		
Negative predictive value (rule out)	98.9 (97.3–99.7)	99.3 (97.9–99.9)
Sensitivity	88.2 (72.5–96.7)	80.0 (51.9–95.7)
Specificity	80.0 (76.1–83.6)	78.3 (74.6–81.7)
Preeclampsia within 4 weeks, % (95% CI)		
Positive predictive value (rule in)	40.7 (31.9–49.9)	36.7 (28.4–45.7)
Sensitivity	74.6 (62.5–84.5)	66.2 (54.0–77.0)
Specificity	83.1 (79.3–86.5)	83.1 (79.4–86.3)

Calculations of sensitivity were defined based on participants who developed preeclampsia within 1 or 4 weeks.
Calculations of specificity were defined based on participants who did not develop preeclampsia within 1 or 4 weeks.
CI denotes confidence interval.

Table 8. Validation of a sFlt-1/PlGF ratio cutoff of 38 for rule out and rule in in preeclampsia ([171]; From New England Journal of Medicine, Zeisler H, Llurba E, Chantraine F, Vatish M, Staff AC, Sennström M, Olovsson M, Brennecke SP, Stepan H, Allegranza D, Dilba P, Schoedl M, Hund M, Verlohren S, Predictive Value of the sFlt-1:PlGF Ratio in Women with Suspected Preeclampsia, 374, 34–42. Copyright © 2016 Massachusetts Medical Society. Reprinted with permission from Massachusetts Medical Society).

To rule out preeclampsia within 1 week, the negative-predictive value (NPV) of the selected level of ≤38 was 99.3%, with a sensitivity and specificity of 80.0 and 78.3%, respectively. To rule in preeclampsia within 4 weeks, an Elecsys® sFlt-1/PlGF ratio of >38 had a positive-predictive value (PPV) of 36.7%, with a sensitivity and specificity of 66.2 and 83.1%, respectively. This PPV is high compared with other predictive tools that have historically been employed: standard clinical and laboratory information (e.g., proteinuria and BP measurements) have PPVs of 20–26% in detecting preeclampsia-related adverse outcomes [179–181]. An Elecsys® sFlt-1/PlGF ratio of ≤38 was also predictive of the absence of fetal adverse outcomes within 1 week (NPV of 99.3% in the validation cohort); a ratio of >38 was associated with a PPV of 47.5% for these outcomes at 4 weeks. The sFlt-1/PlGF ratio is also CE-IVD approved for use as an aid in short-term prediction of preeclampsia in pregnant women with suspicion of preeclampsia in conjunction with other diagnostic and clinical information.

6.9. Tailoring preeclampsia health care using the sFlt-1/PlGF ratio

The Elecsys® sFlt-1/PlGF ratio has only recently been validated for the prediction of preeclampsia, and so its value in tailoring the management of preeclampsia in clinical practice remains to be fully seen. The use of the sFlt-1/PlGF ratio for the short-term prediction of preeclampsia in women with suspected preeclampsia could guide PHC and ensure that the right patients are monitored or referred, and receive appropriate interventions. The ability to rule out preeclampsia could, in theory, prevent the unnecessary hospitalization with economic benefits for health-care providers, although further analyses are needed to establish this [182].

Studies are currently underway to assess the value of the sFlt-1/PlGF ratio in clinical practice. The Preeclampsia Open Study (PreOS), for example, aims to establish whether knowledge of the Elecsys® sFlt-1/PlGF ratio influences a physician's decision making, by assessing intended procedures before and after knowledge of the sFlt-1/PlGF ratio [183].

The utilization of the sFlt-1/PlGF ratio could be used to guide future treatment options. A pilot study examined the safety and efficacy of therapeutic apheresis to remove circulating sFlt-1 in 11 pregnant women (20–38 years of age) with very early-onset preeclampsia. In this study, apheresis reduced the circulating levels of sFlt-1 by 18% (a range of 7–28%). In women who received a single treatment or multiple treatments of apheresis, pregnancy continued for a further 8 days (range 2–11 days) and 15 days (range 11–21 days), respectively. In control patients with preeclampsia ($n = 22$), pregnancy continued for a further 3 days (range 0–14 days). No adverse effects of apheresis were observed in the infants [184]. Further trials are needed to confirm these results; if successful, knowledge of the sFlt-1/PlGF ratio could be used to help identify women who are most likely to benefit from such therapy.

6.10. Current recommendations for the use of preeclampsia biomarkers

In the UK, the National Institute for Health and Care Excellence (NICE) has recommended (as of May 2016) the use of the Elecsys® immunoassay sFlt-1/PlGF ratio and Triage® PlGF test, in combination with standard clinical assessment, to help rule out preeclampsia in women of week 20 + 0 days to 34 weeks + 6 days gestation [174]. NICE suggest that further research is needed before the DELFIA® Xpress PlGF 1-2-3 test and BRAHMS sFlt-1 Kryptor™/BRAHMS PlGF plus Kryptor™ PE ratio can be recommended [174]. In Germany, the sFlt-1/PlGF ratio has been incorporated into guidelines on preeclampsia as a diagnostic aid [185].

A consensus statement has recently been published, providing guidance on the use of the Elecsys® immunoassay sFlt-1/PlGF ratio in women with singleton pregnancies who have signs or symptoms of preeclampsia [154]. According to this guidance, if the ratio is <38, the patient is unlikely to develop preeclampsia within 1 week and further management is at the clinician's discretion. If the ratio is >85 (in women of early gestation) or >110 (in women of late gestation), preeclampsia or placental dysfunction is present, and the patient should be managed according to local guidelines (severely elevated ratios may indicate the need for fetal lung maturation and delivery). If the sFlt-1/PlGF ratio is 38–85 (early gestation) or 38–110 (late gestation), a diagnosis of preeclampsia cannot be definitively made, but the patient is highly likely to develop the condition within 4 weeks. If this occurs in early gestation, a follow-up test within 1–2 weeks should be considered. If this occurs during late gestation, the health-care team should consider lowering the threshold for the induction of delivery.

6.11. Medical value

The sFlt-1/PlGF ratio is a typical example for a medical value test, consisting of two established markers. The medical value component in this case has been established by analyzing how this ratio can contribute to a better patient management. Without this analysis, the clinical value of both markers alone would be somewhat lower. Therefore, the "value" term arises around patients and payers simultaneously describing a framework for performance improvement in health care [186]. The medical value component consists of two pivotal factors and follows a stringent definition:

i. A medical value test must show improved patient outcomes, derived through algorithms, validated in clinical utility studies addressing an unmet medical need.

ii. Deliver actionable and medically relevant information enabling support and guidance in decision making.

Ultimately, such tests may justify a change of the current disease management and thus can help to reduce direct and indirect health-care costs. Medical value is added, when, for example, a test allows patient stratification into responders/non-responders for a given medical treatment or allows a more efficient/more effective allocation of patients to a certain treatment or disease management [187].

7. Closing remarks (summary)

Owing to a complex interaction between genes and proteins in combination with environmental factors that lead to hypertension [188, 189], and despite an increasing body of knowledge regarding genes involved in the pathophysiology of essential hypertension, the commercialization of PHC biomarkers in clinical practice is still at an early stage.

Technologies such as NGS together with computational methods allow us to analyze relationships between genetic and epigenetic factors influencing essential hypertension [188]. Up to now, these technologies have been used mainly for research [79], but in the future such technologies could be used to optimize treatment and primary prevention by combining comprehensive and detailed PHC. Knowing an individual's sequencing data might help to assess the risk for hypertension, while the use of a biosensor to continuously monitor changes in BP would allow physicians to make the treatment decisions at the earliest time point possible and hence avoid organ damage [94]. Arrays of genetic markers, along with clinical factors and/or other biomarkers, could be utilized for the development of mathematical algorithms predicting BP response to a given antihypertensive drug, similar to that used for warfarin pharmacogenetic dosing [190]. "Risk scores" for genetic markers may guide the prediction of the "best drug" avoiding long-term cardiovascular complications (e.g., stroke, atrial fibrillation, etc.).

Contemporary guidelines for the treatment of hypertension mention the potential of pharmacogenomics. An increased uptake of the use of personalized treatments is expected in upcoming years, although more studies are needed to generate a body of clinical evidence before genetic testing can be fully introduced in the treatment of cardiovascular diseases. For the first time, a new scientific statement from the ACC, AHA, and ASH on the treatment of hypertension in patients with coronary artery disease [191] refers to genetic-susceptibility variants for atherosclerotic disease and/or BP response to antihypertensive treatment. The guidelines discuss that the determination of genetic variants may be of some use for selecting appropriate antihypertensive agents to reduce both BP and the risk for coronary artery disease [192]. Thus, with the emergence of pharmacogenetics and other potential "-omics" biomarkers to guide antihypertensive treatment, guidelines are needed for biomarker qualification and clinical validation and to allow translation into clinical tools for clinical application.

The sFlt-1/PlGF ratio is a predictive and diagnostic tool in maternal care that could support the shift toward PHC in preeclampsia management. Measurement of this biomarker ratio in women with suspected preeclampsia can aid physician decision making, and help ensure that the right women receive the monitoring and specialist perinatal care that they require, while avoiding unnecessary hospitalizations.

PHC and pharmacogenomic testing has the potential to predict the response to antihypertensive therapy and to adequately select the appropriate dose that may ensure maximal efficacy, especially in patients with end-stage hypertensive disease, malignant hypertension, or treatment-refractory hypertension. This concept reduces the utilization of cost-intensive drugs in non-responders and avoids costs related to the treatment of side effects or due to the withdrawal of drugs [193]. While physicians must be trained in the handling and interpretation of test results, patients and payers must also be educated on the benefits and limitations of PHC. However, broad acceptance of such tests can only be obtained with a trained clinical workforce and compelling economic evidence for payers that pretreatment testing is efficient.

Acknowledgements

The authors would like to thank Dr. Paul van Haelst for his critical input during the development of this chapter.

Independent medical writing support was provided by Emma McConnell (Gardiner-Caldwell Communications Ltd.) and by Lee Miller (Miller Medical Communications Ltd.). F. Hoffmann-La Roche Ltd. (Diagnostics Division, Basel, Switzerland) provided funding for this writing support.

Author details

Carmen Binder[1], Hans Hendrik Schäfer[2,5], Edelgard Kaiser[3], Martin Hund[3] and Thomas Dieterle[4*]

*Address all correspondence to: Thomas.Dieterle@ksbl.ch

1 Diagnostics Information Solutions, F. Hoffmann-La Roche Ltd., Diagnostics Division, Basel, Switzerland

2 Divisional Medical and Scientific Affairs, F. Hoffmann-La Roche Ltd., Basel, Switzerland

3 Centralized and Point of Care Solutions, Medical and Scientific Affairs, Roche Diagnostics International Ltd., Rotkreuz, Switzerland

4 Kantonsspital Baselland, Liestal, Switzerland

5 Institute of Anatomy II, University Hospital Jena, Friedrich Schiller University, Jena, Germany

References

[1] US President's Council of Advisors on Science and Technology. Priorities for personalized medicine. Washington, DC: Executive Office of the President of United States; September 15, 2008. Available from: https://www.whitehouse.gov/files/documents/ostp/PCAST/pcast_report_v2.pdf. Accessed 04 March 2016.

[2] SPRINT Research Group. A randomized trial of intensive versus standard blood-pressure control. N Engl J Med. 2015;373:2103–2116. DOI: 10.1056/NEJMoa1511939.

[3] Kongkaew C, Noyce PR, Ashcroft DM. Hospital admissions associated with adverse drug reactions: a systematic review of prospective observational studies. Ann Pharmacother. 2008;42:1017–1025.

[4] Zanchetti A, Chalmers JP, Arakawa K, Gyarfas I, Hamet P, Hansson L, et al. The 1993 guidelines for the management of mild hypertension; memorandum from a WHO/ISH meeting. Blood Press. 1993;2:86–100.

[5] Fields LE, Burt VL, Cutler JA, Hughes J, Roccella EJ, Sorlie P. The burden of adult hypertension in the United States 1999 to 2000: a rising tide. Hypertension. 2004;44:398–404. DOI: 10.1161/01.HYP.0000142248.54761.56.

[6] Kearney PM, Whelton M, Reynolds K, Muntner P, Whelton PK, He J. Global burden of hypertension: analysis of worldwide data. Lancet. 2005;365:217–223.

[7] Wolf-Maier K, Cooper RS, Banegas JR, Giampaoli S, Hense HW, Joffres M, et al. Hypertension prevalence and blood pressure levels in 6 European countries, Canada, and the United States. JAMA. 2003;289:2363–2369.

[8] Spear BB, Heath-Chiozzi M, Huff J. Clinical application of pharmacogenetics. Trends Mol Med. 2001;7:201–204. DOI: http://dx.doi.org/10.1016/S1471-4914(01)01986-4.

[9] Aspinall MG, Hamermesh RG. Realizing the promise of personalized Medicine. Harv Bus Rev. 2007;85;108–117, 165.

[10] Arterial hypertension and genetics as a patient-individualized approach: where do we stand? Interview with P. Hamet, Canada. Medicographia. 2012;34:95–99. Available from: http://www.medicographia.com/wp-content/pdf/Medicographia110.pdf. Accessed 04 March 2016.

[11] Aquilante C. Pharmacogenomics: the promise of personalized medicine. Denver, CO: University of Colorado; 2007.

[12] Page IH. The mosaic theory of arterial hypertension—its interpretation. Perspect Biol Med. 1967;10:325–333.

[13] The national high blood pressure education program: 20 years of achievement. Bethesda, MD: National Heart, Lung, and Blood Institute; 1992.

[14] Report of the Joint National Committee on Detection, Evaluation, and Treatment of High Blood Pressure. A cooperative study. JAMA. 1977;237:255–261.

[15] Fan X, Han Y, Sun K, Wang Y, Xin Y, Bai Y, Li W, Yang T, Song X, Wang H, Fu C, Chen J, Shi Y, Zhou X, Wu H, Hui R. Sex differences in blood pressure response to antihypertensive therapy in Chinese patients with hypertension. Ann Pharmacother. 2008;42:1772–1781. DOI: 10.1345/aph.1L036.

[16] Peck RN, Smart LR, Beier R, Liwa AC, Grosskurth H, Fitzgerald DW, Schmidt BM. Difference in blood pressure response to ACE-Inhibitor monotherapy between black

and white adults with arterial hypertension: a meta-analysis of 13 clinical trials. BMC Nephrol. 2013;14:201. DOI: 10.1186/1471-2369-14-201.

[17] Collins FS. Shattuck lecture–medical and societal consequences of the Human Genome Project. N Engl J Med. 1999;341:28–37.

[18] Chan IS, Ginsburg GS. Personalized medicine: progress and promise. Annu Rev Genomics Hum Genet. 2011;12:217–244.

[19] Arnett DK, Claas SA, Glasser SP. Pharmacogenetics of antihypertensive treatment. Vascul Pharmacol. 2006;44:107–118. DOI:10.1016/j.vph.2005.09.010.

[20] Schwartz GL, Turner ST, Chapman AB, Boerwinkle E. Interacting effects of gender and genotype on blood pressure response to hydrochlorothiazide. Kidney Int. 2002;62:1718–1723.

[21] Kircher M, Kelso J*. High-throughput DNA sequencing—concepts and limitations. Article first published online: 18 MAY 2010. DOI: 10.1002/bies.200900181.

[22] Ramani VC, Jeffrey SS. Circulating tumor cell technologies. Mol Oncol. 2016 Mar;10(3): 374–94. DOI: 10.1016/j.molonc.2016.01.007. Epub 2016 Jan 28.

[23] Lewin J. Genetics, your heart and your future, the American College of Cardiology. 2011. Available from: http://www.personalizedmedicinecoalition.org/sites/default/files/files/Jack%20Lewin.pdf Accessed 04 March 2016.

[24] Davis J, Ma P, Sutaria S. The microeconomics of personalized medicine. February 2010. Pharmaceuticals and Medical Products Practice, McKinsey&Company. Available from: http://www.mckinsey.com/industries/pharmaceuticals-and-medical-products/our-insights/the-microeconomics-of-personalized-medicine. Accessed 04 March 2016.

[25] Altshuler D, Brooks LD, Chakravarti A, Collins FS, Daly MJ, Donnelly P. A haplotype map of the human genome. Nature. 2005;437:1299–1320.

[26] Hamburg MA, Collins FS. The path to personalized medicine. N Engl J Med. 2010;363:301–304. DOI: 10.1056/NEJMp1006304.

[27] Bonter K, Desjardins C, Currier N, Pun J, Ashbury FD. Personalised medicine in Canada: a survey of adoption and practice in oncology, cardiology and family medicine. BMJ Open. 2011;1:e000110.

[28] Zineh I, Pebanco GD, Aquilante CL, Gerhard T, Beitelshees AL, Beasley BN, Hartzema AG. Discordance between availability of pharmacogenetics studies and pharmacogenetics-based prescribing information for the top 200 drugs. Ann Pharmacother. 2006;40:639–644. DOI: 10.1345/aph.1G464.

[29] University of Minnesota – Clinical and Translational Science Institute, National Heart, Lung, and Blood Institute (NHLBI). GenHAT—Genetics of Hypertension Associated Treatments. Available from: http://clinicaltrials.gov/show/NCT00006294. NLM Identifier: NCT00006294 Accessed 04 March 2016.

[30] FBPP Investigators. Multi-center genetic study of hypertension: The Family Blood Pressure Program (FBPP). Hypertension. 2002;39:3–9.

[31] Williams RR, Hunt SC, Hasstedt SJ, et al. Genetics of hypertension: what we know and what we don't know. Clin Exp Hypertens. 1990;A12:865–870.

[32] Williams RR, Hunt SC, Hasstedt SJ, et al. Are there interactions and relations between genetic and environmental factors in predisposing to high blood pressure? Hypertension. 1991;18 (suppl I):I-29–I-37.

[33] An P, Rice T, Gagnon J, Borecki IB, et al. Familial aggregation of resting blood pressure and heart rate in a sedentary population: the Heritage Study. Am J Hypertens. 1999;12:264–270.

[34] Levy D, De Stefano AL, Larson MG, et al. Evidence for a blood pressure gene on chromosome 17: genome scan results for longitudinal blood pressure phenotypes in subjects from the Framingham Heart Study. Hypertension. 2000;36:477–483.

[35] Svetkey LP, McKeown SP, Wilson AF. Heritability of salt sensitivity in black Americans. Hypertension. 1996;28:854–858.

[36] Burke W, Motulsky AG. Hypertension. In: King RA, Rotter JI, Motulsky AG, eds. *The Genetic Basis of Human Diseases*. New York, NY: Oxford University Press; 1992: 170–191.

[37] Kurtz TW, Spence MA. Genetics of essential hypertension. Am J Med. 1993;94:77–84.

[38] Koivukoski L, Fisher SA, Kanninen T, et al. Meta-analysis of genome-wide scans for hypertension and blood pressure in Caucasians shows evidence of susceptibility regions on chromosomes 2 and 3. Hum Mol Genet. 2004;13:2325–2332.

[39] Hirschhorn JN, Lohmueller K, Byrne E, et al. A comprehensive review of genetic association studies. Genet Med. 2002;4:45–61.

[40] Chang YP, Liu X, Kim JD, Ikeda MA, et al. Multiple genes for essential hypertension susceptibility on chromosome 1q. Am J Hum Genet. 2007;80:253–264.

[41] Lifton RP. Genetic determinants of human hypertension. Proc Natl Acad Sci. 1995;92:8545–8551.

[42] Tobin MD, Tomaszewski M, Braund PS, et al. Common variants in genes underlying monogenic hypertension and hypotension and blood pressure in the general population. Hypertension. 2008;51:1658–1664.

[43] Levy D, Ehret GB, Rice K, et al. Genome-wide association study of blood pressure and hypertension. Nat Genet. 2009;41:677–687.

[44] Ehret GB, Munroe PB, Rice KM, et al. Genetic variants in novel pathways influence blood pressure and cardiovascular risk. Nature. 2011;478:103–109.

[45] Huan T, Esko T, Peters MJ, et al. A meta-analysis of gene expression signatures of blood pressure and hypertension. PLoS Genet. 2015;11(3):e1005035.

[46] Psaty BM, O'Connell CJ, Gudnason VL, et al. Cohorts for Heart and Aging Research in Genomic Epidemiology (CHARGE) Consortium: design of prospective meta-analyses of genome-wide association studies from five cohorts. Circ Cardiovasc Genet. 2009;2:73–80.

[47] Handschin A, Henny-Fullin K, Buess D, et al. Cardiovascular risk stratification and therapeutic implications. Ther Umschau. 2015;72:361–368.

[48] Ruben RJ. Otitis media; the application of personalized medicine. Otolaryngol Head Neck Surg. 2011;145:707–712.

[49] Lee M-S, Flammer AJ, Lerman LO, et al. Personalized medicine in cardiovascular disease. Korean Circ J. 2012;42:583–591.

[50] Caulfield M, Munroe P, Pembroke J, et al. Genome-wide mapping of human loci for essential hypertension. Lancet. 2003;361:2118–2123.

[51] Cabrera CP, Ng FL, Warren HR, et al. Exploring hypertension genome-wide association studies findings and impact on pathophysiology, pathways, and pharmacogenetics. WIREs Syst Biol Med. 2015;7:73–90.

[52] Abraham G, Kowalczyk A, Zobel J, et al. Performance and robustness of penalized methods for genetic prediction of complex human disease. Genet Epidemiol. 2013;37:184–195.

[53] Chobanian AV. Shattuck lecture. The hypertension paradox—more uncontrolled disease despite improved therapy. N Engl J Med. 2009;361:878–887.

[54] Johnson JA. Advancing management of hypertension through pharmacogenomics. Ann Med. 2012;44:S17–S22.

[55] Chobanian AV, Bakris GL, Black HR, et al. The seventh report of the Joint National Committee on prevention, detection, and treatment of high blood pressure. JAMA. 2003;289:2560–2572.

[56] Turner ST, Bailey KR, Fridley BL, et al. Genomic association analysis suggests chromosome 12 locus influencing antihypertensive response to thiazide diuretics. Hypertension. 2008;52:359–365.

[57] Duarte JD, Turner ST, Tran B, et al. Association of chromosome 12 locus with antihypertensive response to hydrochlorothiazide may involve differential YEATS4 expression. Pharmacogenomics J. 2013 Jun;13(3):257-263. doi: 10.1038/tpj.2012.4. Epub 2012 Feb 21.

[58] Turner, ST, Boerwinkle E, O'Connell JR, et al. Genomic association analysis of common variants influencing antihypertensive response to hydrochlorothizide. Hypertension. 2013;62:391–397.

[59] Svensson-Färbom P, Wahlstrand B, Almgren P, et al. A functional variant of the NEDD4L gene is associated with beneficial treatment response with β-blockers and diuretics in hypertensive patients. J Hypertens. 2011;29:388–395.

[60] McDonough CW, Burbage SE, Duarte JD, et al. Association of variants in NEDD4L with blood pressure response and adverse cardiovascular outcomes in hypertensive patients treated with thiazide diuretics. J Hypertens. 2013;31:698–704.

[61] Gong Y, McDonough CW, Wang Z, Hou W, et al. Hypertension susceptibility loci and blood pressure response to antihypertensives: results from the pharmacogenomic evaluation of antihypertensive responses study. Circ Cardiovasc Genet. 2012;5:686–691.

[62] Hiltunen TP, Donner KM, Sarin A-P, et al. Pharmacogenomics of hypertension: a genome-wide placebo-controlled cross-over study, using four classes of antihypertensive drugs. J Am Heart Assoc. 2015;4:e001521.

[63] Chittani M, Zaninello R, Lanzani C, et al. CSMD1 genes affect SBP response to hydrochlorothiazide in never-treated essential hypertension. J Hypertens. 2015;33:1301–1309.

[64] Su X, Lee L, Li X, Lv J, et al. Association between angiotensinogen, angiotensin II receptor genes, and blood pressure response to an angiotensin converting enzyme inhibitor. Circulation. 2007;115:725–732.

[65] Yu H, Lin S, Zhong J, et al. A core promoter variant of angiotensinogen gene and interindividual variations in response to angiotensin-converting enzyme inhibitors. J Renin Angiotensin Aldosterone Syst. 2014;15:540–546.

[66] Srivastava K, Chandra S, Bhatia J, et al. Association of angiotensinogen (M235T) gene polymorphism with blood pressure lowering response to angiotensin converting enzyme inhibitor. J Pharm Pharm Sci. 2012;15:399–406.

[67] Luo JQ, Wang LY, He FZ, et al. Effect of NR3C2 genetic polymorphisms on the blood pressure response to enalapril treatment. Pharmacogenomics. 2013;15(2):201–208.

[68] Kamide K, Asayama K, Katsuya T, et al. Genome-wide response to antihypertensive medication using home blood pressure measurements: a pilot study nested within the HOMED-BP study. Pharmacogenomics. 2013;14:1709–1721.

[69] Turner ST, Bailey KR, Schwartz GL, et al. Genomic association analysis identifies multiple loci influencing antihypertensive response to an angiotensin II receptor blocker. Hypertension. 2012;59:1204–1211.

[70] Ortlepp JR, Hanrath P, Mevissen V, et al. Variants of the CYP11B2 gene predict response to therapy with candesartan. Eur J Pharmacol. 2002;445:151–152.

[71] Donner KM, Hiltunen TP, Hannila-Handelberg T, et al. STK39 variation predicts the ambulatory blood pressure response to losartan in hypertensive men. Hypertens Res. 2012;35:107–114.

[72] Glorioso N, Argiolas G, Filigheddu F, et al. Genome-wide association study identifies CAMK1D variants involved in blood pressure response to losartan: the SOPHIA study. Pharmacogenomics. 2007;15:1643–1652.

[73] Sanada H, Yoneda M, Yatabe J, et al. Common variants of the G-protein coupled receptor type 4 are associated with human essential hypertension and predict the blood pressure response to angiotensin receptor blockade. Pharmacogenomics. 2015. doi: 10.1038/tpj.2015.6.

[74] Felder RA, sanada H, Xu J, et al. G protein-coupled receptor kinase 4 gene variants in human essential hypertension. Proc Natl Acad Sci U S A. 2002;99:3872–3877.

[75] Harris RC. Abnormalities in renal dopamine signaling and hypertension. Curr Opin Nephrol Hypertens. 2012;21:61–65.

[76] Johnson JA, Zineh I, Puckett BJ, et al. Beta 1-adrenergic receptor polymorphisms and antihypertensive response to metoprolol. Clin Pharmacol Ther. 2003;74:44–52.

[77] Filigheddu F, Argiolas G, Degortes S, et al. Haplotypes of the adrenergic system predict the blood pressure response to beta-blockers in women with essential hypertension. Pharmacogenomics. 2010;11:319–325.

[78] Vandell AG, Lobmeyer MT, Gawronski BE, et al. G protein receptor kinase 4 polymorphisms: β-blocker pharmacogenetics and treatment-related outcomes in hypertension. Hypertension. 2012;60:957–964.

[79] Polimanti R, Iorio A, Piacentini S, et al. Human pharmacogenomics variation of antihypertensive drugs: from population genetics to personalized medicine. Pharmacogenomics. 2014;15:157–167.

[80] Beitelshees AL, Gong Y, Wang D, et al. KCNMB1 genotype influences response to verapamil SR and adverse outcomes in the INternational VErapamil SR/Trandolapril STudy (INVEST). Pharmacogenet Genomics.2007;17:719–729.

[81] Beitelshees AL, Navare H, Wang D, et al. CACNA1C gene polymorphisms, cardiovascular disease outcomes, and treatment response. Circ Cardiovasc Genet.2009;2:362–370.

[82] Hamrefors V, Sjögren M, Almgren P, et al. Pharmacogenetic implications for eight common blood pressure-associated single-nucleotide polymorphisms. J Hypertens. 2012;30(6):1151–1160.

[83] Basson J, Simino J, Rao DC. Between candidate genes and whole genomes: time for alternative approaches in blood pressure genetics. Curr Hypertens Rep. 2012;14:46–61. DOI: 10.1007/s11906-011-0241-8.

[84] Klein D. Quantification using real-time PCR technology: applications and limitations. Trends Mol Med. 2002;8:257–260. DOI: http://dx.doi.org/10.1016/S1471-4914(02)02355-9.

[85] Bernard PS, Wittwer CT. Real-time PCR technology for cancer diagnostics. Clin Chem. 2002;48:1178–1185.

[86] Bengra C, Mifflin TE, Khripin Y, Manunta P, Williams SM, Jose PA, Felder RA. Genotyping of essential hypertension single-nucleotide polymorphisms by a homogeneous PCR method with universal energy transfer primers. Clin Chem. 2002;48:2131–2140.

[87] Whale AS, Huggett JF, Cowen S, Speirs V, Shaw J, Ellison S, Foy CA, Scott DJ. Comparison of microfluidic digital PCR and conventional quantitative PCR for measuring copy number variation. Nucleic Acids Res. 2012;40:e82. DOI: 10.1093/nar/gks203.

[88] Hudecova I. Digital PCR analysis of circulating nucleic acids. Clin Biochem. 2015;48:948–956. DOI: 10.1016/j.clinbiochem.2015.03.015.

[89] Pekin D, Skhiri Y, Baret JC, Le Corre D, Mazutis L, Salem CB, Millot F, El Harrak A, Hutchison JB, Larson JW, Link DR, Laurent-Puig P, Griffiths AD, Taly V. Quantitative and sensitive detection of rare mutations using droplet-based microfluidics. Lab Chip. 2011;11:2156–2166. DOI: 10.1039/c1lc20128j.

[90] Hayden EC. Technology: the $1,000 genome. Nature. 2014;507:294–295. DOI: 10.1038/507294a.

[91] Illumina Inc. HiSeq X Ten System. 2016. Available from: http://www.illumina.com/systems/hiseq-x-sequencing-system/system.html. Accessed 04 March 2016

[92] Bahassi el M, Stambrook PJ. Next-generation sequencing technologies: breaking the sound barrier of human genetics. Mutagenesis. 2014;29:303–310. DOI: 10.1093/mutage/geu031.

[93] Trapnell C, Salzberg SL. How to map billions of short reads onto genomes. Nat Biotechnol. 2009;27:455–457. DOI: 10.1038/nbt0509-455.

[94] Topol EJ. Individualized medicine from prewomb to tomb. Cell. 2014;157:241–253. DOI: 10.1016/j.cell.2014.02.012.

[95] Roche Sequencing [Home page]. 2015. Available from: http://sequencing.roche.com/. Accessed 04 March 2016.

[96] Illumina Inc. Understanding the genetic code: NGS technology enables massively parallel DNA analysis for a deeper understanding of biology. 2016. Available from: http://www.illumina.com/techniques/sequencing/dna-sequencing.html. Accessed 04 March 2016

[97] Stewart WC, Huang Y, Greenberg DA, Vieland VJ. Next-generation linkage and association methods applied to hypertension: a multifaceted approach to the analysis of sequence data. BMC Proc. 2014;8(Suppl 1 Genetic Analysis Workshop 18Vanessa Olmo):S111. DOI: 10.1186/1753-6561-8-S1-S111. eCollection 2014.

[98] Zhao X, Sha Q, Zhang S, Wang X. Testing optimally weighted combination of variants for hypertension. BMC Proc. 2014;8(Suppl 1 Genetic Analysis Workshop 18Vanessa Olmo):S59. DOI: 10.1186/1753-6561-8-S1-S59. eCollection 2014.

[99] Turner ST, Schwartz GL, Boerwinkle E. Personalized medicine for high blood pressure. Hypertension. 2007;50:1–5. DOI: 10.1161/HYPERTENSIONAHA.107.087049

[100] Edwards JS, Atlas SR, Wilson SM, Cooper CF, Luo L, Stidley CA. Integrated statistical and pathway approach to next-generation sequencing analysis: a family-based study of hypertension. BMC Proc. 2014;8(Suppl 1 Genetic Analysis Workshop 18Vanessa Olmo):S104. DOI: 10.1186/1753-6561-8-S1-S104. eCollection 2014.

[101] Wang X, Prins BP, Sõber S, Laan M, Snieder H. Beyond genome-wide association studies: new strategies for identifying genetic determinants of hypertension. Curr Hypertens Rep. 2011;13:442–451. DOI: 10.1007/s11906-011-0230-y.

[102] Murakami K. Non-coding RNAs and hypertension-unveiling unexpected mechanisms of hypertension by the dark matter of the genome. Curr Hypertens Rev. 2015;11:80–90. DOI: 10.2174/1573402111666150401105317.

[103] ENCODE Project Consortium. An integrated encyclopedia of DNA elements in the human genome. Nature. 2012;489:57–74. DOI: 10.1038/nature11247.

[104] Fratkin E, Bercovici S, Stephan DA. The implications of ENCODE for diagnostics. Nat Biotechnol. 2012;30:1064–1065. DOI: 10.1038/nbt.2418.

[105] Kontaraki JE, Marketou ME, Zacharis EA, Parthenakis FI, Vardas PE. Differential expression of vascular smooth muscle-modulating microRNAs in human peripheral blood mononuclear cells: novel targets in essential hypertension. J Hum Hypertens. 2014;28:510–516. DOI: 10.1038/jhh.2013.117.

[106] Archer K, Broskova Z, Bayoumi AS, Teoh JP, Davila A, Tang Y, Su H, Kim IM. Long non-coding RNAs as master regulators in cardiovascular diseases. Int J Mol Sci. 2015;16:23651–23667. DOI: 10.3390/ijms161023651.

[107] Marques FZ, Booth SA, Charchar FJ. The emerging role of non-coding RNA in essential hypertension and blood pressure regulation. J Hum Hypertens. 2015;29:459–467. DOI: 10.1038/jhh.2014.99.

[108] Churchill GA. Fundamentals of experimental design for cDNA microarrays. Nat Genet. 2002;32(Suppl.):490–495.

[109] Bos JM, Towbin JA, Ackerman MJ. Diagnostic, prognostic, and therapeutic implications of genetic testing for hypertrophic cardiomyopathy. J Am Coll Cardiol. 2009;54:201–211. DOI: 10.1016/j.jacc.2009.02.075.

[110] Matafora V, Zagato L, Ferrandi M, Molinari I, Zerbini G, Casamassima N, Lanzani C, Delli Carpini S, Trepiccione F, Manunta P, Bachi A, Capasso G. Quantitative proteomics

reveals novel therapeutic and diagnostic markers in hypertension. BBA Clin. 2014;2:79–87. DOI: 10.1016/j.bbacli.2014.10.001. eCollection 2014.

[111] Ren J, Sun J, Ning F, Pang Z, Qie L, Qiao Q; Qingdao Diabetes Survey Group in 2006 and 2009. Gender differences in the association of hypertension with gamma-glutamyltransferase and alanine aminotransferase levels in Chinese adults in Qingdao, China. J Am Soc Hypertens. 2015;9:951–958. DOI: 10.1016/j.jash.2015.09.014.

[112] van Deventer CA, Lindeque JZ, van Rensburg PJ, Malan L, van der Westhuizen FH, Louw R. Use of metabolomics to elucidate the metabolic perturbation associated with hypertension in a black South African male cohort: the SABPA study. J Am Soc Hypertens. 2015;9:104–114. DOI: 10.1016/j.jash.2014.11.007.

[113] Wang L, Hou E, Wang L, Wang Y, Yang L, Zheng X, Xie G, Sun Q, Liang M, Tian Z. Reconstruction and analysis of correlation networks based on GC–MS metabolomics data for young hypertensive men. Anal Chim Acta. 2015;854:95–105. DOI: 10.1016/j.aca.2014.11.009.

[114] Zhong L, Zhang JP, Nuermaimaiti AG, Yunusi KX. Study on plasmatic metabolomics of Uygur patients with essential hypertension based on nuclear magnetic resonance technique. Eur Rev Med Pharmacol Sci. 2014;18:3673–3680.

[115] Jankowski V, Meyer AA, Schlattmann P, Gui Y, Zheng XL, Stamcou I, Radtke K, Tran TN, van der Giet M, Tölle M, Zidek W, Jankowski J. Increased uridine adenosine tetraphosphate concentrations in plasma of juvenile hypertensives. Arterioscler Thromb Vasc Biol. 2007;27:1776–1781. DOI: 10.1161/ATVBAHA.107.143958.

[116] Zheng Y, Yu B, Alexander D, Mosley TH, Heiss G, Nettleton JA, Boerwinkle E. Metabolomics and incident hypertension among blacks: the atherosclerosis risk in communities study. Hypertension. 2013;62:398–403. DOI: 10.1161/HYPERTENSIONAHA.113.01166.

[117] Best Fitness Tracker Reviews. Best trackers for…heart health data. 2013. Available from: http://www.bestfitnesstrackerreviews.com/fitness-trackers-for-heart-health.html. Accessed 04 March 2016.

[118] O'Donnell AJ, Bogner HR, Cronholm PF, Kellom K, Miller-Day M, McClintock HF, Kaye EM, Gabbay R. Stakeholder perspectives on changes in hypertension care under the patient-centered medical home. Prev Chronic Dis. 2016;13:E28. DOI: 10.5888/pcd13.150383.

[119] Glynn L, Casey M, Walsh J, Hayes PS, Harte RP, Heaney D. Patients' views and experiences of technology based self-management tools for the treatment of hypertension in the community: a qualitative study. BMC Fam Pract. 2015;16:119. DOI: 10.1186/s12875-015-0333-7.

[120] U.S. Food and Drug Administration. Examples of pre-market submissions that include MMAs cleared or approved by FDA. 2016. Available from: http://www.fda.gov/

MedicalDevices/DigitalHealth/MobileMedicalApplications/ucm368784.htm. Accessed 04 March 2016.

[121] Mancia G, Fagard R, Narkiewicz K, Redon J, Zanchetti A, Böhm M, Christiaens T, Cifkova R, De Backer G, Dominiczak A, Galderisi M, Grobbee DE, et al. 2013 ESH/ESC guidelines for the management of arterial hypertension: the Task Force for the Management of Arterial Hypertension of the European Society of Hypertension (ESH) and of the European Society of Cardiology (ESC). Eur Heart J. 2013;34:2159–2219. DOI: 10.1093/eurheartj/eht151.

[122] James PA, Oparil S, Carter BL, Cushman WC, Dennison-Himmelfarb C, Handler J, Lackland DT, LeFevre ML, MacKenzie TD, Ogedegbe O, Smith SC Jr, Svetkey LP, Taler SJ, Townsend RR, Wright JT Jr, Narva AS, Ortiz E. 2014 evidence-based guideline for the management of high blood pressure in adults: report from the panel members appointed to the Eighth Joint National Committee (JNC 8). JAMA. 2014;311:507–520. DOI: 10.1001/jama.2013.284427. Erratum in: JAMA. 2014;311:1809.

[123] Daskalopoulou SS, Rabi DM, Zarnke KB, Dasgupta K, Nerenberg K, Cloutier L, Gelfer M, Lamarre-Cliche M, Milot A, Bolli P, McKay DW, Tremblay G, et al. The 2015 Canadian Hypertension Education Program recommendations for blood pressure measurement, diagnosis, assessment of risk, prevention, and treatment of hypertension. Can J Cardiol. 2015;31:549–568. DOI: 10.1016/j.cjca.2015.02.016.

[124] Go AS, Bauman MA, Coleman King SM, Fonarow GC, Lawrence W, Williams KA, Sanchez E; American Heart Association; American College of Cardiology; Centers for Disease Control and Prevention. An effective approach to high blood pressure control: a science advisory from the American Heart Association, the American College of Cardiology, and the Centers for Disease Control and Prevention. Hypertension. 2014;63:878–885. DOI: 10.1161/HYP.0000000000000003. Erratum in: Hypertension. 2014;63:e175.

[125] Weber MA, Schiffrin EL, White WB, Mann S, Lindholm LH, Kenerson JG, Flack JM, Carter BL, Materson BJ, Ram CV, Cohen DL, Cadet JC, Jean-Charles RR, Taler S, Kountz D, Townsend RR, Chalmers J, Ramirez AJ, Bakris GL, Wang J, Schutte AE, Bisognano JD, Touyz RM, Sica D, Harrap SB. Clinical practice guidelines for the management of hypertension in the community: a statement by the American Society of Hypertension and the International Society of Hypertension. J Clin Hypertens (Greenwich). 2014;16:14–26. DOI: 10.1111/jch.12237.

[126] Rhonda et al., Cooper-DeHoff RM, Johnson JA. Hypertension pharmacogenomics: in search of personalized treatment approaches. Nat Rev Nephrol. 2016;12:110–122. DOI: 10.1038/nrneph.2015.176.

[127] Zanchetti A, Thomopoulos C, Parati G. Randomized controlled trials of blood pressure lowering in hypertension: a critical reappraisal. Circ Res. 2015;116:1058–1073. DOI: 10.1161/CIRCRESAHA.116.303641.

[128] Relling MV, Klein TE. PharmGKB. CPIC: Clinical Pharmacogenetics Implementation Consortium. 2016. Available from: https://www.pharmgkb.org/page/cpic. Accessed 07 March 2016.

[129] Scott SA, Sangkuhl K, Stein CM, Hulot JS, Mega JL, Roden DM, Klein TE, Sabatine MS, Johnson JA, Shuldiner AR; Clinical Pharmacogenetics Implementation Consortium. Clinical Pharmacogenetics Implementation Consortium guidelines for CYP2C19 genotype and clopidogrel therapy: 2013 update. Clin Pharmacol Ther. 2013;94:317–323. DOI: 10.1038/clpt.2013.105.

[130] Johnson JA, Gong L, Whirl-Carrillo M, Gage BF, Scott SA, Stein CM, Anderson JL, Kimmel SE, Lee MT, Pirmohamed M, Wadelius M, Klein TE, Altman RB; Clinical Pharmacogenetics Implementation Consortium. Clinical Pharmacogenetics Implementation Consortium guidelines for CYP2C9 and VKORC1 genotypes and warfarin dosing. Clin Pharmacol Ther. 2011;90:625–629. DOI: 10.1038/clpt.2011.185.

[131] Ramsey LB, Johnson SG, Caudle KE, Haidar CE, Voora D, Wilke RA, Maxwell WD, McLeod HL, Krauss RM, Roden DM, Feng Q, Cooper-DeHoff RM, Gong L, Klein TE, Wadelius M, Niemi M. The clinical pharmacogenetics implementation consortium guideline for SLCO1B1 and simvastatin-induced myopathy: 2014 update. Clin Pharmacol Ther. 2014;96:423–428. DOI: 10.1038/clpt.2014.125.

[132] Collins FS, Varmus H. A new initiative on precision medicine. N Engl J Med. 2015;372:793–795. DOI: 10.1056/NEJMp1500523.

[133] Chasman D, Posada D, Subrahmanyan L, Cook NR, Stanton VP Jr, Ridker PM. Pharmacogenetic study of statin therapy and cholesterol reduction. JAMA. 2004;291:2821–2827. doi:10.1001/jama.291.23.2821.

[134] Hulot JS, Bura A, Villard E, Azizi M, Remones V, Goyenvalle C, Aiach M, Lechat P, Gaussem P. Cytochrome P450 2C19 loss-of-function polymorphism is a major determinant of clopidogrel responsiveness in healthy subjects. Blood. 2006;108:2244–2247.

[135] Simon T, Verstuyft C, Mary-Krause M, Quteineh L, Drouet E, Méneveau N, Steg PG, Ferrières J, Danchin N, Becquemont L; French Registry of Acute ST-Elevation and Non-ST-Elevation Myocardial Infarction (FAST-MI) Investigators. Genetic determinants of response to clopidogrel and cardiovascular events. N Engl J Med. 2009;360:363–375. DOI: 10.1056/NEJMoa0808227.

[136] U.S. Food and Drug Administration. FDA announces new boxed warning on Plavix: Alerts patients, health care professionals to potential for reduced effectiveness. 2010. Available from: http://www.fda.gov/NewsEvents/Newsroom/PressAnnouncements/ucm204253.htm. Accessed 04 March 2016.

[137] Kangelaris KN, Bent S, Nussbaum RL, Garcia DA, Tice JA. Genetic testing before anticoagulation? A systematic review of pharmacogenetic dosing of warfarin. J Gen Intern Med. 2009;24:656–664. DOI: 10.1007/s11606-009-0949-1.

[138] Bussey HI, Wittkowsky AK, Hylek EM, Walker MB. Genetic testing for warfarin dosing? Not yet ready for prime time. Pharmacotherapy. 2008;28:141–143. DOI: 10.1592/phco.28.2.141.

[139] McWilliam A, Letter R, Nardinelli C. Health care savings from personalized medicine using genetic testing: the case of warfarin. Working Paper 06-23. 2006. AEI-Brookings Joint Center for Regulatory Studies.

[140] Rohr UP, Binder C, Dieterle T, Giusti F, Messina CG, Toerien E, Moch H, Schäfer HH. The value of in vitro diagnostic testing in medical practice: a status report. PLoS One. 2016;11:e0149856. DOI: 10.1371/journal.pone.0149856

[141] Roberts JD, Wells GA, Le May MR, Labinaz M, Glover C, Froeschl M, Dick A, Marquis JF, O'Brien E, Goncalves S, Druce I, Stewart A, Gollob MH, So DY. Point-of-care genetic testing for personalisation of antiplatelet treatment (RAPID GENE): a prospective, randomised, proof-of-concept trial. Lancet. 2012;379:1705–1711. DOI: 10.1016/S0140-6736(12)60161-5.

[142] Drummond MF, O'Brien B, Stoddart GL, Torrance GW. Methods for the economic evaluation of health care programmes. 2nd ed. ISBN: 0 19 262773 2. Oxford: Oxford University Press; 1997.

[143] Seely EW, Ecker J. Chronic hypertension in pregnancy. Circulation. 2014;129:1254–1261.DOI: 10.1161/CIRCULATIONAHA.113.003904

[144] Mammaro A, Carrara S, Cavaliere A, et al. Hypertensive disorders of pregnancy. J Prenat Med. 2009;3(1):1–5.

[145] Duley L. The global impact of pre-eclampsia and eclampsia. Semin Perinatol. 2009;33(3):130–137.

[146] Ghulmiyyah L, Sibai B. Maternal mortality from preeclampsia/eclampsia. Semin Perinatol. 2012;36(1):56–9.

[147] Ananth CV, Keyes KM, Wapner RJ. Pre-eclampsia rates in the United States, 1980–2010: age-period-cohort analysis. BMJ. 2013;347:f6564.

[148] Hernandez-Diaz S, Toh S, Cnattingius S. Risk of pre-eclampsia in first and subsequent pregnancies: prospective cohort study. BMJ. 2009;338:b2255.

[149] Goldenberg RL, Culhane JF, Iams JD, Romero R. Preterm birth 1 –epidemiology and causes of preterm birth. Lancet. 2008;371(9606):75–84.

[150] WHO. The World Health Report 2005 Make every mother and child count. http://www.who.int/whr/2005/en/ Accessed March 2016.

[151] McClure JH, Cooper GM, Clutton-Brock TH. Saving mothers' Lives: reviewing maternal deaths to make motherhood safer: 2006–8: a review. Br J Anaesth. 2011;107(2): 127–132.

[152] Duley L, Gulmezoglu AM, Henderson-Smart DJ, Chou D. Magnesium sulphate and other anticonvulsants for women with pre-eclampsia. Cochrane Database Syst Rev. 2010 Nov 10;(11):CD000025. doi: 10.1002/14651858.CD000025.pub2.

[153] Wang A, Rana S, Karumanchi SA. Preeclampsia: the role of angiogenic factors in its pathogenesis. Physiology (Bethesda). 2009;24:147–158.

[154] Stepan H, Herraiz I, Schlembach D, et al. Implementation of the sFlt-1/PlGF ratio for prediction and diagnosis of pre-eclampsia in singleton pregnancy: implications for clinical practice. Ultrasound Obstet Gynecol. 2015;45(3):241–246.

[155] Dekker GA. Management of preeclampsia. Pregnancy Hypertens. 2014;4(3):246–247.

[156] ACOG Task Force on Hypertension in Pregnancy: Hypertension in Pregnancy. American College of Obstetricians and Gynecologists 2013. http://www.acog.org/Resources-And-Publications/Task-Force-and-Work-Group-Reports/Hypertension-in-Pregnancy. Accessed March 2016.

[157] Staff AC, Benton SJ, von Dadelszen P, et al. Redefining preeclampsia using placenta-derived biomarkers. Hypertension. 2013;61(5):932–942.

[158] Karumanchi SA, Epstein FH. Placental ischemia and soluble fms-like tyrosine kinase 1: cause or consequence of preeclampsia? Kidney Int. 2007;71(10):959–961.

[159] Kendall RL, Thomas KA. Inhibition of vascular endothelial-cell growth-factor activity by an endogenously encoded soluble receptor. Proc Natl Acad Sci USA. 1993;90(22): 10705–10709.

[160] Lu F, Bytautiene E, Tamayo E, et al. Gender-specific effect of overexpression of sFlt-1 in pregnant mice on fetal programming of blood pressure in the offspring later in life. Am J Obstet Gynecol. 2007;197(4):418.e1–418.e5.

[161] Chappell LC, Duckworth S, Seed PT, et al. Diagnostic accuracy of placental growth factor in women with suspected preeclampsia: a prospective multicenter study. Circulation. 2013;128(19):2121–2131.

[162] Akolekar R, Syngelaki A, Poon L, et al. Competing risks model in early screening for preeclampsia by biophysical and biochemical markers. Fetal Diagn Ther. 2013;33(1):8–15.

[163] Lai J, Pinas A, Poon LC, et al. Maternal serum placental growth factor, pregnancy-associated plasma protein-a and free beta-human chorionic gonadotrophin at 30–33 weeks in the prediction of pre-eclampsia. Fetal Diagn Ther. 2013;33(3):164–172.

[164] Levine RJ, Maynard SE, Qian C, et al. Circulating angiogenic factors and the risk of preeclampsia. N Engl J Med. 2004;350(7):672–683.

[165] Levine RJ, Lam C, Qian C, Yu KF, Maynard SE, Sachs BP, et al. Soluble endoglin and other circulating antiangiogenic factors in preeclampsia. N Engl J Med. 2006;355(10): 992–1005.

[166] Vatten LJ, Eskild A, Nilsen TI, et al. Changes in circulating level of angiogenic factors from the first to second trimester as predictors of preeclampsia. Am J Obstet Gynecol. 2007;196(3):239.e1–239.e6.

[167] Verlohren S, Herraiz I, Lapaire O, et al. The sFlt-1/PlGF ratio in different types of hypertensive pregnancy disorders and its prognostic potential in preeclamptic patients. Am J Obstet Gynecol. 2012;206(1):58.e1–58.e8.

[168] Villa PM, Hamalainen E, Maki A, et al. Vasoactive agents for the prediction of early- and late-onset preeclampsia in a high-risk cohort. BMC Pregnancy Childbirth. 2013;13:110.

[169] Verlohren S, Galindo A, Schlembach D, et al. An automated method for the determination of the sFlt-1/PIGF ratio in the assessment of preeclampsia. Am J Obstet Gynecol. 2010;202(2):161.e1–161.e11.

[170] Rana S, Powe CE, Salahuddin S, et al. Angiogenic factors and the risk of adverse outcomes in women with suspected preeclampsia. Circulation. 2012;125(7):911–919.

[171] Zeisler H, Llurba E, Chantraine F, et al. Predictive value of the sFlt-1:PlGFratio in women with suspected preeclampsia. N Engl J Med. 2016;374(1):13–22.

[172] Roche Diagnostics. Elecsys®PlGF method sheet. 2015.

[173] Benton SJ, Hu YX, Xie F, Kupfer K, Lee SW, Magee LA, et al. Angiogenic factors as diagnostic tests for preeclampsia: a performance comparison between two commercial immunoassays. Am J Obstet Gynecol. 2011 Nov; 205(5):469.e1–8. doi: 10.1016/j.ajog. 2011.06.058. Epub 2011 Jun 21.

[174] NICE.Diagnostics guidance [DG23]. PlGF-based testing to help diagnose suspected pre-eclampsia (Triage PlGF test, Elecsys immunoassay sFlt-1/PlGF ratio, DELFIA Xpress PlGF 1-2-3 test, and BRAHMS sFlt-1 Kryptor/BRAHMS PlGF plus Kryptor PE ratio). 2016. https://www.nice.org.uk/guidance/DG23. Accessed May 2016.

[175] Roche Diagnostics. Elecsys®sFlt-1 method sheet. 2015.

[176] Stepan H, Hund M, Gencay M, et al. A comparison of the diagnostic utility of thesFlt-1/ PlGF ratio versus PlGF alone for the detection of preeclampsia/HELLPsyndrome. Hypertens Pregnancy. 2016 Mar 30:1–11.

[177] Verlohren S, Herraiz I, Lapaire O, et al. New gestational phase-specific cutoff values for the use of the soluble fms-like tyrosine kinase-1/placental growth factor ratio as a diagnostic test for preeclampsia. Hypertension. 2014;63(2):346–352.

[178] Andersen LB, Frederiksen-Moller B, Work Havelund K, et al. Diagnosis of preeclampsia with soluble Fms-like tyrosine kinase 1/placental growth factor ratio: an inter-assay comparison. J Am Soc Hypertens. 2015;9(2):86–96.

[179] Zhang J, Klebanoff MA, Roberts JM. Prediction of adverse outcomes by common definitions of hypertension in pregnancy. Obstet Gynecol. 2001;97(2):261–267.

[180] von Dadelszen P, Magee LA, Roberts JM. Subclassification of preeclampsia. Hypertens Pregnancy. 2003;22(2):143–148.

[181] Payne B, Hodgson S, Hutcheon JA, et al. Performance of the fullPIERS model in predicting adverse maternal outcomes in pre-eclampsia using patient data from the PIERS (Pre-eclampsia Integrated Estimate of RiSk) cohort, collected on admission. Bjogan Int J Obstet Gynaecol. 2013;120(1):113–118.

[182] Seely EW, Solomon CG. Improving the prediction of preeclampsia. N Engl J Med. 2016;374(1):83–84.

[183] Hund M, Verhagen-Kamerbeek W, Reim M, Messinger D, Van der Does R, Stepan H. Influence of the sFlt-1/PlGF ratio on clinical decision-making in women with suspected preeclampsia – the PreOS study protocol. Hypertens Pregnancy. 2015;34(1):102–115.

[184] Thadhani R, Hagmann H, Schaarschmidt W, et al. Removal of soluble fms-like tyrosine kinase-1 by dextran Sulfate Apheresis in Preeclampsia. J Am Soc Nephrol. 2016 Mar; 27(3):903–913. doi: 10.1681/ASN.2015020157. Epub 2015 Sep 24.

[185] http://www.awmf.org/uploads/tx_szleitlinien/015-018l_S1_Diagnostik_Therapie_hypertensiver_Schwangerschaftserkrankungen_2014-01.pdf Accessed 01 March 2016.

[186] Porter ME, Teisberg EO. Redefining health care: creating value-based cmpetition on results. Boston: Harvard Business School Press; 2006.

[187] Schäfer HH, Filser L, Rohr UP, Laubender RP, Dieterle T, Maitland R, Zaugg CE. Medical value as a new strategy to increase corporate viability: market chances and limitations in the diagnostic industry. J Entrepren Organ Manag.2015;4:131. doi: 10.4172/2169-026X.1000131

[188] Natekar A, Olds RL, Lau MW, Min K, Imoto K, Slavin TP. Elevated blood pressure: Our family's fault? The genetics of essential hypertension. World J Cardiol. 2014;6:327–337. DOI: 10.4330/wjc.v6.i5.327.

[189] Kullo IJ, Leeper NJ. The genetic basis of peripheral arterial disease: current knowledge, challenges, and future directions. Circ Res. 2015;116:1551–1560. DOI: 10.1161/CIRCRESAHA.116.303518.

[190] Klein et al. International Warfarin Pharmacogenetics Consortium, Klein TE, Altman RB, Eriksson N, Gage BF, Kimmel SE, Lee MT, Limdi NA, Page D, Roden DM, Wagner MJ, Caldwell MD, Johnson JA. Estimation of the warfarin dose with clinical and pharmacogenetic data. N Engl J Med. 2009;360:753–764. DOI: 10.1056/NEJMoa0809329. Erratum in: N Engl J Med. 2009;361:1613.

[191] Rosendorff C, Lackland DT, Allison M, Aronow WS, Black HR, Blumenthal RS, Cannon CP, de Lemos JA, Elliott WJ, Findeiss L, Gersh BJ, Gore JM, Levy D, Long JB, O'Connor CM, O'Gara PT, Ogedegbe G, Oparil S, White WB; American Heart Association, American College of Cardiology, and American Society of Hypertension. Treatment of

hypertension in patients with coronary artery disease: a scientific statement from the American Heart Association, American College of Cardiology, and American Society of Hypertension. Circulation. 2015;131:e435–e470. DOI: 10.1161/CIR.0000000000000207.

[192] Tanner RM, Lynch AI, Brophy VH, Eckfeldt JH, Davis BR, Ford CE, Boerwinkle E, Arnett DK. Pharmacogenetic associations of MMP9 and MMP12 variants with cardiovascular disease in patients with hypertension. PLoS One. 2011;6:e23609. DOI: 10.1371/journal.pone.0023609.

[193] Faulkner E, Annemans L, Garrison L, Helfand M, Holtorf AP, Hornberger J, Hughes D, Li T, Malone D, Payne K, Siebert U, Towse A, Veenstra D, Watkins J; Personalized Medicine Development and Reimbursement Working Group. Challenges in the development and reimbursement of personalized medicine-payer and manufacturer perspectives and implications for health economics and outcomes research: a report of the ISPOR personalized medicine special interest group. Value Health. 2012;15:1162–1171. DOI: http://dx.doi.org/10.1016/j.jval.2012.05.006.

Chapter 9

Myocardial Connexin-43 is Implicated in the Prevention of Malignant Arrhythmia in Rats Suffering from Essential Hypertension

Tamara Egan Benova, Barbara Szeiffova Bacova,
Csilla Viczenczova, Miroslav Barancik and
Narcis Tribulova

Additional information is available at the end of the chapter

http://dx.doi.org/10.5772/63456

Abstract

Gap-junction connexin (Cx) channels are important determinants of myocardial conduction and synchronization that is crucial for heart function. Hypertension-induced structural remodeling is associated with an increased risk of life-threatening arrhythmias and heart failure in both humans and experimental animals. Recent studies suggest that abnormal distribution and/or downregulation of Cx43 accompanied with altered protein kinase C (PKC)ε signaling in spontaneously hypertensive rats were linked with increased propensity to ventricular fibrillation compared to normotensive rats. By contrast, the long-term treatment of hypertensive rats with cardioprotective compounds such as melatonin, omega-3 fatty acids, or red palm oil resulted in protection from lethal arrhythmia. Their antiarrhythmic effect was attributed to the attenuation of abnormal Cx43 topology and modulation of Cx43 mRNA as well as protein expression and its functional phosphorylated forms. The latter might be attributed to upregulation of PKCε. It appears that maladaptive consequences of hypertension resulting in abnormal myocardial distribution of Cx43 and its downregulation can contribute to arrhythmogenesis and occurrence of malignant arrhythmias. On the other hand, the attenuation of myocardial Cx43 abnormalities by treatment with melatonin, omega-3 fatty acids, or red palm oil confers arrhythmia protection in rodent model of essential hypertension. Findings uncover novel mechanisms of cardioprotective effects of melatonin, omega-3 fatty acids, and red palm oil. Well-designed clinical trials are needed to explore antiarrhythmic potential of these compounds in human essential hypertension.

Keywords: hypertension, arrhythmias, connexin-43, melatonin, omega-3 fatty acids

1. Introduction

Different types of epidemiologic studies, including a growing number of large cohort studies and interventional trials in different population groups, have consistently shown that there is a strong positive association between hypertension and cardiovascular diseases (CVDs), and that lowering the blood pressure helps to improve cardiovascular health. Hypertension is the leading risk factor for the development of CVD, with men exhibiting a higher arterial pressure than women during the ages from 20 to 65. Up until menopause, there are significant sex differences in blood pressure, vascular reactivity, and renal function [1].

Hypertension is a multifactorial process. Environmental factors and the genetic component as well as epigenetic inheritance contribute significantly to essential hypertension [2] that is known to be on rise in the human population. Sympathetic nervous system plays a major role in the maintenance of hypertension and the rostral ventrolateral medulla is the main source of this sympathetic activation. It is proposed that melatonin-induced epigenetic modifications in the neurons of area postrema are implicated in this process [3]. Sympathetic activation in hypertension is accompanied by oxidative stress and inflammation as by-product [4]. These undesired processes might be ameliorated by interventions with compounds possessing antioxidant and free radical-scavenging ability, for example, melatonin, statins, adrenergic beta receptor blockers, and omega-3 fatty acids. Patients with uncontrolled essential hypertension have elevated concentrations of superoxide anion, hydrogen peroxide, lipid peroxides, endothelin, and transforming growth factor-beta with a simultaneous decrease in endothelial nitric oxide, superoxide dismutase, vitamin E, and long-chain polyunsaturated fatty acids (PUFAs) [5–7]. The implication of redox signaling and lower omega-3 index is suggested in the pathogenesis of essential hypertension in animal models as well [8, 9]. Omega-3 fatty acids exhibit wide-ranging biological actions [6] that include the regulation of renal sodium excretion and vasomotor tone, partly by decreasing the production of vasocostrincting and anti-inflammatory eicosanoids. Omega-3 fatty acids also activate the parasympathetic nervous system. It is proposed that the availability of adequate amount of omega-3 fatty acids during the critical periods of growth prevents the development of hypertension in adulthood [10].

Hypertension is a major risk factor for cardiovascular injury resulting in heart attack, congestive heart failure, stroke, as well as sudden arrhythmic death [11, 12]. The latter is associated with myocardial structural remodeling that follows hypertension, such as hypertrophy and fibrosis. This remodeling is accompanied by changes in expression, distribution, and function of cell membrane ion channels, intercellular gap-junction connexin-43 (Cx43) channels, Ca^{2+}-cycling proteins, and extracellular matrix composition [13–16]. Mentioned remodeling predisposes to arrhythmogenic mechanisms including early or delayed after-depolarization and reentry of excitation, facilitating life-threatening ventricular tachycardia (VT) and ventricular fibrillation (VF).

2. Hypertension-related gap junctions and connexin-43 remodeling

Changes in cardiac workload due to pressure or volume overload induce hypertrophic growth of individual myocytes. Hypertrophy of cardiomyocytes counteracts the increased wall tension (Laplace's law), and is therefore often considered as compensated hypertrophy [17]. However, prolonged state of hypertrophy is accompanied by maladaptation that promotes progression into heart failure (decompensated hypertrophy). Typical ultrastructural alterations of cardiomyocytes from the left ventricle of old spontaneously hypertensive rats (frequently used model mimicking essential hypertension in humans) are demonstrated in

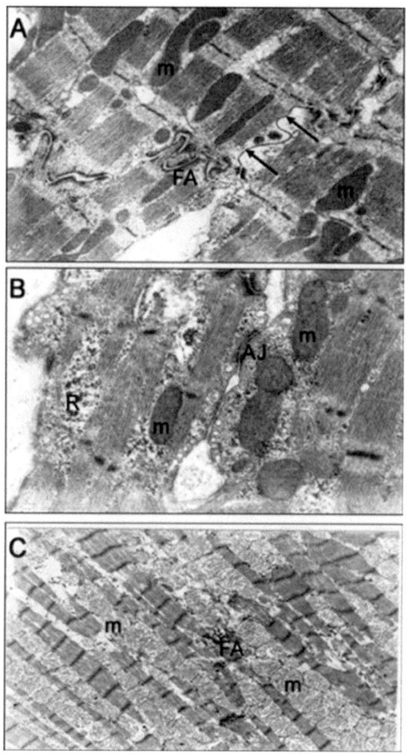

Figure 1. Representative electron microscopic images demonstrating cardiomyocytes and intercellular junctions in the left ventricles of spontaneously hypertensive rat hearts. (**A**) Conventional ultrastructure showing electron-dense mitochondria (m), adhesive fascia adherens (FA) junctions at the intercalated disk, and peripheral gap junction (arrows) on the lateral sides of the cardiomyocytes. (**B**) Development of lateral gap junctions following the formation of adhesive junctions (AJs) and high amounts of ribosomes (R) and dense mitochondria (m) are seen in young hypertensive rat heart at compensate stage of hypertrophy. (**C**) Severely injured cardiomyocytes exhibiting edematous mitochondria, myocytolysis, pronounced reduction of adhesive fascia adherens (FA) junctions, and loss of gap junctions are sporadically seen in the myocardium of old hypertensive rats at early decompensate stage of hypertrophy.

Figure 1. The cardiac remodeling process is characterized by both structural and electrical disorders that decrease the electrical stability of the heart [16, 18]. A hallmark of the electrical changes with regard to impulse conduction is an impairment of electrical coupling due to abnormal expression of Cx43-constituted gap junctions. Available data suggest that particularly spatial heterogeneity and severity of Cx43 channels dysfunction throughout myocardium affects myocardial conduction and electrical properties of the heart. In addition to structural remodeling, hypertension likewise other systemic or heart disease and proarrhythmogenic conditions are linked with oxidative stress and/or inflammation [4, 7, 9]. This pathology contributes to the impairment of intercellular junctions and communication due to the acceleration of Cx43 degradation and/or dysfunction as well as other Cx43-interacting proteins [19]. Cascade events induced by hypertension resulting in an increased risk for malignant arrhythmias are demonstrated in **Figure 2**.

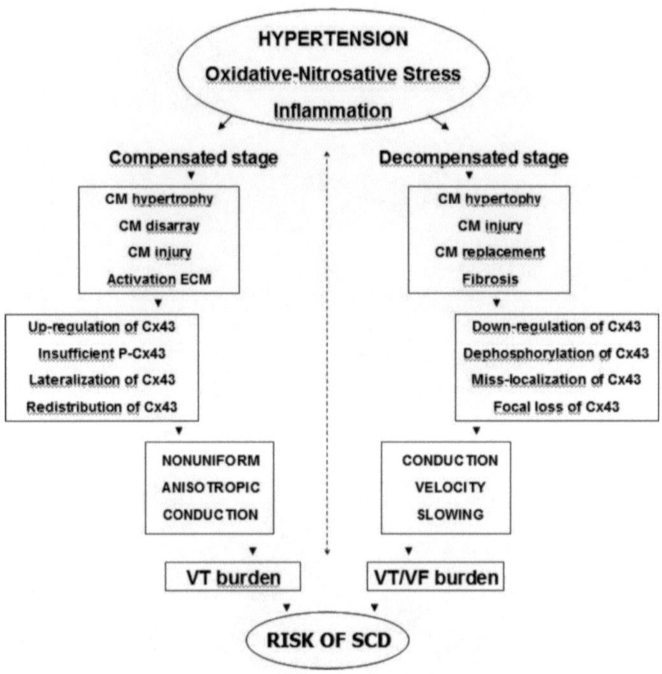

Figure 2. Scheme showing possible myocardial alterations of cardiomyocytes as well as Cx43 expression and distribution that might increase a risk for SCD in spontaneously hypertensive rats and also most likely in patients suffering from essential hypertension.

Several studies have described changes in the number, size, and distribution of myocardial gap junctions during hypertrophic heart disease. In general, Cx43 expression appears to be unaltered or upregulated during the initial and compensatory phase of hypertrophy but they are always redistributed along the cardiomyocyte surface (**Figures 3** and **4**). Cx43 expression and the number of intercalated disk-related gap junctions are reduced when the hypertrophy becomes maladaptive, accompanied by severe cardiomyocyte injury (**Figures 3** and **4**) and interstitial fibrosis resulting in progression to heart failure [16]. Kostin et al. [15] reported that in the left ventricles of pressure-overloaded human hearts with aortic stenosis, Cx43 expression was increased in the compensated hypertrophic stage, but was decreased and heterogeneously distributed throughout the ventricles in the period of decompensated hypertensive heart. The decreased expression of Cx43 at the protein level is accompanied by a reduction of Cx43 mRNA, suggesting that the downregulation of Cx43 in hypertrophic heart disease is regulated at the transcriptional level. Downregulation and/or heterogeneous redistribution of Cx43 channels is often associated with abnormal conduction that facilitates arrhythmias (**Figure 2**), although there seems to be a large reserve before reduced intercellular coupling becomes arrhythmogenic [18]. Interestingly, hypertrophic cardiomyopathy, the most common genetic disease of the myocardium, is also characterized by cardiomyocyte hypertrophy, myofibrillar disarray, fibrosis, and miss-localization of Cx43 linked with changes in myocardial conduction and prolonged QRS interval [20]. Consequently, there is a high risk of sudden arrhythmic death, especially in young adults (including competitive athletes).

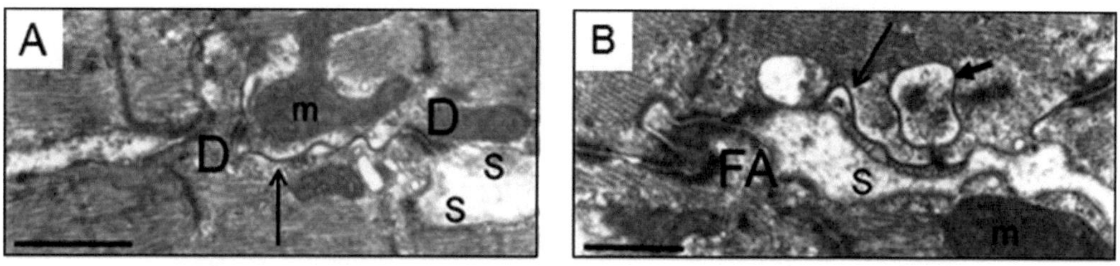

Figure 3. Representative electron microscopic images demonstrating altered topology of myocardial gap junctions in hypertensive rat hearts. (**A**) Lateraly situated gap junctions in the vicinity of adhesive junctions are seen in young rats frequently at compensated stage of hypertrophy. (**B**) Internalization of intercalated disk-related gap junctions (arrows) is often seen in old rats at decompensated stage of hypertrophy. Abbreviations: s – sarcolemma, D – desmosome, FA – fascia adherens junction, m – mitochondria, bar 1 μm.

In the context of myocardial remodeling and Cx43 alterations, it is important to note that microRNA-1 has an essential regulatory impact in cardiogenesis, cardiac hypertrophy, and cardiac electrophysiology. The latter is due to its ability to modulate the expression levels of molecular targets that modulate the electrical properties of cardiac cells. These targets are GJA1-encoding Cx43 and KCNJ2-encoding potassium channel protein that determine myocardial conduction velocity and repolarization [21]. Downregulation of microRNA-1 at the early stage of cardiac hypertrophy was associated with an increased Cx43 protein levels and enhanced Cx43 phosphorylation. The latter correlated with the displacement of Cx43 from the gap junctions that facilitated ventricular tachyarrhythmias [22]. In turn, it is most likely that decompensated hypertrophic stage accompanied by a decrease of Cx43 gene transcripts and protein levels might result from upregulation of microRNA-1. This view is supported by findings that inflammation (known to be implicated in the pathogenesis of hypertension) represses Cx43 expression via upregulation of microRNA-1 and potentiates arrhythmogenesis by targeting GJA1 [23, 24].

Taken together, it can be hypothesized that the prevention or attenuation of maladaptive myocardial Cx43 remodeling and dysfunction induced by hypertension could decrease a risk of arrhythmic death and heart failure [18, 25].

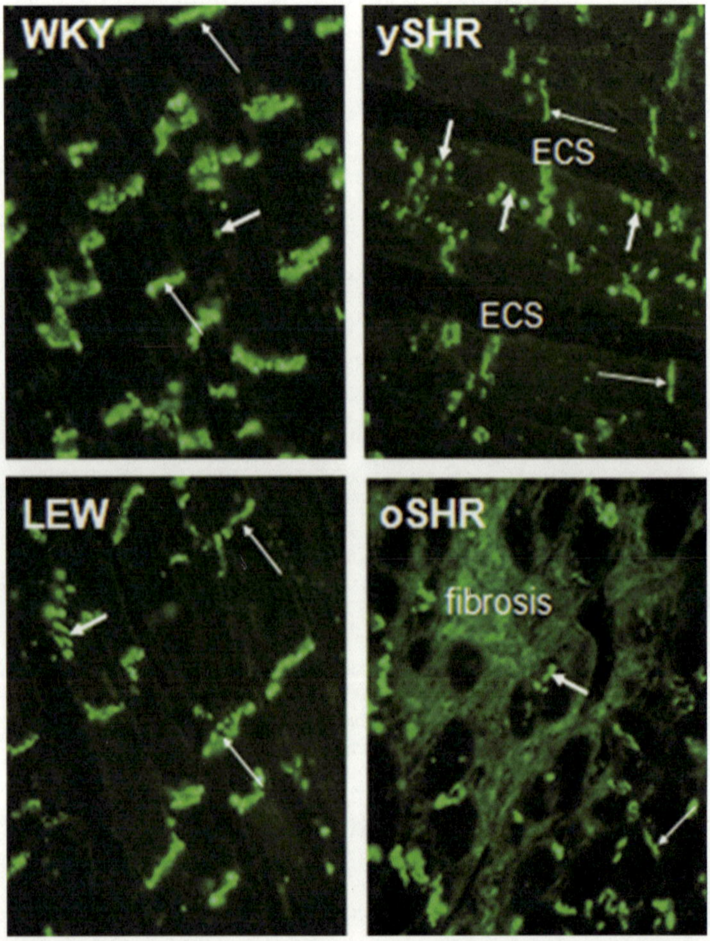

Figure 4. Representative images of myocardial Cx43-immunofluorescence in the left ventricles of young (WKY) and old (LEW) normotensive rats as well as young (ySHR) and old (oSHR) spontaneously hypertensive rat hearts. Note: conventional topology of Cx43-positive gap junctions at the intercalated disks (thin arrows) and enhanced expression of Cx43 on lateral surfaces (short arrows) of the cardiomyocytes in young rats at compensate stage of hypertrophy and pronounced mislocalization of Cx43 due to fibrosis in old rats at decompensate stage of hypertrophy. ESC, extracellular space. Magnification, objective ×40.

3. The role of myocardial Cx43 in protecting from malignant arrhythmias

Therapy to prevent death due to arrhythmias involves invasive procedures, that is, implantable cardioverter defibrillator to protect from sudden cardiac death when VF occurs, catheter ablation of arrhythmogenic loci, and resynchronization devices for supporting myocardial synchronization and thereby reducing arrhythmia risk. Blockade of ion current by antiarrhythmic drugs is often ineffective and may even cause proarrhythmia that can increase mortality. As a result, the effort to develop new antiarrhythmic drugs directed at specific ion channels has decreased dramatically. However, mentioned invasive treatment did not prevent the occurrence and/or recurrence of life-threatening arrhythmias. Moreover, these interventions decrease the quality of life and can also be accompanied by various complications. Therefore, novel approach fighting arrhythmia-related sudden cardiac death and stroke is warranted. Considering the crucial role of intercellular coupling and communication to ensure synchronized myocardial contraction, it seems relevant to suggest the implication of these factors in the prevention of arrhythmias.

The novel approach is based on a prevention or attenuation of the development of arrhythmogenic substrates in relation to Cx43 channel function to reduce a risk of arrhythmia occurrence [25, 26]. Taking into consideration, events involved in the development of malignant arrhythmias include oxidative/nitrosative stress, myocardial hypertrophy and/or fibrosis, Cx43 remodeling, and conduction disturbances; the action of antiarrhythmic compounds is expected to include one or more steps in cascade of events [25]. Consistent with it, the "upstream" drug therapy is of great interest aiming to prevent or eliminate arrhythmogenic substrates and triggers. Lipid-lowering drugs, statins, and some antihypertensive drugs are known to exhibit antiarrhythmic effects likely due to the attenuation of myocardial remodeling (hypertrophy, fibrosis) that affects intercellular coupling mediated by Cx43 channels. In addition, these pharmacological compounds exert antioxidant and anti-inflammatory efficacy. All these actions seem to preserve the adequate myocardial Cx43 levels and topology. Direct and/or indirect salutary modulation of Cx43 channel function may confer protection from malignant arrhythmias. Despite the increasing number of experimental studies supporting this idea, there are still many questions to be answered by further research. The topic is challenging to address in experimental as well as in clinical settings or when considering the development of new antiarrhythmic drugs. This article focuses on the benefit of non-pharmacological compounds in spontaneously hypertensive rats, a rodent model mimicking human essential hypertension. It demonstrates novel pleiotropic effects of melatonin and new mechanisms of omega-3 fatty acids and antioxidant-rich red palm oil (RPO) actions that are associated with the modulation of myocardial Cx43.

3.1. Antihypertensive and antiarrhytmic effects of melatonin

Melatonin can reduce blood pressure through the (1) direct effect on hypothalamus, (2) by its antioxidant properties that lower blood pressure, and (3) by decreasing the amount of catecholamines [27]. Hypotensive effect of melatonin could also be mediated by its direct effect on blood vessels or by decreasing serotonin production that is crucial in the inhibition of sympathetic and stimulation of parasympathetic system [28]. Melatonin could affect changes in blood pressure also through its specific melatonin receptors localized in the peripheral vessels or in parts of central nervous system that directly participate in the control of blood pressure [29].

It appears that melatonin in addition to its circadian rhythm regulation exerts a hypotensive effect, and it can modulate cellular redox state and improve the function of the cardiovascular system in pathological conditions. Elderly population has reduced circulating melatonin levels [30, 31]. Decrease of melatonin was also registered in patients suffering from primary hypertension compared with normotensive individuals [32]. Increased melatonin concentration in elderly patients suffering from hypertension may thus be of crucial therapeutic importance. Patients suffering from coronary heart disease, the most typical complication of chronic hypertension, exhibited over fivefold lower level of serum melatonin at night compared with the control group [33]. Likewise, patients demonstrating a "non-dipping profile" of nocturnal arterial pressure exhibited decreased nocturnal melatonin secretion compared with the patients showing a "dipping profile" [34, 35]. The study of Kedziora-Kornatowska et al. [36] confirms the benefit of melatonin supplementation on parameters of oxidative stress in elderly patients suffering from primary hypertension and suggests that melatonin supplementation can be considered as a supporting therapy in the treatment of hypertension. In "non-dippers," a significant hypotensive effect was observed [37]. Melatonin is effective in lowering blood pressure in essential hypertensive patients [38] and in patients with nocturnal hypertension [39]. Antihypertensive effect of exogenous melatonin is reported in numerous experimental studies [29, 39–43].

In addition to antihypertensive effects of melatonin, in vitro and in vivo experimental studies demonstrate its acute antiarrhythmic effects [44–46]. Melatonin appears to be effective even in physiological concentrations. On the other hand, arrhythmias score was significantly higher after coronary artery ligation in pinealectomized rats compared with controls [47, 48]. In almost all of the above mentioned studies, melatonin-induced cardioprotection and antiarrhythmic effects are attributed to its free radical-scavenging potential [44, 49, 50]. Of note, melatonin has several features that are of clinical interest. It has low toxicity, crosses all types of biological barriers (i.e., blood-/brain barrier and placenta), and it can easily enter into all cell compartments including mitochondrias, producers of free radicals [50].

3.2. Antihypertensive and antiarrhythmic effects of omega-3 PUFA

Numerous studies report salutary effects of omega-3 PUFA, that is, eicosapentaenoic acid (EPA) and docosahexaenoic acid (DHA) on CVD risk factors [51]. These effects include (1) lowering of serum triglycerides via reduction in hepatic triglycerides production, (2) lowering blood pressure via improved endothelial cell function, (3) decreasing platelet aggregation via reduction in prothrombotic prostanoids, (4) decreasing inflammation via reduction in four-series leukotriene production, and (5) protection from arrhythmia via modulation of electrophysiological properties of cardiac myocytes. Beneficial effects of omega-3 PUFA on CVD risk factors in children including regulation of blood pressure, during childhood, and adolescence are recently reviewed [52]. Systematic meta-analysis suggests that high doses of omega-3 PUFA (~3 g/day) produce a small but significant decrease in systolic blood pressure in older and hypertensive subjects [53].

Observational and interventional studies indicate that dietary omega-3 PUFA may be effective in preventing cardiac arrhythmias and sudden cardiac death. The strongest evidence suggesting an antiarrhythmic effect of omega-3 PUFA, resulting in significant reduction of sudden cardiac death, provides large GISSI-Prevenzione trial [54]. Antiarrhythmic actions observed in both clinical and experimental conditions are mostly associated with myocardial infarction or post-infarction-related malignant arrhythmias. Some studies, in particular clinical trials, do not clearly demonstrate the antiarrhythmic effects of omega-3 PUFA [55–57]. To explain the discrepancy of the results, it is suggested that the effectiveness of omega-3 PUFA treatment might depend on the mechanism of cardiac arrhythmia, dose, and the route of omega-3 PUFA administration [58]. Moreover, the efficacy of omega-3 PUFA supplementation in clinical trials should be adjusted to initial basal levels of omega-3 PUFA as well as medical treatment regimen of patients. Multiple mechanisms of cardioprotective and antiarrhythmic effects of omega-3 PUFA are suggested, including ion channel function modulation and prevention of pressure overload-related cardiac remodeling [59].

3.3. Cardioprotective and antiarrhythmic effects of red palm oil

The link between dietary fats and cardiovascular diseases has initiated a growing interest in a dietary red palm oil research. RPO is obtained from the orange-red mesocarp of the fruit of a tropical plant known as oil palm *(Elaeis guineensis)* [60]. Besides unsaturated and saturated fatty acids, it contains high concentration of antioxidants such as vitamin A (carotenes), pro-vitamin E—namely tocotrienols, tocopherols, coenzyme Q10, and lycopene [61–63]. In spite of its high level of saturated fatty acid content, RPO intake does not promote vascular disease. On the contrary, the benefits of RPO on health include reduction in the risk of arterial thrombosis and/or atherosclerosis, platelet aggregation, reduction in blood pressure [61], inhibition of endogenous cholesterol biosynthesis, and a reduction in oxidative stress [62]. Oxidative stress and the severity or progression of disease have stimulated further interest in the potential role of RPO (a cocktail of natural antioxidants) to improve redox status. Experimental studies suggest that the cardioprotective effects of RPO may not only be due to the high antioxidant content but could also be mediated by the ability of RPO to modulate signaling events during ischemia and reperfusion [63, 64]. The cardioprotective effects of the tocotrienol-rich fraction have been attributed to the effect of tocotrienol to modulate the Akt signaling, thus generating a survival signal during reperfusion [62]. Beneficial effects of RPO are partially mediated via the phosphatidylinositol 3-kinase (PI3K) and protein kinase B (Akt) signaling pathway [64]. These findings strongly suggest that PI3K-Akt pathway may play an important role in the RPO-induced cardioprotection. However, this evidence is circumstantial since PI3K has several downstream targets other than Akt. Specific inhibition of Akt will allow to elucidate the importance of Akt on post-ischemic functional recovery in RPO-supplemented animals. RPO supplementation is associated with an increased dual phosphorylation of Akt on Ser473 and Thr308 residues indicating that the optimal activation of Akt requires phosphorylation on both Ser473 and Thr308 residues [65, 66]. Recent experimental studies demonstrate that RPO supplementation offers protection against ischemia/reperfusion injury by improved cardiac output recovery. Evidence strongly suggests that mitogen-activated protein kinases (MAPKs), NO-cGMP, and pro-survival PI3K-Akt signaling pathway may be involved in [63, 64, 66–68]. Further studies are needed to explore novel cellular and molecular mechanisms that might be involved in RPO-related cardioprotection. Data about antiarrhythmic potential of RPO are rare. According to the recent study [8], increased susceptibility of hyperthyroid rats to malignant arrhythmias is partially ameliorated by supplementation with red palm oil and related mainly to the upregulation of Cx43 and protein kinase C (PKC)ε.

4. Modulation of myocardial Cx43 expression by melatonin

In addition to antiarrhythmic effects of acute administration of melatonin in the setting of ischemia/reperfusion, its antiarrhythmic efficacy has been recently demonstrated in spontaneously hypertensive rats after long-term administration [43]. Several studies showed that compared to normotensive rats, spontaneously hypertensive rats are much prone to develop VF [25]. Consistent with it, the threshold to electrically inducible VF is significantly lower in hypertensive versus normotensive rats but it is increased in response to melatonin treatment. This antiarrhythmic effect of melatonin is associated with the enhancement of myocardial Cx43 gene expression (**Figure 5A**) as well as the total levels of Cx43 protein and its functional phosphorylated forms in hypertensive and to lesser extent in normotensive Wistar rat hearts (**Figure 6**, left panel). Increase of Cx43 phosphorylation could be in part attributed to the increase of PKCε isoform resulting from melatonin treatment. Moreover, Cx43 immunofluorescence labeling and quantitative image analysis reveal an attenuation of abnormal Cx43 distribution and enhanced myocardial Cx43-positive signal in hypertensive rats treated with melatonin. These findings strongly indicate that melatonin may modulate Cx43 expression and distribution in the remodeled heart of hypertensive rats.

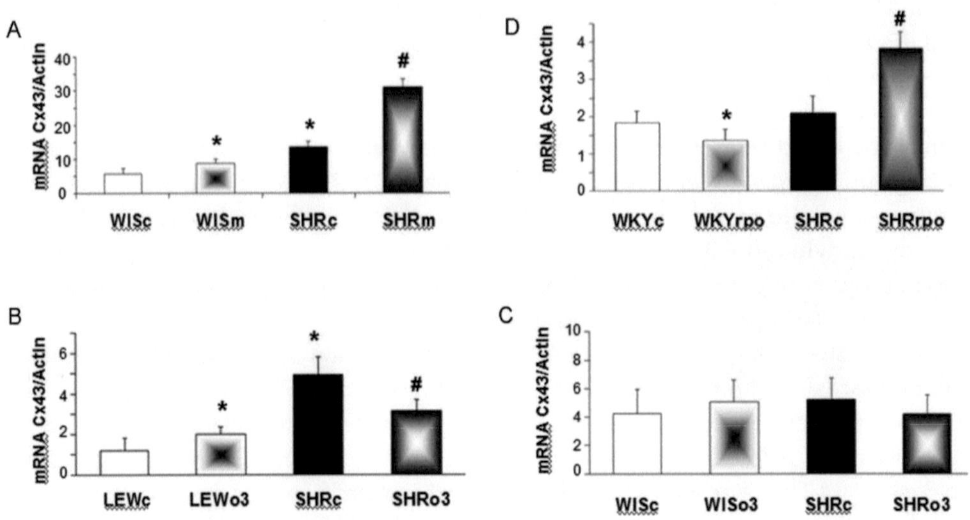

Figure 5. Cx43 mRNA expression normalized to actin in the left ventricles of young (**A**) and old (**B**) untreated and omega-3-treated young SHR and normotensive rat hearts. WKYc, untreated WKY rats; WKYo3, WKY rats treated with omega-3; LEWc, untreated Lewis rats; LEWo3, Lewis rats treated with omega-3; SHRc, untreated SHR; SHRo3, SHR treated with omega-3 PUFA.Results are mean ± SD of eight hearts,significant difference ($P < 0.05$) * from WKYc (WISc, LEWc resp.),and # from SHRc.* Modified with permission from [82]; [43]; [78].

http://dx.doi.org/10.5772/63456

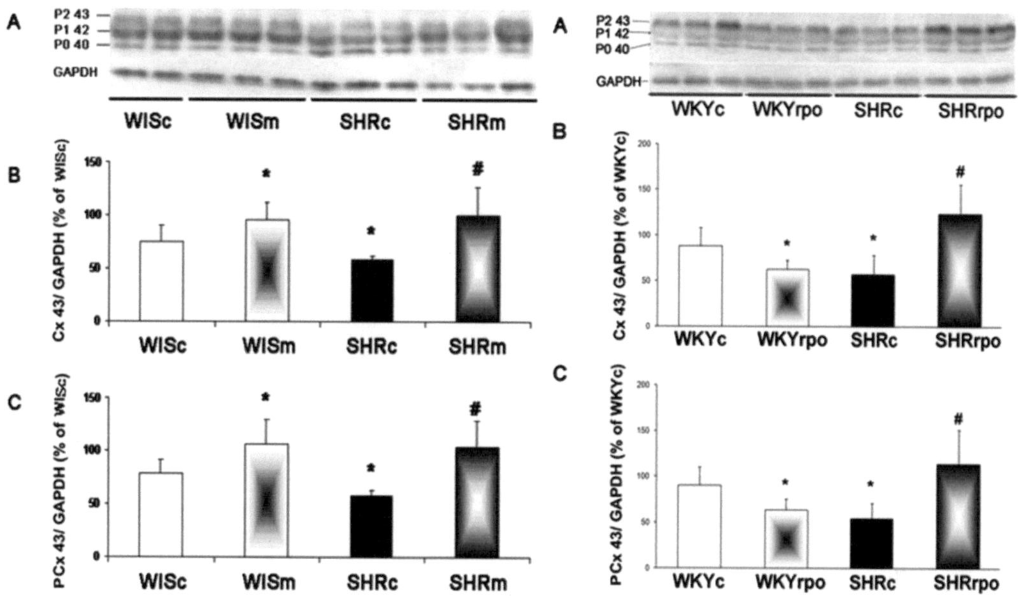

Figure 6. Representative immunoblot (**A**) showing two phosphorylated and one non-phosphorylated form of Cx43 and densitometric quantification of total Cx43 expression (**B**) and its functional phosphorylated forms (**C**) normalized to GAPDH in the left ventricles of untreated and melatonin-treated (left panel), and red palm oil-treated (right panel) hypertensive (SHR) and normotensive (WIS or WKY) rat hearts. Significant difference ($P < 0.05$) * from WKYc (WISc resp.), and # from SHRc. *Modified with permission from [82]; [43].

However, molecular mechanisms of melatonin effects on myocardial Cx43 are not elucidated yet. It has been reported that melatonin upregulates Cx43 (mRNA and protein) and enhances cell-to-cell coupling in human myometrial smooth muscle cells via MT_2 receptor and protein kinase C-dependent manner [69]. It is proposed that melatonin activates phospholipase C followed by the generation of inositol triphosphate and diacylglycerol. The latter activates PKC, which can affect transcription factors c-fos and c-jun that are important in the regulation of Cx43 expression in myometrial cells [70]. Further studies are needed to explore whether this pathway might be involved in the upregulation of Cx43 in heart muscle as well. The cardioprotective and antiarrhythmic effects of acute melatonin treatment in condition of Ischemia/reperfusion were attributed mainly to its antioxidant and free radical-scavenging activity. It is most likely that these cardioprotective actions of melatonin are involved in the condition of oxidative stress induced by hypertension. Consequently, it might result in the preservation of myocardial Cx43 proteins and protection from its downregulation. Melatonin may be classified as a naturally occurring, mitochondrial-targeted antioxidant [71]. This fact is important when considering the most recent studies [26, 72] showing that arrhythmias could be prevented by mitochondria-targeted antioxidants rather than by general antioxidants. It also seems possible that melatonin could protect myocardial Cx43 via inhibiting the activity of cyclooxygenase 2 and inducible NO synthase caused by chronic inflammation [73]. Hypothetical mechanisms of the modulation of cardiac Cx43 channels and protection from malignant arrhythmias by melatonin are depicted on **Figure 7**.

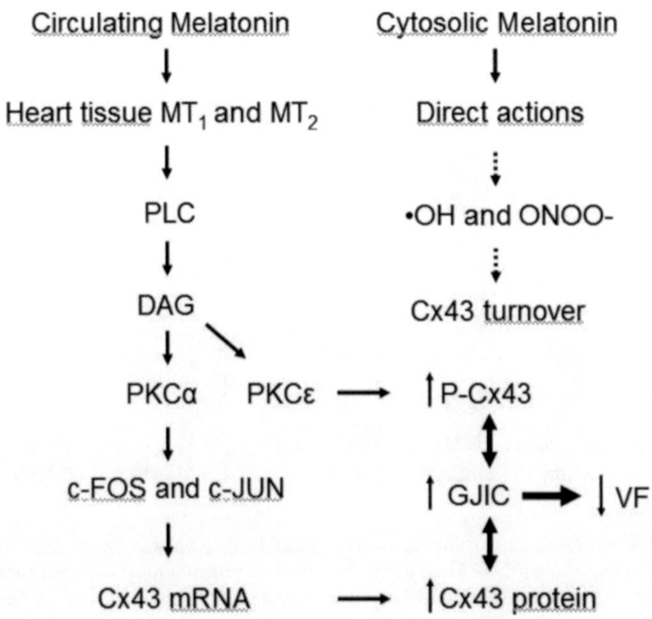

Figure 7. Proposed mechanisms of melatonin action on myocardial Cx43 expression and distribution in spontaneusly hypertensive rat heart. Circulating melatonin via its receptors, MT_1 and MT_2, activates phospholipase C (PLC) followed by the production of diacylglycerol (DAG), which activates protein kinase C (PKC). PKCε by phosphorylation of Cx43 can modulate the channel's function as well as its myocardial distribution and subsequently gap-junctional intercellular communication (GJIC). Activation of PKCα also affects transcription factors c-FOS and cJUN, which bind to conserved activator protein-1 in the promoter region of Cx43 and hence can increase Cx43 expression. In addition, melatonin exhibits receptor-independent actions due to its ability to scavenge free radicals. Free radicals enhance the degradation of Cx43 and melatonin can attenuate this process and preserve myocardial Cx43 levels. Altogether, the protection of functional Cx43 by melatonin can affect GJIC and improve electrical stability resulting in the decrease of inducible VF.

5. Modulation of myocardial Cx43 expression by omega-3 PUFA

A direct renin inhibitor, aliskiren, and dietary omega-3 PUFA attenuate electrical remodeling in renin-angiotensin transgenic rats (another model mimicking human hypertension) most likely due to the restoration of normal topology of Cx43 [74]. Both treatments also reduce the QRS and QT interval suggesting an improvement in conduction that could be attributed to reduced fibrosis and the elimination of lateral distribution of Cx43. Consequently, it results in the decline of tachyarrhythmia induction. In addition, aliskiren and omega-3 PUFA prevent hypertension-related inflammation that is generally known to downregulate Cx43 [75].

Antiarrhythmic effects of both omega-3 PUFA and atorvastatin (a hypolipidemic drug with anti-inflammatory and antioxidant properties) are demonstrated in hereditary hypertriglyceridemic rats with elevated blood pressure [76]. The decrease of VF inducibility is associated with the suppression of hyper-phosphorylation of Cx43 and the restoration of its normal myocardial topology. Electron microscopy examination reveals that both omega-3 PUFA and atorvastatin improve the structural integrity of mitochondria, plasma membrane, and intercellular junctions when compared to untreated diseased rats. This membrane protective effect may be partially explained by changes in membrane composition [77], that is, increased incorporation of omega-3 PUFA and decreased cholesterol levels due to treatments. It would be interesting to know whether atorvastatin affects properties of ion and Cx43 channels as well as well as myocardial conduction, (likewise omega-3 PUFA), to understand better its antiarrhythmic effect in relation to myocardial Cx43 alterations.

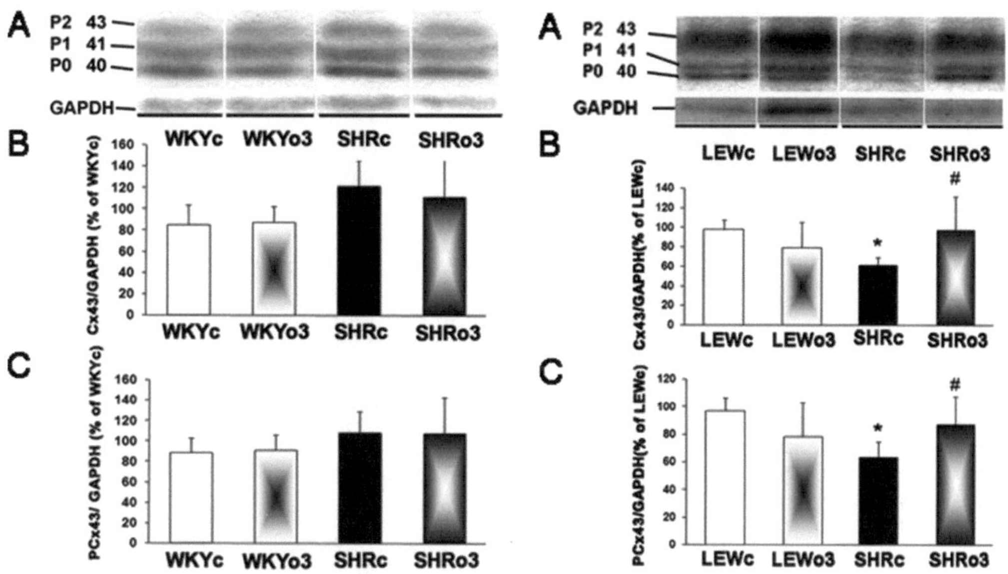

Figure 8. Representative immunoblot (**A**) showing three forms of Cx43 and densitometric quantification of total Cx43 expression (**B**) and its functional phosphorylated forms (**C**), normalized to GAPDH in the left ventricles of untreated and omega-3-treated young SHR and WKY rat hearts (left panel) as well as in the left ventricles of untreated and omega-3-treated old SHR and Lewis rat hearts (right panel). Results are mean ± SD of eight hearts, Significant difference ($P < 0.05$) * from LEWc, and # from SHRc. *Modified with permission from [78].

Protection from VF due to intake of omega-3 PUFA (i.e., DHA and EPA) and the implication of myocardial Cx43 are demonstrated in another study [78] using young (compensated stage of hypertrophy) and old spontaneously hypertensive rats (early decompensated stage of hypertrophy). Findings show that omega-3 PUFA intake normalizes myocardial Cx43 mRNA levels in old rats (**Figure 5C, D**) and Cx43 protein expression as well as its functional phosphorylated status in both young and old hypertensive animals (**Figure 8**). Enhanced Cx43 phosphorylation might be in part attributed to PKCε that is upregulated by omega-3 PUFA. The treatment significantly eliminates abnormal Cx43 distribution (**Figure 9**), diminishes the internalization of gap junctions, and improves ultrastructure (integrity) of the mitochondria in cardiomyocytes of hypertensive rats. These findings clearly indicate that the modulation of Cx43 channel function and myocardial cell-to-cell coupling by omega-3 PUFA might be possible.

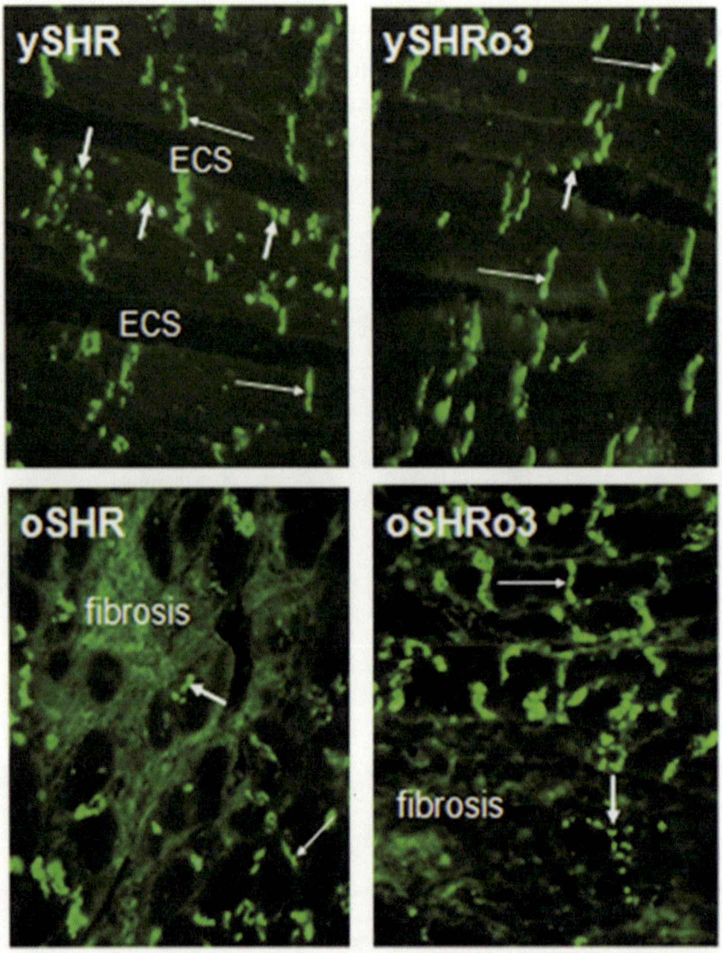

Figure 9. Representative images of myocardial Cx43-immunofluorescence in the left ventricles of untreated young (ySHR) and old (oSHR) and omega-3 fatty acid-treated young (ySHRo3) and old (oSHRo3) spontaneously hypertensive rat hearts. Note: prevalent normal Cx43 distribution at the intercalated disks (thin arrows) and apparent attenuation of disordered Cx43 distribution (short arrows) as well as reduced fibrosis due to supplementation with omega-3 fatty acids. ESC, extracellular space. Magnification, objective ×40.

Nevertheless, the question arises as to how omega-3 affects myocardial Cx43 expression and its phosphorylation. It is known that omega-3 PUFA are ligands for the nuclear transcription factor, peroxisome proliferator-activated receptor (PPAR). It is also known that omega-3 PUFA might regulate numerous gene expressions and consequently intracellular pathways involved in protein expression and phosphorylation [79, 80]. The discovery of omega-3 PUFA signaling pathways linked with Cx43 modulation may reveal new candidates for antiarrhythmic drug development. Antiarrhythmic properties of omega-3 PUFA may also include the modulation of membrane ion current densities and intracellular Ca^{2+} handling [81]. Available data suggest that possible mechanisms of omega-3 PUFA (shown in **Figure 10**) could prevent downregulation and mislocalization of cardiac Cx43. Consequently, it could lead to suppression in the incidence of life-threatening arrhythmias.

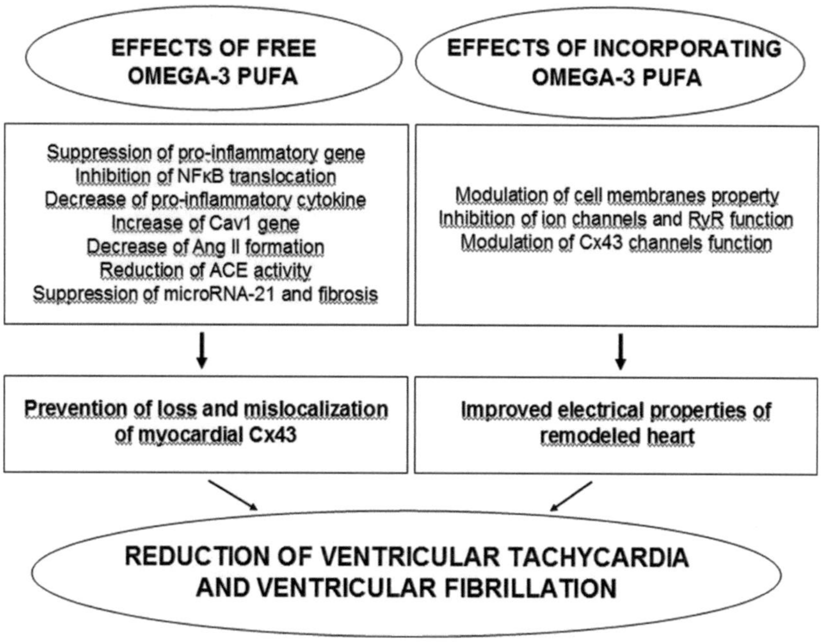

Figure 10. Diagram for the proposed mechanisms of omega-3 PUFA that could prevent downregulation and mislocalization of cardiac Cx43. Consequently, it could lead to a reduction in the incidence of life-threatening arrhythmias.

6. Modulation of myocardial Cx43 by red palm oil

It has been, for the first time, demonstrated that there is upregulation of myocardial Cx43 and suppression of PKCε activation in response to RPO supplementation of male, adult spontaneously hypertensive rats [82]. In this study, Cx43-mRNA (**Figure 5D**), total Cx43 proteins, and its phosphorylated forms are increased. Moreover, disordered localization of Cx43 is attenuated in the left ventricle of RPO-fed hypertensive rats compared with untreated rats. These alterations are associated with the suppression of early post-ischemic-reperfusion-related VT and electrically inducible VF. Moreover, it is linked with the improvement of functional recovery of the heart during post-ischemic reperfusion. However, the treatment dose of RPO (200 mg/day for 5 weeks) causes downregulation of myocardial Cx43 in normotensive age-matched rats. It results in poor arrhythmia protection, suggesting overdosing of

RPO in healthy rats. Findings indicate that hypertensive rats benefit from RPO intake, particularly because of its apparent antiarrhythmic effects. This protection can be, in part, attributed to the upregulation of myocardial Cx43 but not with PKCε activation. In addition, RPO supplementation reduced blood pressure in hypertensive rats and blood glucose in both hypertensive and normotensive rats. Taken together, the results indicate that hypertensive rats benefit from RPO supplementation, particularly due to its apparent antiarrhythmic and post-ischemic-reperfusion-related cardioprotective effects that can be, in part, explained by the upregulation of myocardial Cx43. This view is supported by findings that the downregulation of Cx43 in response to RPO intake of healthy normotensive rats is associated with poor antiarrhythmic effect.

7. Conclusions and perspectives

Data included in this comprehensive article suggest that the attenuation of hypertension-induced abnormal and/or restoration of normal myocardial expression and distribution of Cx43 as well as enhancement of its functional phosphorylated forms along with positive modulation of PKC signaling by melatonin, omega-3 fatty acids, and red palm oil may be crucial in their antiarrhythmic mechanisms. Despite "optimal" therapy of patients suffering from hypertension, there is still urgent need for preventing severe rhythm disorders. In view of the many missed potential targets for preventing adverse myocardial remodeling, it appears that the beneficial modulation of Cx43 by melatonin, omega-3 fatty acids, and red palm oil might be a useful approach in current therapy. Our findings support the prophylactic use of these non-pharmacological compounds to minimize cardiovascular risk and sudden arrhythmic death. A novel approach is needed since despite a plethora of available treatment options, a substantial portion of the hypertensive population has uncontrolled blood pressure. Further studies should elucidate more in detail mechanisms of myocardial Cx43 modulation in the context of electrical properties of the heart in response to treatment of hypertension

Acknowledgements

This study was supported by APVV 0348/12, VEGA 2/0076/16, 2/0167/15, and SKS grants.

Author details

Tamara Egan Benova, Barbara Szeiffova Bacova, Csilla Viczenczova, Miroslav Barancik and Narcis Tribulova*

*Address all correspondence to: narcisa.tribulova@savba.sk

Institute for Heart Research, SAS, Bratislava, Slovakia

References

[1] Sampson AK, Jennings GL, Chin-Dusting JP. Y are males so difficult to understand? A case where X does not mark the spot. Hypertension. 2012;59:525–531. DOI: 10.1161/HYPERTENSIONAHA.111.187880

[2] Kunes J, Zicha J. The interaction of genetic and environmental factors in the etiology of hypertension. Physiol Res. 2009;58:33–41.

[3] Irmak MK, Sizlan A. Essential hypertension seems to result from melatonin-induced epigenetic modifications in area postrema. Med Hypotheses. 2006;66:1000–1007. DOI: 10.1016/j.mehy.2005.10.016

[4] Hirooka Y. Oxidative stress in the cardiovascular center has a pivotal role in the sympathetic activation in hypertension. Hypertens Res. 2011;34:407–412. DOI: 10.1038/hr.2011.14

[5] Wolf G. Free radical production and angiotensin. Curr Hypert Res. 2000;2:167–173.

[6] Borghi C, Cicero AF. Omega-3 polyunsaturated fatty acids: Their potential role in blood pressure prevention and management. Heart Int. 2006;2:98–105. DOI: 10.4081/hi.2006.98

[7] Rodrigo R, González J, Paoletto F. The role of oxidative stress in the pathophysiology of hypertension. Hypertens Res. 2011;34:431–440. DOI: 10.1038/hr.2010.264

[8] Bačová B, Seč P, Radošinská J, Certík M, Vachulová A, Tribulová N. Lower omega-3 index is a marker of increased propensity of hypertensive rat heart to malignant arrhythmias. Physiol Res. 2013;62:201–208.

[9] Majzunova M, Dovinova I, Barancik M, Chan JY. Redox signaling in pathophysiology of hypertension. J Biomed Sci. 2013;20:69. DOI: 10.1186/1423-0127-20-69

[10] Das UN. Long-chain polyunsaturated fatty acids interact with nitric oxide, superoxide anion, and transforming growth factor-beta to prevent human essential hypertension. Eur J Clin Nutr. 2004;58:195–203. DOI: 10.1038/sj.ejcn.1601766

[11] Diamond JA, Phillips RA. Hypertensive heart disease. Hypertens Res. 2005;28:191–202. DOI:10.1291/hypres.28.191

[12] Zanchetti A. Is hypertension a fatal disease today? Proceedings of a satellite symposium held during the 21st European Meeting on Hypertension and Cardiovascular Prevention Milan (Italy). Foreword. J Hypertens. 2011;29:1. DOI: 10.1097/01.hjh.0000410245.51597.04

[13] Hill JA. Electrical remodeling in cardiac hypertrophy. Trends Cardiovasc Med. 2003;13:316–322. DOI: 10.1016/j.tcm.2003.08.002

[14] Tribulova N, Okruhlicova L, Imanaga I, Hirosawa N, Ogawa K and Weismann P. Factors involved in the susceptibility of spontaneously hypertensive rats to low K+-induced arrhythmias. Gen Physiol Biophys. 2003;22:369–382.

[15] Kostin S, Dammer S and Hein S. Connexin 43 expression and distribution in compensated and decompensated cardiac hypetrophy in patients with aortic stenosis. Cardiovas Res. 2004;62:426–436. DOI: http://dx.doi.org/10.1016/j.cardiores.2003.12.010

[16] Teunissen BEJ, Jongsma HJ and Bierhuizen MFA. Regulation of myocardial connexins during hypertrophic remodelling. Eur Heart J. 2004;25:1979–1989. DOI: http://dx.doi.org/10.1016/j.ehj.2004.08.007

[17] Lorell BH, Carabello BA. Left ventricular hypertrophy: pathogenesis, detection, and prognosis. Circulation. 2000;102:470–479. DOI: 10.1161/01.CIR.102.4.470

[18] Fontes MS, van Veen TA, de Bakker JM, van Rijen HV. Functional consequences of abnormal Cx43 expression in the heart. Biochim Biophys Acta. 2012;1818:2020–2029. DOI: 10.1016/j.bbamem.2011.07.039

[19] Smyth JW, Hong TT, Gao D, Vogan JM, Jensen BC, Fong TS et al. Limited forward trafficking of connexin 43 reduces cell-cell coupling in stressed human and mouse myocardium. J Clin Invest. 2010;120:266–279. DOI: 10.1172/JCI39740

[20] Calore C, Zorzi A, Corrado D. Clinical meaning of isolated increase of QRS voltages in hypertrophic cardiomyopathy versus athlete's heart. J Electrocardiol. 2015;48:373–379. DOI: 10.1016/j.jelectrocard.2014.12.016

[21] Zhao Y, Ransom JF, Li A, Vedantham V, von Drehle M, Muth AN, Tsuchihashi T, McManus MT, Schwartz RJ, Srivastava D. Dysregulation of cardiogenesis, cardiac conduction, and cell cycle in mice lacking miRNA-1-2. Cell. 2007;129:303–317. DOI: 10.1016/j.cell.2007.03.030

[22] Curcio A, Torella D, Iaconetti C, Pasceri E, Sabatino J, Sorrentino S, Giampà S, Micieli M, Polimeni A, Henning BJ, Leone A, Catalucci D, Ellison GM, Condorelli G, Indolfi C. MicroRNA-1 downregulation increases connexin 43 displacement and induces ventricular tachyarrhythmias in rodent hypertrophic hearts. PLoS One. 2013;8:e70158. DOI: 10.1371/journal.pone.0070158

[23] Yang B, Lin H, Xiao J, Lu Y, Luo X, Li B, et al. The muscle-specific microRNA miR-1 regulates cardiac arrhythmogenic potential by targeting GJA1 and KCNJ2. Nat Med. 2007;13:486–491. DOI:10.1038/nm1569

[24] Xu HF, Ding YJ, Shen YW, Xue AM, Xu HM, Luo CL,et al. MicroRNA-1 represses Cx43 expression in viral myocarditis. Mol Cell Biochem. 2012;362:141–148. DOI: 10.1007/s11010-011-1136-3

[25] Tribulova N, Szeiffova Bacova B, Benova T, Viczenczova C. Can we protect from malignant arrhythmias by modulation of cardiac cell-to-cell coupling? J Electrocardiol. 2015;48:434–440. DOI: 10.1016/j.jelectrocard.2015.02.006

[26] Sovari AA, Rutledge CA, Jeong EM, Dolmatova E, Arasu D, Liu H, Vahdani N, Gu L, Zandieh S, Xiao L, Bonini MG, Duffy HS, Dudley SC Jr. Mitochondria oxidative stress, connexin43 remodeling, and sudden arrhythmic death. Circ Arrhythm Electrophysiol. 2013;6:623–631. DOI: 10.1161/CIRCEP.112.976787

[27] Sewerynek, E. Melatonin and the cardiovascular system. Neuro Endocrinol Lett. 2002;23:79–83.

[28] Benova M, Herichova I, Stebelova K, Paulis L, Krajcirovicova K, Simko F, Zeman M. Effect of L-NAME-induced hypertension on melatonin receptors and melatonin levels in the pineal gland and the peripheral organs of rats. Hypertens Res. 2009;32:242–247. DOI: 10.1038/hr.2009.12

[29] Simko F, Paulis L. Melatonin as a potential antihypertensive treatment. J Pineal Res. 2007;42:319–322. DOI: 10.1111/j.1600-079X.2007.00436.x

[30] Reiter RJ. The pineal gland and melatonin in relation to aging: a summary of the theories and of the data. Exp Gerontol. 1995;30:199–212.

[31] Kedziora-Kornatowska K, Szewczyk-Golec K, Czuczejko J, van Marke de Lumen K, Pawluk H, Motyl J, Karasek M, Kedziora J. Effect of melatonin on the oxidative stress in erythrocytes of healthy young and elderly subjects. J Pineal Res. 2007;42:153–158. DOI: 10.1111/j.1600-079X.2006.00394.x

[32] Das R, Balonan L, Ballard HJ, Ho S. Chronic hypoxia inhibits the antihypertensive effect of melatonin on pulmonary artery. Int J Cardiol. 2008;126:340–345. DOI: 10.1016/j.ijcard.2007.04.030

[33] Brugger P, Marktl W, Herold M. Impaired nocturnal secretion of melatonin in coronary heart disease. Lancet. 1995;345:1408. DOI: 10.1016/S0140-6736(95)92600-3

[34] Jonas M, Garfinkel D, Zisapel N, Laudon M, Grossman E. Impaired nocturnal melatonin secretion in non-dipper hypertensive patients. Blood Press. 2003;12:19–24.

[35] Zeman M, Dulková K, Bada V, Herichová I. Plasma melatonin concentrations in hypertensive patients with the dipping and non-dipping blood pressure profile. Life Sci. 2005;76:1795–1803. DOI:10.1016/j.lfs.2004.08.034

[36] Kedziora-Kornatowska K, Szewczyk-Golec K, Czuczejko J, Pawluk H, van Marke de Lumen K, Kozakiewicz M, Bartosz G, Kedziora J. Antioxidative effects of melatonin administration in elderly primary essential hypertension patients. J Pineal Res. 2008;45:312–317. DOI: 10.1111/j.1600-079X.2008.00592.x

[37] Możdżan M, Możdżan M, Chałubiński M, Wojdan K, Broncel M. The effect of melatonin on circadian blood pressure in patients with type 2 diabetes and essential hypertension. Arch Med Sci. 2014;4:669–675. DOI: 10.5114/aoms.2014.44858

[38] Scheer FA, Van Montfrans GA, Van Someren EJ, Mairuhu G, Buijs RM. Daily nighttime melatonin reduces blood pressure in male patients with essential hypertension. Hypertension. 2004;43:192–197. DOI: 10.1161/01.HYP.0000113293.151 86.3b

[39] Grossman E, Laudon M, Yalcin R, Zengil H, Peleg E, Sharabi Y, Kamari Y, Shen-Orr Z, Zisapel N. Melatonin reduces night blood pressure in patients with nocturnal hypertension. Am J Med. 2006;119:898–902. DOI: 10.1016/j.amjmed.2006.02.002

[40] Simko F, Pechanova O. Recent trends in hypertension treatment: perspectives from animal studies. J Hypertens. 2009;27:1–4. DOI: 10.1097/01.hjh.0000358829.87815.d4

[41] Rechciński T, Trzos E, Wierzbowska-Drabik K, Krzemińska-Pakula M, Kurpesa M. Melatonin for nondippers with coronary artery disease: assessment of blood pressure profile and heart rate variability. Hypertens Res. 2010;33:56–61. DOI: 10.1038/hr. 2009.174

[42] Paulis L, Simko F, Laudon M. Cardiovascular effects of melatonin receptor agonists. Expert Opin Investig Drugs. 2012;21:1661–1678. DOI: 10.1517/13543784.2012.714771

[43] Benova T, Viczenczova C, Radosinska J, Bacova B, Knezl V, Dosenko V, Weismann P, Zeman M, Navarova J, Tribulova N: Melatonin attenuates hypertension-related proarrhythmic myocardial maladaptation of connexin 43 and propensity of the heart to lethal arrhythmias. Can J Physiol Pharmacol. 2013;91:633–639. DOI: 10.1139/ cjpp-2012-0393

[44] Kaneko S, Okumura K, Numaguchi Y, Matsui H, Murase K, Mokuno S, Morishima I, Hira K, Toki Y, Ito T, Hayakawa T. Melatonin scavenges hydroxyl radical and protects isolated rat hearts from ischemic reperfusion injury. Life Sci. 2000;67:101–112. DOI: 10.1016/S0024-3205(00)00607-X

[45] Szarszoi O, Asemu G, Vanecek J et al. Effects of melatonin on ischemia and reperfusion injury of the rat heart. Cardiovasc Drugs Ther. 2001;5:251–257.

[46] Benova T, Knezl V, Viczenczova C, Bacova BS, Radosinska J, Tribulova N. Acute antifibrillating and defibrillating potential of atorvastatin, melatonin, eicosapentaenoic acid and docosahexaenoic acid demonstrated in isolated heart model. J Physiol Pharmacol. 2015;66:83–89.

[47] Sahna E, Olmez E, Acet A. Effects of physiological and pharmacological concentrations of melatonin on ischemiareperfusion arrhythmias in rats: can the incidence of complete sudden cardiac death be reduced? J Pineal Res. 2002;32:194–198. DOI: 10.1034/j. 1600-079x.2002.1o853.x

[48] Sahna E, Acet A, Ozer MK et al. Myocardial ischemiareperfusion in rats: reduction of infarct size by either supplemental physiological or pharmacological doses of melatonin. J Pineal Res. 2002;33:324–328.

[49] Lee YM, Chen HR, Hsiao G et al. Protective effects of melatonin on myocardial ischemia/reperfusion injury in vivo. J Pineal Res. 2002;33:72–80. DOI: 10.1034/j.1600-079X.2002.01869.x

[50] Dobsak P, Siegelova J, Eicher JC, Jancik J, Svacinova H, Vasku J, Kuchtickova S, Horky M, Wolf JE. Melatonin protects against ischemia-reperfusion injury and inhibits apoptosis in isolated working rat heart. Pathophysiology. 2003;9:179–187. DOI:10.1016/S0928-4680(02)00080-9

[51] Allayee H, Roth N, Hodis HN. Polyunsaturated fatty acids and cardiovascular disease: implications for nutrigenetics. J Nutrigenet Nutrigenomics. 2009;2:140–148. DOI: 10.1159/000235562

[52] Bonafini S, Antoniazzi F, Maffeis C, Minuz P, Fava C. Beneficial effects of -3 PUFA in children on cardiovascular risk factors during childhood and adolescence. Prostaglandins Other Lipid Mediat. 2015;120:72–79. DOI: 10.1016/j.prostaglandins.2015.03.006

[53] Cabo J, Alonso R, Mata P. Omega-3 fatty acids and blood pressure. Br J Nutr. 2012;107:195–200. DOI: 10.1017/S0007114512001584

[54] Marchioli R, Marfisi RM, Borrelli G, Chieffo C, Franzosi MG, Levantesi G, Maggioni AP, Nicolosi GL, Scarano M, Silletta MG, Schweiger C, Tavazzi L, Tognoni G. Efficacy of n-3 polyunsaturated fatty acids according to clinical characteristics of patients with recent myocardial infarction: insights from the GISSI-Prevenzione trial. J Cardiovasc Med (Hagerstown). 2007;8:34–37. DOI: 10.2459/01.JCM.0000289271.80180.b6

[55] Rauch B, Senges J. The effects of supplementation with omega-3 polyunsaturated Fatty acids on cardiac rhythm: anti-arrhythmic, pro-arrhythmic, both or neither? It depends… Front Physiol. 2012;3:57. DOI: 10.3389/fphys.2012.00057

[56] Rizos EC, Ntzani EE, Bika E, Kostapanos MS, Elisaf MS. Association between omega-3 fatty acid supplementation and risk of major cardiovascular disease events: a systematic review and meta-analysis. JAMA. 2012;308:1024–1033. DOI: 10.1001/2012.jama.11374

[57] Calò L, Martino A, Tota C. The anti-arrhythmic effects of n–3 PUFAs. Int J Cardiol. 2013;170:21–27. DOI: 10.1016/j.ijcard.2013.06.043

[58] Richardson ES, Iaizzo PA, Xiao YF. Electrophysiological mechanisms of the anti-arrhythmic effects of omega-3 fatty acids. J Cardiovasc Transl Res. 2011;4:42–52. DOI: 10.1007/s12265-010-9243-1

[59] Endo J, Arita M. Cardioprotective mechanism of omega-3 polyunsaturated fatty acids. J Cardiol. 2016;67:22–27. DOI: 10.1016/j.jjcc.2015.08.002

[60] Edem DO. Haematological and histological alterations induced in rats by palm oil – containing diets. Eur J Sci Res. 2009;32:405–518.

[61] Edem DO. Palm oil: biochemical, physiological, nutritional, hematological, and toxicological aspects: a review. Plant Foods Hum Nutr. 2002;57:319–341.

[62] Das S, Lekli I, Das M, Szabo G, Varadi J, Juhasz B, Bak I, Nesaretam K, Tosaki A, Powell SR, Das DK. Cardioprotection with palm oil tocotrienols: comparision of di erent isomers. Am J Physiol Heart Circ Physiol. 2008;294:970–978. DOI: 10.1152/ajpheart. 01200.2007

[63] Van Rooyen J, Esterhuyse AJ, Engelbrecht AM, Du Toit EF. Health benefits of a natural carotenoid rich oil: a proposed mechanism of protection against ischaemia/reperfusion injury. Asia Pac J Clin Nutr. 2008;17:316–319.

[64] Engelbrecht AM, Odendaal L, Du Toit EF, Kupai K, Csont T, Ferdinandy P, Van Rooyen J. The effect of dietary red palm oil on the functional recovery of the ischaemic/ reperfused isolated rat heart: the involvement of the PI3-kinase signaling pathway. Lipids Health Dis. 2009;8:18. DOI: 10.1186/1476-511X-8-18

[65] Esterhuyse JS, Van Rooyen J, Strijdom H, Bester D, du Toit EF. Proposed mechanisms for red palm oil induced cardioprotection in a model of hyperlipidaemia in the rat. Prostaglandins Leukot Essent Fat Acids. 2006;75:375–384. DOI: 10.1016/j.plefa. 2006.07.001

[66] Engelbrecht AM, Esterhuyse J, Du Toit EF, Lochner A, Van Rooyen J. p38-MAPK and PKB/Akt, possible role players in red palm oil-induced protection of the isolated perfused rat heart? J Nutritional Biochem. 2006;17:265–271. DOI: 10.1016/j.jnutbio. 2005.05.001

[67] Bester DJ, Kupai K, Csont T, Szucs G, Csonka C, Esterhuyse AJ, Ferdinandy P, Van Rooyen J. Dietary red palm oil supplementation reduces myocardial infarct size in an isolated perfused rat heart model. Lipids Health Dis. 2010;9:64. DOI: 10.1186/1476-511X-9-64

[68] Szucs G, Bester DJ, Kupai K et al. Dietary red palm oil supplementation decreases infarct size in cholesterol fed rats. Lipids Health Dis. 2011;10:103. DOI: 10.1186/1476-511X-10-103

[69] Sharkey JT, Puttaramu R, Word RA, Olcese J. Melatonin synergizes with oxytocin to enhance contractility of human myometrial smooth muscle cells. J Clin Endocrinol Metab. 2009;94:421–427. DOI: 10.1210/jc.2008-1723

[70] Mitchell JA, Lye SJ. Regulation of connexin 43 expression by c-fos and c-jun in myometrial cells. Cell Commun Adhes. 2001;8:299–302.

[71] Reiter RJ, Tan DX, Galano A. Melatonin: exceeding expectations. Physiology (Bethesda), 2014;29:325–333. DOI: 10.1152/physiol.00011.2014

[72] Yang KC, Bonini MG, Dudley SC Jr. Mitochondria and arrhythmias. Free Radic Biol Med. 2014;71:351–361. DOI: 10.1016/j.freeradbiomed.2014.03.033

[73] Deng WG, Tang ST, Tseng HP, Wu KK. Melatonin suppresses macrophage cyclooxygenase-2 and inducible nitric oxide synthase expression by inhibiting p52 acetylation and binding. Blood. 2006;108:518–524. DOI: 10.1182/blood-2005-09-3691

[74] Fischer R, Dechend R, Qadri F, Markovic M, Feldt S, Herse F, Park JK, Gapelyuk A, Schwarz I, Zacharzowsky UB, Plehm R, Safak E, Heuser A, Schirdewan A, Luft FC, Schunck WH, Muller DN. Dietary n-3 polyunsaturated fatty acids and direct renin inhibition improve electrical remodeling in a model of high human renin hypertension. Hypertension. 2008;51:540–546. DOI: 10.1161/HYPERTENSIONAHA.107.103143

[75] Reiffel JA, McDonald A. Antiarrhythmic effects of omega-3 fatty acids. Am J Cardiol. 2006;21:50i–60i. DOI: 10.1016/j.amjcard.2005.12.027

[76] Bacova B, Radosinska J, Knezl V, Kolenova L, Weismann P, Navarova J, Barancik M, Mitasikova M, Tribulova N. Omega-3 fatty acids and atorvastatin suppress ventricular fibrillation inducibility in hypertriglyceridemic rat hearts: implication of intracellular coupling protein, connexin-43. J Physiol Pharmacol. 2010;61:717–723.

[77] Nair SS, Leitch JW, Falconer J, Garg ML. Prevention of cardiac arrythmia by dietary (n-3) polyunsaturated fatty acids and their mechanism of action. J Nutr. 1997;127:383–393.

[78] Radosinska J, Bacova B, Knezl V, Benova T, Zurmanova J, Soukup T, Arnostova P, Slezak J, Gonçalvesova E, Tribulova N. Dietary omega-3 fatty acids attenuate myocardial arrhythmogenic factors and propensity of the heart to lethalarrhythmias in a rodent model of human essential hypertension. J Hypertens. 2013;31:1876–1885. DOI: 10.1097/HJH.0b013e328362215d

[79] Deckelbaum RJ, Worgall TS, Seo T. n3 Fatty acids and gene expression. Am J Clin Nutr. 2006;83:1520–1525.

[80] Baum JR, Dolmatova E, Tan A, Duffy HS. Omega 3 fatty acid inhibition of inflammatory cytokine-mediated Connexin43 regulation in the heart. Front Physiol. 2012;3:1–8. DOI: 10.3389/fphys.2012.00272

[81] Den Ruijter HM, Berecki G, Opthof T, Verkerk AO, Zock PL, Coronel R. Pro- and antiarrhythmic properties of diet rich in fish oil. Cardiovasc Res. 2007;73:316–325. DOI: http://dx.doi.org/10.1016/j.cardiores.2006.06.014

[82] Bačová B, Radošinská J, Viczenczová C, Knezl V, Dosenko V, Beňova T, Navarová J, Gonçalvesová E, van Rooyen J, Weismann P, Slezák J, Tribulová N. Up-regulation of myocardial connexin-43 in spontaneously hypertensive rats fed red palm oil is most likely implicated in its antiarrhythmic effects. Can J Physiol Pharmacol. 2012;90:1235–1245. DOI: 10.1139/y2012-103

Chapter 10

Hypertension and Hypertension-Related Disparities in Underrepresented Minorities

Carlos J. Rodriguez

Additional information is available at the end of the chapter

http://dx.doi.org/10.5772/64510

Abstract

Racial-ethnic disparities in cardiovascular disease (CVD) have been evident over the past few decades. As such, addressing these disparities have been a part of national programs such as Health People 2020 and the Million Heart initiative. Hypertension (HTN) has been a primary focus of these initiatives due to the significant contribution of HTN as a risk factor for CVD and its role in CVD racial/ethnic disparities. HTN is common among various racial/ethnic groups, in particular non-Hispanic blacks and certain groups of Hispanics. Additionally, both non-Hispanic black and Hispanic adults have been known to have higher prevalence of poorly controlled blood pressure (BP) compared to non-Hispanic whites. Long-standing HTN leads to increased risk of end-organ damage, development of coronary heart disease, stroke, end-stage kidney disease, and increased overall CVD-specific mortality. This chapter provides an update of available data on the prevalence of HTN in various racial/ethnic groups and prevalence of awareness, treatment, and control of HTN in attempts to further demonstrate the significant role HTN plays in racial/ethnic disparities in CVD. We also discuss the most recently published HTN guidelines that has led to debate regarding the potential impact on worsening CVD disparities, through disproportionate effects on the elderly, women, and non-Hispanic blacks.

Keywords: hypertension, disparities, hypertensive heart disease, African Americans, Hispanics

1. Introduction

Race-ethnic disparities in cardiovascular disease (CVD) have been evident over the past several decades in the United States (US). Despite an overall decline in deaths from CVD, the declines in CVD mortality have not been as great for US ethnic minorities. CVD age-adjusted death rates are 33% higher for blacks than for the overall population in the US. The overall CVD death rate in 2011 was 230 per 100,000. In black males and females, the rates were 352 and 249 per 100,000 compared to 272 and 188 per 100,000 for white males and females, respectively with similar disparities mirrored in hypertension (HTN) related mortality rates (**Figure 1**) [1]. In 2009, age-adjusted estimates reported by the CDC showed that the rate of premature death from coronary heart disease (CHD) among non-Hispanic blacks was 66% compared to 43% in non-Hispanic whites. Similar findings were reported for premature death due to stroke for non-Hispanic blacks compared to whites (25 and 10%, respectively) [2].

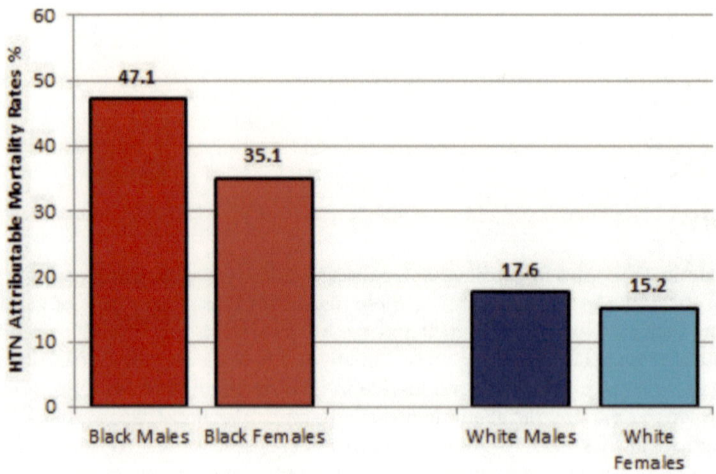

Figure 1. Overall mortality rates from causes related to hypertension.

The public health burden from CVD racial/ethnic disparities that exist is in large part due to modifiable risk factors. Ninety percent of CVD events among black participants in the Atherosclerosis Risk in Communities (ARIC) study were explained by having elevated or borderline CV risk factors compared to 65% among white participants [3]. The American Heart Association (AHA) has adopted the new concept of CV health based on seven health metrics, including smoking status, physical activity, healthy diet, body weight, along with optimal blood pressure (BP), blood glucose, and total cholesterol levels [4]. Non-Hispanic blacks (10%) and Mexican Americans (12%) were less likely than whites (19%) to have ≥5 metrics at ideal levels defined by the AHA [1, 5]. Similarly, the 2009 Behavioral Risk Factor Surveillance System (BRFSS) survey analyzed CV health metrics of US adults demonstrating racial/ethnic disparities. Non-Hispanic blacks, Hispanics, and American Indian/Alaska Native adults were all less likely than non-Hispanic whites to have ideal CV health and had the highest prevalence CV risk factors [6]. Poor CV health (0–2 ideal health metrics) was significantly more prevalent among non-Hispanic blacks (17%), American Indians/Alaska Natives (15%), and Hispanics (13%) when compared to non-Hispanic whites (11%) [5]. Previous data from the 2003 BRFSS demonstrated disparities in both self-reported and measured CVD risk factors which most

http://dx.doi.org/10.5772/64510

adversely affected non-Hispanic blacks, Mexican Americans, and American Indian/Alaska Natives [6].

In particular, HTN or high blood pressure is more prevalent among certain racial/ethnic minority groups in the US, especially African American adults [1]. In addition, the population attributable risk for CVD mortality was estimated to be 41% for HTN, compared to 14% for smoking, 13% for poor diet, and 9% for abnormal blood glucose levels [3, 7]. This means that hypothetically, 41% of CVD mortality is explained by and could be avoided by optimal blood pressure. Since hypertension is significantly more prevalent among race/ethnic minorities, the proportion of CVD mortality that could be avoided in these populations by optimal BP control is much higher. Furthermore, the sequela of HTN morbidity such as heart failure, stroke, renal disease, and coronary heart disease are disproportionate among race/ethnic minorities. As such, HTN plays a major role in the race/ethnic CVD disparities given the various ethnic/racial groups who suffer disproportionately from the condition and the significant contribution of HTN to CVD morbidity and mortality.

2. Epidemiology of HTN

According to NHANES 2009–2010 data, the prevalence of HTN was highest among non-Hispanic blacks (40%), followed by non-Hispanic whites (27%) and Hispanics (26%), respectively [8]. Data from the 2012 National Health Interview Survey (NHIS) demonstrated that black adults were more likely to have self-reported hypertension than white adults [9]. In the Multi-Ethnic Study of Atherosclerosis (MESA), measured systolic and diastolic blood pressure was higher among African Americans and Hispanics compared to their white counterparts [10].

Although Hispanics have been reported to have rates not significantly different from non-Hispanic whites, the majority of data has been extrapolated primarily from Mexican Americans [11]. The Hispanic/Latino population is currently the largest ethnic minority in the US with a growing heterogeneous subgroup population as evident by recent census updates [11]. In the Hispanic Community Health Study/Study of Latinos (HCHS/SOL), a cohort of 16,415 Hispanics representative of the major Hispanic subgroups, Sorlie et al. report that the overall age-adjusted prevalence of HTN for Hispanic men and women was 26% and 25%, respectively [12]. There was however variation among Hispanic subgroups with HTN prevalence being higher at upwards of 32% among Hispanics of Caribbean descent (Dominican, Puerto Rican, and Cuban adults). Interestingly, Hispanics of Mexican descent had significantly lower HTN prevalence when compared to all other Hispanic subgroups except South Americans [12]. NHIS data demonstrated that Hispanic blacks had a higher HTN prevalence than Hispanic whites. This disparity remained even for Hispanic blacks with higher income and higher education levels when compared to Hispanic whites of lower socioeconomic status [13].

Analyses from NHANES 1998 to 1994 and 1999 to 2004 data showed an increased in HTN prevalence over the past few decades among both men and women and non-Hispanic blacks and whites. However, non-Hispanic blacks had greater increases in prevalence when compared to non-Hispanic whites during both time periods and the greatest increase was seen among non-Hispanic black women [14]. According to NHANES data from the period 2003 to 2010, among adults with hypertension, non-Hispanic blacks (74%) and Mexican American (72%) were more likely to be aged <65 years, compared with non-Hispanic whites (57%) [15]. Similar data were shown from NHANES 1999–2002 data, where 63% of non-Hispanic blacks and 45% of non-Hispanic whites with HTN were ≤60 years of age.

In addition to US non-Hispanic black adults having the highest HTN prevalence rates in the world, they have been reported to develop HTN earlier in life when compared to non-Hispanic whites [16]. The incidence of HTN among racial/ethnic groups has been examined in the MESA. After a median follow-up of approximately 5 years, blacks had the highest HTN incidence rate (85 per 1000 person-years) followed by Hispanics (66 per 1000 person-years), whites (57 per 1000 person-years), and then Chinese (52 per 1000 person-years). After adjustment for MESA study site, age and sex, blacks and Hispanics had increased incidence rate ratios when compared to whites [16]. A prospective cohort study of 18,865 participants examined the progression of non-Hispanic blacks and whites in the normotensive (28%) and prehypertensive (27%) stages at baseline to the hypertensive stage [17]. After adjustment for multiple covariates, results demonstrated that non-Hispanic blacks had a 35% increased risk of conversion to hypertension when compared to non-Hispanic whites. Additionally, the median conversion time when 50% became hypertensive was significantly shorter for non-Hispanic blacks compared to whites (626 vs 991 days; $p < 0.001$). Non-Hispanic blacks in this sample had accelerated risk of new-onset hypertension [17].

3. Hypertension disparities: awareness, treatment, and control

An important aspect regarding the racial/ethnic disparities has been the focus on awareness, treatment, and control of HTN. Overall in 2009–2010, approximately 82, 76, and 53% of adults with hypertension were aware of their condition, taking medication, and HTN was controlled, respectively [9]. There were also no significant changes seen from the periods 2007–2008 and 2009–2010 in the US. There were several differences, however, reported between racial and ethnic groups. According to 2009–2010 National Centers for Health Statistics (NCHS), Hispanic adults were least likely to be aware of their hypertension (78%), when compared to Non-Hispanic whites (81%) and non-Hispanic blacks (87%) [9]. In addition, Hispanic adults were least likely to take medication for their hypertension (70%), compared with non-Hispanic whites (77%) and non-Hispanic black adults (80%). Further NCHS analysis demonstrated that age-adjusted control of hypertension was least likely in Hispanic adults (41%) compared to non-Hispanic black (48%) and non-Hispanic white adults (56%) [9]. Even with the highest rates of hypertension awareness and treatment, non-Hispanic blacks were less likely to have adequate control of their blood pressure compared to their white counterparts. It is important to note that this disparity remains even with increased overall rates of hypertension control in US adults from 48% in 2007–2008 to 53% in 2009–2010 [9].

HCHS/SOL reported notable variation in the rates of awareness, treatment, and control among Hispanic subgroups. Awareness of HTN ranged from as low as 59% among men of Central

American descent to 78% among men of Cuban descent; to as low as 72% among women of South American descent; and to 79% among women of Cuban and Dominican descent. The percentage of those treated for HTN were highest in Cuban men (65%); whereas rates of HTN control were low for all subgroups and lowest among both Central American men and women (12 and 32%, respectively) with the highest rates of control being seen among Cuban men (40%) [12].

Similar racial/ethnic disparities regarding hypertension awareness, treatment, and control have been demonstrated in additional NHANES reports along with population-based cohorts such as MESA, and the REasons for Geographic and Racial Differences in stroke Study (REGARDS). According to NHANES data from 2003–2010, HTN awareness, treatment, and control were lowest among Mexican Americans compared to non-Hispanic blacks and whites [15]. In the REGARDS cohort, awareness was significantly higher in blacks compared to whites [18]. In addition, blacks were more likely to be treated for HTN compared to whites but were significantly less likely to have controlled HTN when compared to whites [18]. In the MESA, non-Hispanic blacks (35%) and Hispanic (32%) adults had a significantly higher prevalence of treated but uncontrolled HTN compared to non-Hispanic white (24%) adults [10].

NHANES has also reported a trend analysis through exam periods 1988–1994 and 1999–2008. Overall hypertension control increased from 27% in 1988–1994 to 50% in 2007–2008, these gains were not seen equally among all US race-ethnic groups, thus race-ethnic disparities remain. The prevalence of adults with uncontrolled hypertension on treatment was reported to be significantly higher among blacks ($p < 0.001$) and Hispanics ($p = 0.02$) compared to whites [19]. Egan and colleagues analyzed NHANES data over 3 survey time periods (1988–1994, 1999–2004, and 2005–2008) to specifically address the prevalence of uncontrolled and treatment-resistant hypertension (TRH). Uncontrolled hypertension was defined by a blood pressure ≥140/90 mm Hg while treatment-resistant hypertension (TRH) included participants reported taking ≥3 medications for hypertension. Non-Hispanic blacks and Hispanics had higher prevalence of uncontrolled HTN compared to non-Hispanic whites. Non-Hispanic black race was reported to be independently associated with TRH in the 2005–2008 survey period [20].

4. Hypertension categorization

"Uncontrolled hypertension" signifies blood pressure (BP) that is inadequately treated rather than blood pressure that is refractory to treatment. Refractory hypertension is defined by a blood pressure ≥140/90 mm Hg or ≥130/80 mm Hg in patients with diabetes or renal disease despite adherence to at least three antihypertensive medications, including a diuretic [21]. The Health Plan Employer Data and Information Set, as well as the National Center for Health Statistics who orchestrated the National Health and Nutrition Examination Survey serve as a repository for the most comprehensive information concerning the prevalence of uncontrolled hypertension both in the general population as well as those groups deemed at high risk of cardiovascular disease [22].

5. Prevalence of refractory hypertension

The best estimates of refractory hypertension prevalence is provided by large outcome studies such as The Antihypertensive and Lipid-Lowering Treatment to Prevent Heart Attack Trial from which we can extrapolate the prevalence of patients with refractory hypertension where despite some participants on three medications and approximately 8% who were on receiving four or more medications at the end of the study, approximately 15% of that entire cohort could be classified as having refractory hypertension [23]. In the Controlled Onset Verapamil Investigation of Cardiovascular Endpoints trial, 18% of participants being treated with three or more medications remained with uncontrolled BP (≥140/90 mm Hg) [24]. These two studies suggest that approximately 15–18% of patients with uncontrolled hypertension have refractory hypertension.

A small study in the specialty hypertension clinic setting suggested that among diabetics, African Americans, older patients and men, systolic blood pressure remained difficult to control and fewer patients in those groups achieved HTN goals despite careful drug titration on three or more agents [25]. Additionally, others have found that refractory hypertension is more prevalent in patients over 60 years of age [26]. In the REGARDS study, ~14% of the 14,809 participants had resistant hypertension (defined as being on ≥4 antihypertensive medications) and only 0.5% had refractory hypertension (defined as being on ≥5 antihypertensive medications) with a greater proportion of African Americans residing in both categories [27]. Further literature by Meissner and Berlowitz has shown that over 10% of all hypertensive patients remain uncontrolled despite the administration of three or more drugs with good adherence to therapy after excluding causes of secondary systemic arterial hypertension [28, 29]. Importantly these studies also highlight the underuse of spironolactone and long-acting thiazide diuretics such as chlorthalidone as an opportunity to reduce the occurrence of refractory, resistant, and uncontrolled HTN particularly among African Americans.

6. Hypertension complications

HTN remains a major risk factor for coronary heart disease, congestive heart failure, stroke, chronic kidney disease, and CV death. Data from NCHS/NHANES surveys showed that HTN was the single largest risk factor for CV mortality in the US, responsible for an estimated 45% of all CV deaths [7]. In 2010, HTN was reported as the 13th leading cause of death in the US. The rate deaths attributed to HTN in 2010 was 50.2 per 100,000 for non-Hispanic black men and 37.1 per 100,000 for non-Hispanic black women compared to 17.2 per 100,000 for non-Hispanic white men, and 15 per 100,000 for non-Hispanic white women [30]. In addition, non-Hispanic blacks have 1.3 and 1.8-times the increased rate of fatal and nonfatal strokes, and 4.2-times the increased rate of end-stage kidney disease compared to non-Hispanic whites [1].

In 2010, HTN, coronary heart disease, and stroke accounted for 56% of preventable deaths which occurred in adults aged <65 years. Death rates were significantly higher for non-Hispanic blacks (83.7 per 100,000) and American Indians/Alaska Natives when compared to

http://dx.doi.org/10.5772/64510

whites. However, death rates were found to be significantly lower for Hispanics and Asian/Pacific islanders compared to whites [31]. As previously stated, age-adjusted HTN prevalence rates for Hispanics have been demonstrated to be similar to that of non-Hispanic whites, although with higher HTN prevalence among Hispanics of Caribbean descent, with lower rates of HTN awareness, treatment, and control. CDC data demonstrates further hypertension-related mortality (HRM) disparities among the Hispanic subgroups. While age-standardized HRM was similar for Hispanics (127.3 per 100,000) compared to non-Hispanic whites (135.9), Hispanics of Puerto Rican background had 13% higher rates ($p < 0.01$) than non-Hispanic whites. Hispanics of Mexican descent had similar and Hispanics of Cuban background had lower HRM rates compared to non-Hispanic whites [32].

7. Hypertension guidelines – implications for racial/ethnic minorities

This chapter has attempted to outline the role of HTN among racial/ethnic groups. HTN is a very common, yet modifiable disease that contributes significantly to both CVD morbidity and mortality. Management guidelines for HTN among racial/ethnic groups have been a focus for many national and international organizations such as the Association of Black Cardiologists (ABC), American Heart Association (AHA), American College of Cardiology (ACC), and the International Society of Hypertension in Blacks (ISHIB). One of the major changes in recent guidelines providing recommendations on the management of HTN from the Eight Joint National Committee (JNC8) in 2014 [33] has gained attention due to concerns for the implications on particular subgroup populations including African-Americans, the elderly, and women. This change increased the treatment threshold for the general population age ≥60 years to SBP ≥ 150 mm Hg or DBP ≥ 90 mm Hg and to treat to goal SBP <150 mm Hg and DBP <90 mm Hg [33]. The JNC8 panel concluded that this recommendation was strongly supported by several reviewed randomized controlled trials (**Table 1**).

Modification	Recommendation	Approximate SBP reduction range
Weight reduction	Maintain normal body weight (BMI 18.5–24.9 kg/m^2)	5–20 mm Hg/10 kg
DASH-like eating plan	Diet rich in fruits, vegetables, low-fat dairy, and reduced fat	8–14 mm Hg
Restrict sodium intake	Consume no more than 2.4 g of sodium per day	2–8 mm Hg
Physical activity	Regular aerobic exercise for at least 30 minutes most days of the week	4–9 mm Hg
Moderate alcohol consumption	≤2 drinks/day for men and ≤1 drink/day for women	2–4 mm Hg

Table 1. Lifestyle modifications for hypertension control in adults.

However, a recent review highlights a summary of the debate regarding the potential implications of the recent guideline changes on African Americans and women [34]. The ABC stated that the proposed guidelines would put African Americans, who suffer disproportionately from HTN, at further increased risk for HTN-related morbidity and mortality [34]. The 2014 JNC8 recommendations are also discordant with the ISHIB consensus statement on the management of HTN in blacks in 2010. ISHIB recommendations include a lower threshold for SBP (<135/85 mm Hg) in blacks and for black individuals with evidence of target organ damage, preclinical or overt CVD, the threshold is even lower at SBP <130/80 mm Hg [35]. The ABC suggests that clinicians treating high-risk populations, such as African Americans, maintain the previously accepted standard of care and await further guideline recommendations from major professional organizations particularly in light of the recent Systolic Blood Pressure Intervention Trial results [34, 36].

Similarly, the Working Group on Women's Cardiovascular Health was in discordance with the JNC8 HTN recommendations [34] stating that women would be disproportionately affected by changes in treatment target goals as women make up the majority of those with HTN ≥60 years of age and older. Further, women are already known to have poor BP control with African American women constituting 40% of those with poor BP control and being already at highest risk for target end organ damage [34]. In addition, results from the Women's Health Initiative demonstrate a 93% increased stroke risk in older women who were prehypertensive compared to those that were normotensive.

8. Reducing health disparities in hypertension

Hypertension is a major modifiable risk factor for CVD, and thus a significant contributor to premature death [1]. Importantly, there are race-ethnic disparities that remain evident in the US. Several national health initiatives and programs at the individual, community, health system, and population level have attempted to address the goal of decreasing existing HTN disparities through primary and secondary prevention efforts [37].

A major population-based intervention approach is the Million Hearts (MH) public health campaign [37, 38]. The MH initiative, sponsored by the US Department of Health and Human Services, consists of comprehensive evidence-based interventions and strategies aimed at preventing one million heart attacks and strokes over the years of 2012–2016. A central component to this initiative promotes the use of standardized HTN treatment protocols, effective use of health information technology and self-measure blood pressure monitoring with clinical support [37, 38].

Community-based interventions are also instrumental in reducing the public health burden of HTN and reducing HTN-related disparities. Community-based outreach programs such as the Healthy Heart Community Prevention Project (HHCPP) and the Barber-Assisted Reduction in Blood Pressure in Ethnic Residents (BARBER-1) have utilized barbershops and churches to provided HTN education and screening among racial/ethnic groups suffering HTN

http://dx.doi.org/10.5772/64510

disparities [39, 40]. The use of black and Hispanic owned barbershops and beauty salons as part of community outreach programs to increase hypertension awareness and control among non-Hispanic blacks and Hispanics has been an effective screening, monitoring, and referral program shown to increase health-care access and HTN knowledge in risk minority communities [40, 41]. In Hispanic communities, outreach programs utilizing lay community health workers (CHWs), known as *Promotoras de Salud*, share the same ethnicity, culture, language, and life experiences as the people they serve and have been shown to improve hypertension awareness [39].

Health-care system-based approaches are equally as important in reducing HTN disparities given the differences in health outcomes that persist among race-ethnic groups secondary to institutional barriers. Effective approaches to reducing disparities due to institutional barriers include cultural competency training and data-based quality improvement (QI) efforts [42]. Health-care provider cultural competency training may improve health-care quality, along with patient satisfaction and health. Hospital-based QI programs such as the Robert Wood Johnson Foundation-supported Expecting Success and national ACC-supported Get With The Guidelines initiative have shown overall improvement in health-care quality and reduction of racial/ethnic disparities [42]. The use of big data health information technology and electronic medical records (EMRs) can also play an important role in reducing HTN disparities. The Kaiser Permanente large-scale hypertension program included the use of EMR and clinical decision support tools in the development, sharing, and incorporation of HTN performance metrics, evidence-based guidelines, clinic visit blood pressure measurements, and HTN treatment therapies [43] into a successful program that demonstrated high rates of HTN control improvement in adversely affected populations.

9. Conclusion

Despite overall decline in CVD morbidity and mortality, racial/ethnic disparities continue to exist in the US. Several racial/ethnic groups are known to suffer disproportionately from many modifiable CVD risk factors. In addition, these high-risk groups are less likely to have markers of ideal CV health. HTN remains a common risk factor that significantly contributes to overall and CVD mortality. Although HTN awareness has increased, non-Hispanic blacks in the US remain with a significantly higher prevalence of HTN when compared to non-Hispanic whites. In addition, non-Hispanic blacks are still more likely to have poor blood pressure control. Certain groups of Hispanics appear to have higher HTN prevalence rates to non-Hispanic whites, and Hispanic adults are least likely to be aware, treated, and have controlled HTN when compared to non-Hispanic blacks and whites. Continuing to move forward in research, clinical, and preventative effort to understand and intervene upon the multifaceted reasons as to why HTN disparities exist among certain populations is central to providing HTN specialty care.

Author details

Carlos J. Rodriguez*

Address all correspondence to: crodrigu@wakehealth.edu

Department of Epidemiology and Prevention, Division of Public Health Sciences, Wake Forest School of Medicine, Medical Center Boulevard, Winston-Salem, NC, USA

Department of Medicine, Section of Cardiovascular Medicine, Division of Public Health Sciences, Wake Forest School of Medicine, Medical Center Boulevard, Winston-Salem, NC, USA

References

[1] Mozaffarian D, Benjamin EJ, Go AS, Arnett DK, Blaha MJ, Cushman M, de Ferranti S, Després J-P, Fullerton HJ, Howard VJ, Huffman MD, Judd SE, Kissela BM, Lackland DT, Lichtman JH, Lisabeth LD, Liu S, Mackey RH, Matchar DB, McGuire DK, Mohler ER, Moy CS, Muntner P, Mussolino ME, Nasir K, Neumar RW, Nichol G, Palaniappan L, Pandey DK, Reeves MJ, Rodriguez CJ, Sorlie PD, Stein J, Towfighi A, Turan TN, Virani SS, Willey JZ, Woo D, Yeh RW, Turner MB. Heart disease and stroke statistics —2015 update: a report from the American Heart Association. Circulation. 2015;131:e29-e322. doi: 10.1161/cir.0000000000000152.

[2] CDC. Health disparities and inequalities report – United States. Mortal Wkly Rep. 2013;62 Suppl 3:157–160.

[3] Hozawa A, Folsom AR, Sharrett AR, Chambless LE. Absolute and attributable risks of cardiovascular disease incidence in relation to optimal and borderline risk factors: comparison of African American with white subjects – Atherosclerosis Risk in Communities Study. Arch Intern Med. 2007;167(6):573–579. doi: 10.1001/archinte.167.6.573. PubMed PMID: 17389288.

[4] Lloyd-Jones DM, Hong Y, Labarthe D, Mozaffarian D, Appel LJ, Van Horn L, Greenlund K, Daniels S, Nichol G, Tomaselli GF, Arnett DK, Fonarow GC, Ho PM, Lauer MS, Masoudi FA, Robertson RM, Roger V, Schwamm LH, Sorlie P, Yancy CW, Rosamond WD, American Heart Association Strategic Planning Task F, Statistics C. Defining and setting national goals for cardiovascular health promotion and disease reduction: the American Heart Association's strategic impact goal through 2020 and beyond. Circulation. 2010;121(4):586–613. doi: 10.1161/CIRCULATIONAHA.109.192703. PubMed PMID: 20089546.

[5] Fang J, Yang Q, Hong Y, Loustalot F. Status of cardiovascular health among adult Americans in the 50 States and the District of Columbia, 2009. J Am Heart Assoc.

2012;1(6):e005371. doi: 10.1161/JAHA.112.005371. PubMed PMID: 23316331; PMCID: PMC3540670.

[6] Centers for Disease C, Prevention. Racial/ethnic and socioeconomic disparities in multiple risk factors for heart disease and stroke – United States, 2003. MMWR Morb Mortal Wkly Rep. 2005;54(5):113–117. PubMed PMID: 15703691.

[7] Danaei G, Ding EL, Mozaffarian D, Taylor B, Rehm J, Murray CJ, Ezzati M. The preventable causes of death in the United States: comparative risk assessment of dietary, lifestyle, and metabolic risk factors. PLoS Med. 2009;6(4):e1000058. doi: 10.1371/journal.pmed.1000058. PubMed PMID: 19399161; PMCID: PMC2667673.

[8] Yoon SS, Burt V, Louis T, Carroll MD. Hypertension among adults in the United States, 2009–2010. NCHS Data Brief. 2012(107):1–8. PubMed PMID: 23102115.

[9] Blackwell DL, Lucas JW, Clarke TC. Summary health statistics for U.S. adults: national health interview survey, 2012. Vital Health Stat 10. 2014(260):1–161. PubMed PMID: 24819891.

[10] Kramer H, Han C, Post W, Goff D, Diez-Roux A, Cooper R, Jinagouda S, Shea S. Racial/ethnic differences in hypertension and hypertension treatment and control in the multi-ethnic study of atherosclerosis (MESA). Am J Hypertens. 2004;17(10):963–970. doi: 10.1016/j.amjhyper.2004.06.001. PubMed PMID: 15485761.

[11] Rodriguez CJ, Allison M, Daviglus ML, Isasi CR, Keller C, Leira EC, Palaniappan L, Pina IL, Ramirez SM, Rodriguez B, Sims M. Status of cardiovascular disease and stroke in Hispanics/Latinos in the United States: a science advisory from the American Heart Association. Circulation. 2014;130(7):593–625. doi: 10.1161/CIR.0000000000000071. PubMed PMID: 25098323; PMCID: PMC4577282.

[12] Sorlie PD, Allison MA, Aviles-Santa ML, Cai J, Daviglus ML, Howard AG, Kaplan R, Lavange LM, Raij L, Schneiderman N, Wassertheil-Smoller S, Talavera GA. Prevalence of hypertension, awareness, treatment, and control in the Hispanic Community Health Study/Study of Latinos. Am J Hypertens. 2014;27(6):793–800. doi: 10.1093/ajh/hpu003. PubMed PMID: 24627442; PMCID: PMC4017932.

[13] Hertz RP, Unger AN, Cornell JA, Saunders E. Racial disparities in hypertension prevalence, awareness, and management. Arch Intern Med. 2005;165(18):2098–2104. doi: 10.1001/archinte.165.18.2098. PubMed PMID: 16216999.

[14] Centers for Disease C, Prevention. Racial/Ethnic disparities in the awareness, treatment, and control of hypertension – United States, 2003–2010. MMWR Morb Mortal Wkly Rep. 2013;62(18):351–355. PubMed PMID: 23657109.

[15] Romero CX, Romero TE, Shlay JC, Ogden LG, Dabelea D. Changing trends in the prevalence and disparities of obesity and other cardiovascular disease risk factors in three racial/ethnic groups of USA adults. Adv Prev Med. 2012;2012:172423. doi: 10.1155/2012/172423. PubMed PMID: 23243516; PMCID: PMC3518078.

[16] Carson AP, Howard G, Burke GL, Shea S, Levitan EB, Muntner P. Ethnic differences in hypertension incidence among middle-aged and older adults: the multi-ethnic study of atherosclerosis. Hypertension. 2011;57(6):1101–1107. doi: 10.1161/HYPERTENSIONAHA.110.168005. PubMed PMID: 21502561; PMCID: PMC3106342.

[17] Selassie A, Wagner CS, Laken ML, Ferguson ML, Ferdinand KC, Egan BM. Progression is accelerated from prehypertension to hypertension in blacks. Hypertension. 2011;58(4):579–587. doi: 10.1161/HYPERTENSIONAHA.111.177410. PubMed PMID: 21911708; PMCID: PMC3186683.

[18] Howard G, Prineas R, Moy C, Cushman M, Kellum M, Temple E, Graham A, Howard V. Racial and geographic differences in awareness, treatment, and control of hypertension: the reasons for geographic and racial differences in stroke study. Stroke. 2006;37(5):1171–1178. doi: 10.1161/01.STR.0000217222.09978.ce. PubMed PMID: 16556884.

[19] Egan BM, Zhao Y, Axon RN. US trends in prevalence, awareness, treatment, and control of hypertension, 1988–2008. JAMA. 2010;303(20):2043–2050. doi: 10.1001/jama.2010.650. PubMed PMID: 20501926.

[20] Egan BM, Zhao Y, Axon RN, Brzezinski WA, Ferdinand KC. Uncontrolled and apparent treatment resistant hypertension in the United States, 1988 to 2008. Circulation. 2011;124(9):1046–1058. doi: 10.1161/CIRCULATIONAHA.111.030189. PubMed PMID: 21824920; PMCID: PMC3210066.

[21] Aram V. Chobanian Seventh Report of the Joint National Committee on prevention, detection, evaluation, and treatment of high blood pressure. Hypertension. 2003;42:1206–1252.

[22] Wang Thomas J, Ramachandran S. Epidemiology of uncontrolled hypertension in the United States. Circulation. 2005;112:1651–1662.

[23] Epstein M. Resistant hypertension: prevalence and evolving concepts. J Clin Hypertens (Greenwich). 2007;9(1 Suppl 1):2–6. PubMed PMID: 17215648.

[24] Black HR. Principal results of the controlled onset verapamil investigation of cardiovascular end points (CONVINCE) trial. JAMA. 2003;289:2073–2082.

[25] Singer GM, Izhar M, Black HR. Goal-oriented hypertension management: translating clinical trials to practice. Hypertension. 2002;40(4):464–469. PubMed PMID: 12364348.

[26] Hyman DJ, Pavlik VN. Characteristics of patients with uncontrolled hypertension in the United States. N Engl J Med. 2001;345(7):479–486. doi: 10.1056/NEJMoa010273. PubMed PMID: 11519501.

[27] Calhoun DA, Booth JN, 3rd, Oparil S, Irvin MR, Shimbo D, Lackland DT, Howard G, Safford MM, Muntner P. Refractory hypertension: determination of prevalence, risk factors, and comorbidities in a large, population-based cohort. Hypertension.

2014;63(3):451–458. doi: 10.1161/HYPERTENSIONAHA.113.02026. PubMed PMID: 24324035; PMCID: PMC4141646.

[28] Meissner I, Whisnant JP, Sheps SG, Schwartz GL, O'Fallon WM, Covalt JL, Sicks JD, Bailey KR, Wiebers DO. Detection and control of high blood pressure in the community: do we need a wake-up call? Hypertension. 1999;34(3):466–471. PubMed PMID: 10489395.

[29] Berlowitz DR, Ash AS, Hickey EC, Friedman RH, Glickman M, Kader B, Moskowitz MA. Inadequate management of blood pressure in a hypertensive population. N Engl J Med. 1998;339(27):1957–1963. doi: 10.1056/NEJM199812313392701. PubMed PMID: 9869666.

[30] Murphy SL, Xu J, Kochanek KD. Deaths: final data for 2010. Natl Vital Stat Rep. 2013;61(4):1–117. PubMed PMID: 24979972.

[31] Centers for Disease C, Prevention. Vital signs: avoidable deaths from heart disease, stroke, and hypertensive disease – United States, 2001–2010. MMWR Morb Mortal Wkly Rep. 2013;62(35):721–727. PubMed PMID: 24005227.

[32] Centers for Disease C, Prevention. Hypertension-related mortality among Hispanic subpopulations – United States, 1995–2002. MMWR Morb Mortal Wkly Rep. 2006;55(7): 177–180. PubMed PMID: 16498382.

[33] James PA, Oparil S, Carter BL, Cushman WC, Dennison-Himmelfarb C, Handler J, Lackland DT, LeFevre ML, MacKenzie TD, Ogedegbe O, Smith SC, Jr., Svetkey LP, Taler SJ, Townsend RR, Wright JT, Jr., Narva AS, Ortiz E. 2014 evidence-based guideline for the management of high blood pressure in adults: report from the panel members appointed to the Eighth Joint National Committee (JNC 8). JAMA. 2014;311(5):507–520. doi: 10.1001/jama.2013.284427. PubMed PMID: 24352797.

[34] Krakoff LR, Gillespie RL, Ferdinand KC, Fergus IV, Akinboboye O, Williams KA, Walsh MN, Bairey Merz CN, Pepine CJ. 2014 hypertension recommendations from the Eighth Joint National Committee panel members raise concerns for elderly black and female populations. J Am Coll Cardiol. 2014;64(4):394–402. doi: 10.1016/j.jacc.2014.06.014. PubMed PMID: 25060376; PMCID: PMC4242519.

[35] Flack JM, Sica DA, Bakris G, Brown AL, Ferdinand KC, Grimm RH, Jr., Hall WD, Jones WE, Kountz DS, Lea JP, Nasser S, Nesbitt SD, Saunders E, Scisney-Matlock M, Jamerson KA, International Society on Hypertension in B. Management of high blood pressure in blacks: an update of the International Society on Hypertension in Blacks consensus statement. Hypertension. 2010;56(5):780–800. doi: 10.1161/HYPERTENSIONAHA.110.152892. PubMed PMID: 20921433.

[36] Group SR, Wright JT, Jr., Williamson JD, Whelton PK, Snyder JK, Sink KM, Rocco MV, Reboussin DM, Rahman M, Oparil S, Lewis CE, Kimmel PL, Johnson KC, Goff DC, Jr., Fine LJ, Cutler JA, Cushman WC, Cheung AK, Ambrosius WT. A randomized trial of

intensive versus standard blood-pressure control. N Engl J Med. 2015;373(22):2103–2116. doi: 10.1056/NEJMoa1511939. PubMed PMID: 26551272; PMCID: PMC4689591.

[37] Ritchey MD, Wall HK, Gillespie C, George MG, Jamal A, Division for Heart Disease, Stroke Prevention CDC. Million hearts: prevalence of leading cardiovascular disease risk factors – United States, 2005–2012. MMWR Morb Mortal Wkly Rep. 2014;63(21): 462–467. PubMed PMID: 24871251.

[38] Centers for Disease C, Prevention. Million hearts: strategies to reduce the prevalence of leading cardiovascular disease risk factors – United States, 2011. MMWR Morb Mortal Wkly Rep. 2011;60(36):1248–1251. PubMed PMID: 21918495.

[39] Ferdinand KC, Patterson KP, Taylor C, Fergus IV, Nasser SA, Ferdinand DP. Community-based approaches to prevention and management of hypertension and cardiovascular disease. J Clin Hypertens (Greenwich). 2012;14(5):336–343. doi: 10.1111/j.1751-7176.2012.00622.x. PubMed PMID: 22533661.

[40] Victor RG, Ravenell JE, Freeman A, Leonard D, Bhat DG, Shafiq M, Knowles P, Storm JS, Adhikari E, Bibbins-Domingo K, Coxson PG, Pletcher MJ, Hannan P, Haley RW. Effectiveness of a barber-based intervention for improving hypertension control in black men: the BARBER-1 study: a cluster randomized trial. Arch Intern Med. 2011;171(4):342–350. doi: 10.1001/archinternmed.2010.390. PubMed PMID: 20975012; PMCID: PMC3365537.

[41] Solomon FM, Linnan LA, Wasilewski Y, Lee AM, Katz ML, Yang J. Observational study in ten beauty salons: results informing development of the North Carolina BEAUTY and Health Project. Health Educ Behav. 2004;31(6):790–807. doi: 10.1177/1090198104264176. PubMed PMID: 15539548.

[42] Yancy CW, Wang TY, Ventura HO, Pina IL, Vijayaraghavan K, Ferdinand KC, Hall LL, credo Advisory G. The coalition to reduce racial and ethnic disparities in cardiovascular disease outcomes (credo): why credo matters to cardiologists. J Am Coll Cardiol. 2011;57(3):245–252. doi: 10.1016/j.jacc.2010.09.027. PubMed PMID: 21232662.

[43] Jaffe MG, Lee GA, Young JD, Sidney S, Go AS. Improved blood pressure control associated with a large-scale hypertension program. JAMA. 2013;310(7):699–705. doi: 10.1001/jama.2013.108769. PubMed PMID: 23989679; PMCID: PMC4270203.